Equine Reproductive Physiology, Breeding and Stud Management

Equine Reproductive Physiology, Breeding and Stud Management

Editor

Nitin Vichare

scitus
academics

Equine Reproductive Physiology, Breeding and Stud Management

Edited by **Nitin Vichare**

ISBN: 978-1-68117-060-2

Library of Congress Control Number: 2015935458

SCITUS Academics LLC,
www.scitusacademics.com
Box No. 4766, 616 Corporate Way,
Suite 2, Valley Cottage,
NY 10989

Printed in United States of America on Acid Free Paper ∞

Contents

Preface

Horses have the potential for high reproductive performance. With an understanding of basic reproductive science, breeders can be better positioned to achieve their goals. This Factsheet presents information on basic anatomy, physiology and management techniques that can assist in improving reproductive performance in the mare. This book coverage includes the reproductive anatomy, endocrine control and selection for breeding of both the mare and stallion, and also pregnancy, parturition and lactation in the mare. This comprehensive text goes on to study how this knowledge can be applied to the successful breeding of horses, maximizing both productivity and animal welfare. It has also been expanded to include more recent experimental work and updated references, including a brand new chapter on the significant developments in embryo technology. This widely popular textbook is an essential addition to the collections of both students in equine science and practicing veterinarians.

Editor

Chapter 1

Analysis of Horse Myostatin Gene and Identification of Single Nucleotide Polymorphisms in Breeds of Different Morphological Types

Stefania Dall'Olio[1], Luca Fontanesi[1], Leonardo Nanni Costa[1], Marco Tassinari[2], Laura Minieri[3], and Adalberto Falaschini[2]

[1]DIPROVAL, Sezione di Allevamenti Zootecnici, Faculty of Agriculture, University of Bologna, 42123 Reggio Emilia, Italy

[2]DIMORFIPA, Sezione di Zootecnia, Faculty of Veterinary Medicine, University of Bologna, 40064 Ozzano Emilia, Italy

[3]Department of Human and General Physiology, Faculty of Medicine, University of Bologna, 40127 Bologna, Italy

ABSTRACT

Myostatin (MSTN) is a negative modulator of muscle mass. We characterized the horse (Equus caballus) MSTN gene and identified and analysed single nucleotide polymorphisms (SNPs) in breeds of different morphological types. Sequencing of coding, untranslated, intronic, and regulatory regions of MSTN gene in 12 horses from 10 breeds revealed seven SNPs: two in the promoter, four in intron 1, and one in intron 2. The SNPs of the promoter (GQ183900:g.26T>C and GQ183900:g.156T>C, the latter located within a conserved TATA-box like motif) were screened in 396 horses from 16 breeds. The g.26C and the g.156C alleles presented higher frequency in heavy (brachymorphic type) than in light breeds (dolichomorphic type such as Italian Trotter breed). The significant difference of allele frequencies for the SNPs at the promoter and analysis of molecular variance (AMOVA) on haplotypes indicates that these polymorphisms could be associated with variability of morphology traits in horse breeds.

INTRODUCTION

Myostatin, encoded by the MSTN gene (previously referred to as GDF8), is a member of the transforming growth factor β superfamily that normally acts to limit skeletal muscle mass by regulating both the number and growth of muscle fibres [1, 2]. MSTN is synthesized as precursor and upon proteolytic processing gives an N-terminal latency-associated peptide, termed myostatin propeptide or LAP-fragment, and a smaller mature peptide at the C-terminus [3]. The MSTN gene, composed of three exons and two introns, has been characterized in rodents [1], humans [4], and several livestock species [3, 5–8]. Natural mutations that decrease the amounts of myostatin and/or inhibit its function have been identified in a human subject [9] and in several cattle [2, 3, 10–13], sheep [14–16], and dog [17] breeds. In Belgian Blue, Piedmontese, Marchigiana, and other cattle breeds, loss-of-function mutations within the coding sequence of the MSTNgene determine increased skeletal muscle mass, relevant in shoulders and thighs, and the produced phenotype is known as "double-muscling" [2, 3, 10–13, 18]. These polymorphisms have, in several cases, effects on growth, reproductive, performances, and carcass quality traits [3, 18, 19]. In the Whippet dog breed a mutation in the third exon determining a premature stop codon causes an increased muscle mass phenotype in homozygous state and enhanced racing performance in heterozygous dogs [17]. In two Norwegian sheep breeds, two different mutations in the MSTN coding region are associated with carcass conformation and fatness [15, 16]. In addition, in other sheep and in pigs, mutations identified in non coding regulatory regions affect the level of MSTN gene expression and/or are associated with growth, muscle mass, and other carcass traits [8, 14, 20, 21].

In horse (Equus caballus), only few studies examined the MSTN gene so far. Hosoyama et al. [22] isolated and sequenced an MSTN cDNA from a Thoroughbred horse and Caetano et al. [23] mapped this gene to equine chromosome 18. Mutations in the equine MSTN gene have been identified only recently in Thoroughbred breed [24].

Different horse breeds present a variety of morphological phenotypes that have been used to group breeds into a few classes. However, no system provides a robust classification in which each breed could have an unequivocal assignment. Based on size traits and build, horse breeds are categorized in draught (or heavy), light, and pony (or animals that mature at less than 148 cm high, usually used as riding school and children's mounts) [25]. Considering skeletal structure, proportions, zoometrical indices, length, and volume of muscling, that, in turn, reflect the selective goals and uses of the horse breeds, they are categorized in brachymorphic, mesomorphic, dolichomorphic, and intermediate types (such as meso-dolichomorphic) [26]. Brachymorphic horses (corresponding to draught horses), traditionally referred to as cold-blooded horses in relation to their quiet and calm temperament, are tall in stature, heavy boned, and extremely muscular with short and thick muscles and slow twitch oxidative fibers for slow contraction. They most likely develop strength and power, and their conformation is well suited for pulling carriage, draught power and meat production. Dolichomorphic horses (corresponding to light horses) are characterized by longer bodies and long and thin muscles mainly constituted by fast twitch glycolytic fibers. They are selected for sport purposes, fast running, and high speeds. Examples of Italian breeds representative of these two extreme phenotypes are reported in Figure 1. Mesomorphic type is characterized by a lighter physical structure than brachymorphic but still powerful and compact with massive muscling. This group also includes some breeds with draft-type qualities and classified as ponies based on their withers height (such as Bardigiano and Haflinger breeds). The mesomorphic horses are usually used for pleasure and riding. In addition, several breeds (like local breeds with influence of Oriental, Thoroughbred, and Iberian halfbreed and descendents) have characteristics of both mesomorphic and dolichomorphic types (referred to as meso-dolichomorphic) [26].

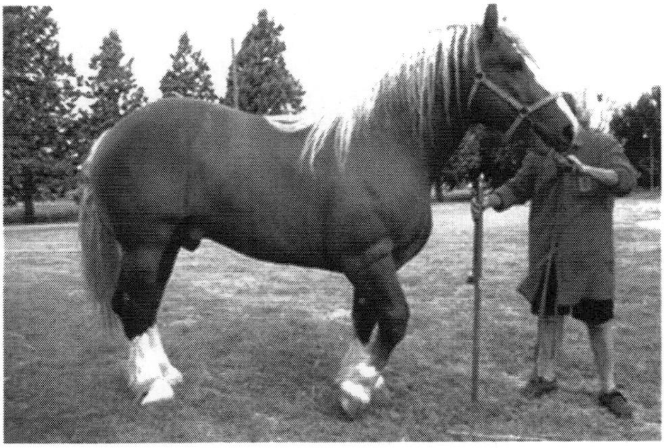

1(a)

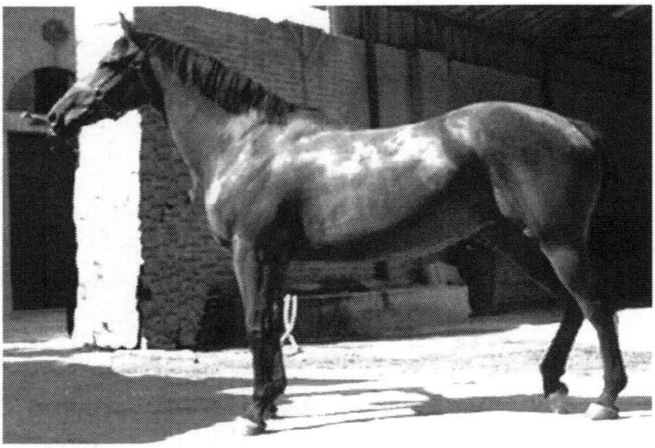

1(b)

Figure 1: Horses of extreme and opposite morphological types:(a) Rapid Heavy Draft (brachymorphic type or heavy) and (b) Italian Trotter (dolichomorphic type or light).

For the important pleiotropic effects of the MSNT gene, including its role on muscle mass development, polymorphisms in this gene could contribute to explain the morphological variability among horse breeds. Here we sequenced the MSTN gene, including regulatory regions, in several horse breeds and identified a few polymorphisms that were used to evaluate their potential association with different morphological types.

MATERIALS AND METHODS

Animals and Horse Breeds Classification Based on Different Morphological Types

A total of 396 minimal related horses belonging to 16 breeds were sampled in different farms or stables. Details of the horse breeds involved in the analysis are given in Table 1.

Table 1: Numbers, types, origin, uses, and morphological information of the analysed horse breeds*

International breed name (Home page of Breed National Associations)	Typesx	Number of horses	Origin of the samples	Uses (adult animals, males/females: withers height, cm; live weight, kg)
Rapid Heavy Draft (http://www.anacaitpr.it/)	B	81	North East of Italy	Meat, draught power (160/155 cm; 700/570 kg)

Noric or Pinzgauer (http://www.aia.it/tecnico/equini/a_norico.htm)	B	26	Alps, Northern Italy	Draught power, driving, carriage, dressage, meat (155/153 cm; 700/650 kg)
Bardigiano (http://www.bardigiano.it/)	M	34	Emilia Romagna region, Northern Italy	Meat, agricultural work, hobby (143/142 cm; 530/480 kg)
Haflinger or Avelignese (http://www.haflinger.it/)	M	31	Northern Italy	Hobby, meat, draught power (142/140 cm; 450/450 kg)
Lipizzan or Lipizzaner(http://www.aia.it/tecnico/equini/a_lipizzano.htm)	M	12	Rome, Central Italy	Dressage, riding, carriage (164/150 cm; 550/480 kg)
Murgese(http://www.aia.it/tecnico/equini/download/DM%20MURGESE.pdf)	M	12	Apulia region, Southern Italy	Riding, equestrian tourism, draught power (164/162 cm; 550/480 kg)
Tolfetano (http://www.aia.it/tecnico/equini/a_tolfetan.htm)	M	7	Latium region, Central Italy	Riding (160/150 cm)
Uruguayan Creole or Criollo(http://www.caballoscriollos.com.uy/homepage_en.php)	M	35	Uruguay	Draught power, government of livestock, endurance (144/144 cm; 420/420 kg)
Italian Saddle (http://www.aia.it/ANACSI/Frame.htm)	M-D	30	Country wide, Italia	Riding, equestrian tourism, drift competitions (jumping, dressage, complete, endurance) (min 156 cm).

Maremmano (http://www.anamcavallomaremmano.com)	M-D	13	Tuscany region, Central Italy	Riding, equestrian tourism, draught power, government of livestock (165/162 cm; 500/450 kg)
Quarter Horse (http://www.aiqh.it)	M-D	15	Emilia Romagna region, Italy	Riding, equestrian tourism (160 cm; 550/350 kg)
Salernitano or Salernitano-Persano(http://www.agraria.org/equini/salernitano.htm)	M-D	4	Campania region, Southern Italy	Riding, equestrian tourism (158/150 cm; 500/450 kg)
Spanish Purebred or Andalusian (http://www.aipre.com)	M-D	10	Emilia Romagna region, Italy	Sport, hobby (160/155 cm; 570 kg)
Ventasso (http://www.aia.it/tecnico/equini/a_ventass.htm)	M-D	8	Emilia-Romagna region, Northern Italy	Equestrian tourism (164/152 cm)
Italian Trotter (http://www.anact.it/)	D	67	Country wide, Italy	Selected for competitive merit as trotter at short and medium distances (160–145 cm)
Throroughbred (http://www.anacpurosangue.com/)	D	11	Country wide, Italy	Racehorses (gallop) and used for genetic improvement of Italian local breeds.

*Based on information obtained from Horse Breeds National Associations, if available. Types^x: B= brachimorphic or heavy, M= mesomorphic, M-D= meso-dolichomorphic, D= dolichomorphic or light.

These horse breeds were classified as brachymorphic (B), mesomorphic, (M), meso-dolichomorphic (M-D), and dolichomorphic (D) (Table 1) as indicated in the homepage of their own Breed National

Associations based on linear measures (height at withers, chest girth, and cannon circumference), structure and anamorphosis index (AI= (chest girth)^2*100/height at wither), and based on bibliographic data [27–30].

All horses were registered in the Stud Books or in the Italian Anagraphic Register constituted for local ethnic groups (Noric, Salernitano, Tolfetano, and Ventasso). The Lipizzan samples (Lipizzan Italian Stud, Monterotondo, Italy) included all six classical stallion lines: Conversano, Favory, Maestoso, Neapolitano, Pluto, and Siglavy.

PCR and Sequencing

Genomic DNA was extracted from hair roots following standard procedures. Ten primer pairs (Table 2) that amplify different MSTN regions were designed using Primer 3 (http://frodo.wi.mit.edu/primer3/input.htm) software. PCR reactions were performed in a final volume of 20 μL containing 10–80 ng of equine genomic DNA, 250 mM of each dNTP, 10 pmol of each primer, 1 U of EuroTaq DNA polymerase (EuroClone Ltd., Paington, Devon, UK), or 1 U of TaKaRa Ex Taq DNA Polymerase (TaKaRa Bio Inc., Shiga, Japan) and 1 × PCR buffer with $MgCl_2$ concentration specific for each primer pair (Table 2). PCR conditions were: an initial step at 95°C for 5 minutes, 35 cycles of 95°C for 30 s, specific annealing temperature for each primer pair for 30 s, 72°C for specific reaction times for different primer pair (Table 2), and a final step at 72°C for 9 minutes. Genomic DNA obtained from 12 horses of 10 breeds (1 Bardigiano, 1 Haflinger, 1 Italian Saddle, 2 Italian Trotter, 1 Noric, 2 Rapid Heavy Draft, 1 Salernitano, 2 Throroughbred, and 1 Ventasso) constituted the sequencing panel. PCR fragments obtained from the sequencing panel with primer pairs 1–10 were purified using the QIAquick PCR Purification Kit (Qiagen, Düsseldorf, Germany) and sequenced on both strands using the BigDye Cycle Sequencing kit v.3.1 (Applied Biosystems, Foster City, CA, USA). Sequencing reactions were electrophoresed in a capillary sequencer (Applied Biosystems).

Table 2: Primers, PCR conditions, amplified regions, and use of the PCR products

Primer pair	F: Forward sequence (5′-3′) R: Reverse sequence (5′-3′)	Primer annealing regions	Amplified region (bp)*	PCR condition sx	Use of the PCR products
1#	1F: TCAGGGAAACAAGTTTCTCAAAT	Promoter	1–484	58/1.5/45/	Sequencing,
	1R: TGCTCCACAATGAATCTCG	Promoter	(484)	E	PCR-RFLP
2#	2F: TGAATCAGCTCACCCTTGAC	Promoter	369–727	62/0.8/45/	Sequencing
	2R: CCAGCAACAATCAGCATAAA	Exon 1	(360)	E	
3{	3F TGTGCTGATTCTTGCTGGTC	Exon 1	710–947	58/1.5/45/	Sequencing
	3R: ATCAATCAGTTCCCGGAGTG	Exon 1	(238)	E	
4{	4F: GACCCGTCAAGACTCCTACA	Exon 2	2982–3226	58/1.0/45/	Sequencing
	4F: TGGGAAGGTTACAGCAAGA	Exon 2	(245)	E	
5{	5F: AGGCCAATTACTGCTCTGGA	Exon 3	5430–5744	58/1.5/45/	Sequencing
	5R: ATACTCTAGGCTTATAGCCT	3′ UTR	(315)	E	
6{	6F: CACTCCGGGAACTGATTGAT	Exon 1	928–3098	58/0.8/130	Sequencing
	6R: CGCCTGGGTTCATGTCAAGT	Exon 2	(2171)	/T	
7{	7F: AGGCAGGCACATTGCTTAAT	Intron 1	1808–2287	58/0.8/45/	Sequencing
	7R: GAATGTTATATTCAGGCTATCTCAA	Intron 1	(480)	E	

8{	8F: AAATGTGACATAAGCAAATGATTAG	Intron 2	5152–5534	62/0.8/45/	Sequencing
	8R: AGCAGGGGCCTGCTGAACCTCTGGG	Exon 3	(383)	E	
9{	9F: TGCAAAATTGGCTCAAACAG	Exon 2	3135–5361	55/0.8/130	Sequencing
	9R: CAGCATCGAGATTCTGTGGA	Exon 3	(2227)	/T	
1 0{	10F: CCCCCAGAAGAGTGTCAAAT	Intron 2	3627–4822	60/0.8/130	Sequencing
	10R: TCTTTACTTGGGGAAACTTGGA	Intron 2	(1196)	/T	
11	1F: TCAGGGAAACAAGTTTCTCAAAT	Promoter	1–204	53/1.2/35/	PCR-RFLP
	11R: ACTTCCTCAGAAATTAAGATTTAAT	Promoter	(204)	E	

*Numbering accoding to GenBank accession number GQ183900. §Annealing temperature (°C), [$MgCl_2$], extension time (s), Taq DNA polymerase (E = EuroTaq; T = TaKaRa). #Primers pairs 1 and 2 were designed based on conserved sequences of the published cattle, pig, and humans MSTN promoter regions (GenBank accession numbers AJ310751, AJ133580, and AX058992, respectively). {Primer pairs 3–10 were designed based on horse MSTN mRNA sequence (GenBank accession number AB033541).

Sequence Analysis, Polymorphism Identification, and Genotyping

Sequences were aligned and processed with the help of the BioEdit software v.7.0.5.2. Polymorphisms were identified by visual inspection of the electropherograms and sequences were aligned with ClustalW2 program (http://www.ebi.ac.uk/Tools/clustalw2/index.html) and using BLASTN (http://blast.ncbi.nlm.nih.gov/Blast.cgi). The horse MSTN promoter sequence was analysed in silico for the presence of putative transcription factor binding sites using MatInspector (http://www.genomatix.de/) bioinformatics tool. This region of horse MSTN gene was aligned with that of cattle (AJ310751), goat (AY827576), human (AX058992), mouse (AY204900), pig (AY8641281), and sheep (DQ530260) to identify evolutionary conserved motifs.

PCR-RFLP protocols were designed to genotype two identified SNPs (g.26T>C and g.156T>C) in the sampled horses. To genotype the g.26T>C SNP, the amplified products of 484 bp obtained with primer pair 1 (Table 2) were digested with RsaI (recognition sequence: GT↓AC). Briefly, 5–10 μL of PCR reaction was restricted with 2.5U of RsaI (Fermentas, Vilnius, Lithuania) at 37°C overnight and the resulting fragments (g.26T allele=484 bp; g.26C allele=437 bp + 47 bp) were resolved on 2.0 % agarose gels stained with ethidium bromide. The g.156T>C SNP was genotyped amplifying a fragment of 204 bp with primer pair 11 (Table 2) that inserted an artificial restriction site (with a mismatched reverse primer) for SspI (recognition sequence: AAT↓ATT) when allele g.156T occurred. The obtained fragments (g.156T allele=179 bp + 25 bp; g.156C allele=204 bp) resulting from digestion of 5–10 μL of PCR reaction with 2.5U of SspI (Fermentas) at 37°C overnight were electrophoresed in 3.5% agarose gels and visualized with ethidium bromide.

Statistical Analysis

Allele and genotype frequencies, observed and expected heterozygosity, and F_{st} were calculated using PopGene software v. 1.32 [31]. F_{st} is a measure of population differentiation based on genotypic data. Allele frequencies among the four groups (B, M, M-D, and D) were compared using Fisher's exact test. The haplotypes of the two promoter SNPs were reconstructed using PHASE program v. 2.0 [32]. ARLEQUIN software v. 3.1 (http://cmpg.unibe.ch/software/arlequin3) was used for the analysis of molecular variance (AMOVA) testing the effect of the morphological types in population differentiation with a model including types (four levels: B, M, M-D and D; and two levels: B + M and M-D + D), types/breeds, individuals/breeds, and individuals.

RESULTS AND DISCUSSION

Horse MSTN Genomic Structure and Sequence Analysis

Sequenced fragments of the horse *MSTN* gene were assembled into one sequence of 5724 bp (submitted to GenBank under accession number GQ183900) that resulted 100% identical with that that was, in the meantime, annotated in the EquCab2 horse genome assembly derived from a Thoroughbred horse (http://www.ensembl.org/Equus caballus/Search/, Ensembl release 52-Dec 2009). Our sequence contained 671 bp upstream from the ATG start codon, 538 bp of the promoter, and the entire 5-untranslated region (UTR) of 133 bp, the three exons (except 33 bp of exon 1), the two intervening introns, and 80 bp of the 3-UTR (Figure 2). The transcription start site of the first exon was deduced from human and bovine *MSTN* exon 1 sequences [4, 6]. The coding regions of exons 1, 2, and 3 of the horse *MSTN* gene contained 373, 374, and 381 bp, respectively. Introns 1 and 2 included 1829 bp and 2016 bp, respectively, almost the same length reported in cattle (1840 bp and 2033 bp, respectively) and pig (1809 bp and 1980 bp, respectively) [6, 8]. Intron 1 is a type 1 intron as it interrupts a codon between the first and second exon whereas intron 2 is a type 0 intron as it divides the coding sequence between two codons as in other species [6, 8]. The analysed proximal promoter region and the 5- UTR of the horse *MSTN* exhibited a degree of identity with the corresponding regions of other species ranging from 77% (mouse) to 90% (pig). Putative consensus DNA sequences known as transcription factor binding sites, DNA-binding motifs, or *cis*-regulatory elements were identified in the positive strand of horse promoter (Figure 3). Considering the general transcription factors, three different putative TATA boxes (TATA-1, TATA-

2, and TATA-3) and one CCAAT box were detected. Among muscle-specific transcription factors, four E-boxes (named E1, E2, E3, and E4 boxes, Figure 3), one putative site for myocyte specific enhancer factor 2 (MEF2 or MEB1) and consensus sequences for FoxO and SMAD binding sites (CAAAATA and CAGACA, respectively) family sequences were identified. The alignment of *MSTN* promoter sequences across different species (horse, cattle, goat, human, mouse, pig, and sheep) revealed that these DNA-binding motives, particularly close to the TATA-1 surrounding sequence, were highly conserved across species. In particular, TATA-1 was conserved in all examined species except mouse, the second TATA sequence (TATA-2) was conserved across all seven species, and TATA-3 was conserved in all species except pig and mouse. The MEF2 and E-boxes were conserved in all the considered mammals except in human and mouse for E-box4. The E-boxes can be activated by the myogenic regulatory factors (MRFs: MyoD, Myf5, myogenin, and MRF4). MyoD upregulates *MSTN* transcription [33] and at the same time MSTN inhibitsMyoD expression and activity regulating the differentiation of myoblasts into myotubes [34]. MyoD and MRF4 play competitive roles in myogenesis and might act as molecular switches to determine myogenic differentiation and cell proliferation, respectively [35]. Additional E-boxes were identified in the analysed region (such as an E-box located near the TATA- 2 in pig and an additional E-box in all mammalian but cattle) and in the distal region of the promoter of the other mammals (not included in Figure 3). In cattle, Spiller et al. [33] showed the importance of three functional E-boxes (E3, E4, and E6) of which the E6, occupied by MyoD *in vitro* and *in vivo*, resulted crucial for the *MSTN* promoter activity. The close position of functional E-boxes suggests that they might function as a cluster to better sustain the stability of DNAprotein. Across the *MSTN* promoter sequences of all considered livestock species we identified the conserved position of sites matching the consensus for FoxO binding and the adjacent SMAD box whose presence was not evidenced in previous works [8, 33, 36]. Recent data demonstrated that these factors appear to act through independent pathways but additively to regulate the expression of *MSTN* and contribute to control muscle cell growth and differentiation [37, 38]. In addition, FoxO transcription factors plays a critical role in development ofmuscle atrophy by stimulating proteolysis and by increasing myostatin expression. Putative E-boxes were identified both in intron 1 (six boxes) and in intron 2 (six boxes) and one putative E-box was located in the 3′-UTR at seven nucleotides downstream of the TGA stop codon (data not shown). The presence of E-boxes in the introns and 3-UTR of equine *MSTN* gene has not been described yet even if their occurrence has been highlighted recently in introns of porcine *MSTN* gene [8].

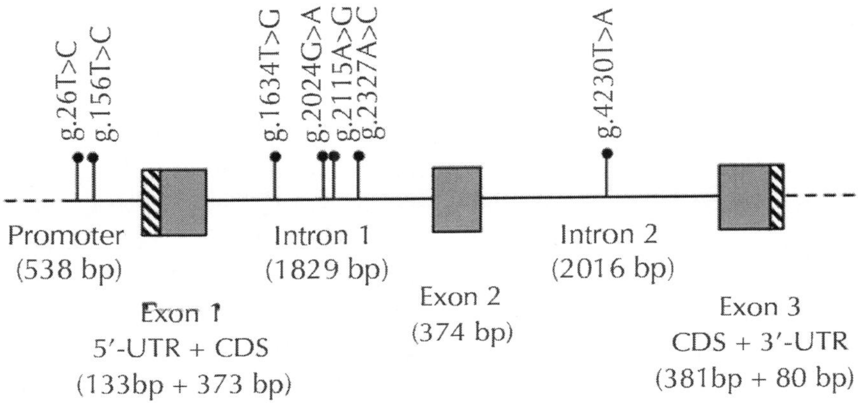

Figure 2: Genomic organization of the horse MSTN gene. Exons are shown as boxes. Solid boxes indicate protein coding regions. Untranslated regions are shown as striped boxes. Size of the sequenced regions of the promoter, exons, and introns is reported. Polymorphisms, indicated according to GenBank accession number GQ183900, are reported on the genomic organization of the gene.

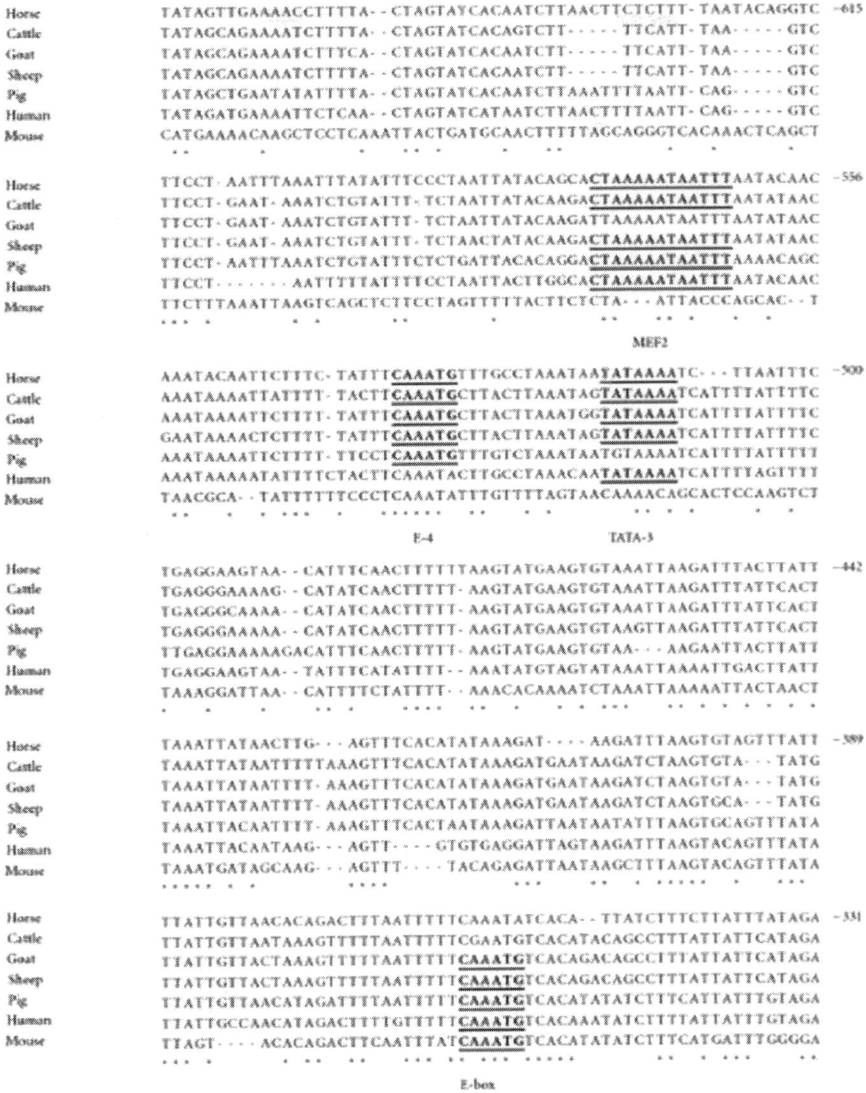
Horse
Cattle
Goat
Sheep
Pig
Human
Mouse
-615
-556
MEF2
-500
E-4
TATA-3
-442
-389
-331
E-box

3(a)

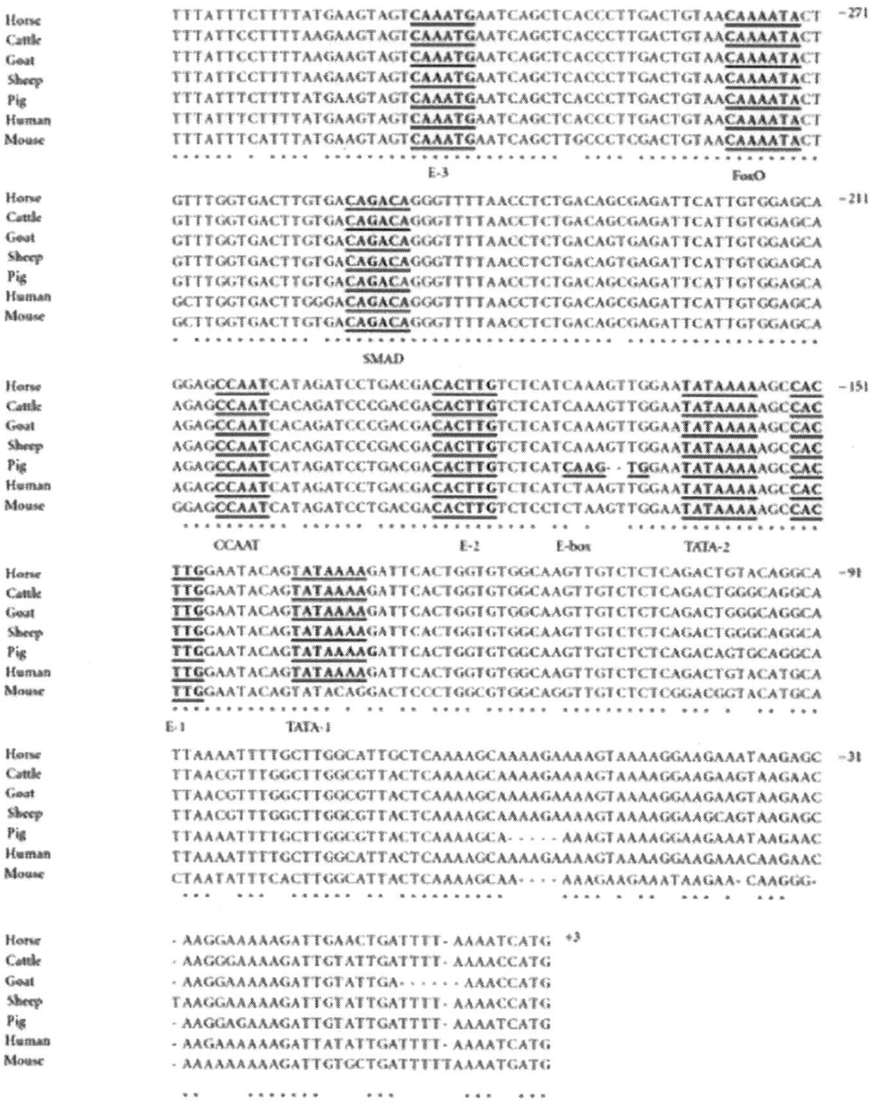

3(b)

Figure 3: Sequence analysis of the proximal promoter region and -UTR of MSTNgene. Approximately 670 bp of the MSTN -flanking region and -UTR from horse, cattle, goat, human, mouse, pig, and sheep is shown. The consensus for transcription factor binding motives is shown in bold text and underlined. Numbering of the horse sequence is relative to the ATG start codon. Numbering of E-boxes is relative to the horse sequence. The two identified SNPs of horse MSTN gene are indicated with Y (T or C according to the IUPAC nomenclature) and in red.

Identification of Polymorphisms in the Horse MSTN Gene

Sequencing of the panel of horses of different morphological types revealed a total of seven single nucleotide polymorphisms (SNPs) (Figure 2). Two transitions were located in the promoter region at -646 (GQ183900:g.26T>C) and -516 (GQ183900:g.156T>C) bp upstream from the start codon. The g.26T>C SNP was within a conserved position (except in mouse) but not within an identified known functional motif while the g.156T>C polymorphism was within a TATA box-like (TATA-3; YATAAA, Figure 3). Sequence alignments of the *MSTN* promoter regions of different species indicate that the g.26T and g.156T alleles derive from an ancestral *MSTN* sequence as most close species present the indicated nucleotides (Figure 3 and data not shown). The other five SNPs were in intronic regions: four were localized in intron 1 and one in intron 2 (Figure 2). Three of the SNPs of intron 1 (g.1634T>G, g.2115A>G, and g.2327A>C) were also recently identified in Thoroughbred breeds [24]. One of which (g.2115A>G; indicated by [24] as g.66493737C>T) has been associated with sprinting ability and racing stamina in Thoroughbred horses [24]. The remaining SNPs were not reported by others and represent new polymorphisms of the horse *MSTN* gene. None of these intronic SNPs resided within splice sites or within particularly conserved sequence elements. No indels and synonymous or nonsynonymous substitutions were identified.

Analysis of Polymorphisms in Breeds with DifferentMorphological Types and Genetic Diversity Parameters

Allele frequencies for the two SNPs located in the promoter region (g.26T>C and g.156T>C) are shown in Table 3. The g.26T>C SNP was polymorphic in 6 out of 16 breeds with higher observed frequency of the g.26C allele in the Lipizzan breed (0.21). For the g.156T>C polymorphism, the mutant g.156C allele, which changes the predicted TATA box3-like, was detected in 11 out 16 breeds and was identified in homozygous condition in a few Bardigiano, Haflinger, Noric, Rapid Heavy Draft, and Uruguayan Creole horses.

Table 3: Minor allele frequency (MAF) and haplotype (Hap*) frequencies of the two promoter SNPs of the MSTN gene in different horse breeds

Horse breeds	Typesx	Number of horses	MAF g.26C	MAF g.156C	Hap [T:T]	Hap [T:C]	Hap [C:T]
Rapid Heavy Draft	B	81	0.12	0.15	0.73	0.15	0.12
Noric	B	26	0.06	0.40	0.54	0.40	0.06
Bardigiano	M	34	—	0.15	0.85	0.15	—
Haflinger	M	31	—	0.37	0.63	0.37	—
Lipizzan	M	12	0.21	—	0.79	—	0.21
Murgese	M	12	—	0.17	0.83	0.17	—
Tolfetano	M	7	—	0.29	0.71	0.29	—
Uruguayan Creole	M	35	—	0.24	0.76	0.24	—
Italian Saddle	M-D	30	0.05	0.10	0.85	0.10	0.05
Maremmano	M-D	13	—	0.12	0.88	0.12	—
Quarter Horse	M-D	15	—	—	1.00	—	—
Salernitano	M-D	4	—	0.25	—	—	—
Spanish Purebred	M-D	10	—	—	1.00	—	—
Ventasso	M-D	8	0.12	—	0.88	—	0.12
Italian Trotter	D	67	0.01	—	0.99	—	0.01
Thoroughbred	D	11	—	0.05	0.95	0.05	—

*Haplotypes for the g.26T>C and g.156T>C polymorphisms. xTypes: B= brachimorphic or heavy, M= mesomorphic, M-D= meso-dolichomorphic, D= dolichomorphic or light.

Haplotype analyses of the twomutations showed the presence of three haplotypes: [g.26T:g.156T], [g.26T:g.156C], and [g.26C:g.156T] (Table 3). The [T:T] haplotype could be the wild type according to its presence in all breeds and higher frequency (from 0.54 to 1.00). The [T:C] haplotype was observed in 10 breeds (frequency from 0.05 to 0.40), whereas the [C:T] haplotype was identified only in 6 breeds (frequency from 0.01 to 0.21) (Table 3). In order to evaluate if the two SNPs in the promoter region could account for a quote of variability related to morphological types, we classified the analysed horse breeds in four groups (brachymorphic, B; mesomorphic, M; mesodolichomorphic, M-D; and dolichomorphic, D) (seeMaterials and Methods). Several descriptive statistics summarizing the genetic diversity of these groups are reported in Table 4. The B group showed the highest observed and expected heterozygosity (0.24 ± 0.09 and 0.26 ± 0.10, respectively), whereas the D group had the lowest values (0.02 ± 0.01 for both measures). For the g.26T>C SNP, differences in allele frequencies were significant between B and the other three groups ($P < .0001$ for B versus M and B versus D; $P < .05$ for B versus M-D). For the g.156T>C polymorphism, only the comparison between B and M groups was not significant. In particular, differences in allele frequencies were highly significant between the B and D groups and between the M and D groups (P = 3.78E − 11 and P = 3.95E − 9, respectively. For the remaining comparisons: $P < .0001$ for B versus M-D and for M versus M-D, $P < .01$ for M-D versus D). The overall *F*st value showed that the genetic differences among the groups accounted for 6.1% (3.6% for the g.26T>C SNP and 7.0% for the g.156T>C SNP) of the genetic variation. The AMOVA on haplotypes confirmed that a proportion of the total molecular variance was associated to morphological types of the horses. Using the four morphological types the molecular variance explained was 6.40% ($P<.05$). Grouping these four types into two groups (B + M and M-D + D) according to their similarities on morphological types the quote of explained molecular variance was 10.6% ($P < .01$). It could be possible that differences of allele and haplotype frequencies among types are influenced by phylogenetic closeness rather than any association with morphological types. This issue should be further investigated as, to our knowledge, there are no studies analyzing this question that include most of the breeds we investigated. However, Di Stasio et al. [39] analysed genetic relationships among only three breeds included in our study and evidenced significant genetic differentiation among Bardigiano, Haflinger, and Maremmano, suggesting that the results we obtained might not be biased by a putative common origin of the breeds. The association of the two promoter SNPs with morphological types could be due to linkage disequilibrium with alleles in other chromosome 18 loci that affect the variability of morphological traits in horses. However, based on our results it cannot be excluded that *MSTN* SNPs could influence morphological traits, that are indirectly related to muscle mass. A few SNPs in the promoter region of the swine *MSTN* gene were associated with muscularity, growth, and meat quality traits [8, 20, 21]. One of them, with high frequency in the muscled Belgian Pietrain breed, was associated with *MSTN* expression level, suggesting that promoter polymorphisms could contribute to muscle mass in this pig breed [8]. To demonstrate the putative functional role of the identified horse *MSTN* promoter SNPs, expression studies in skeletalmuscle of animals with different genotypes should be performed. However, it is worth to point out that *in vivo* RNA *expression* studies in horses are very complicated as it is quite difficult to standardize temporary and permanent environmental factors (i.e. age, sex, management, feeding, etc.) that are major sources of variability in such experiments. For these reasons *in vitro* assays might be needed to clarify if the identified SNPs could alter *MSTN* gene expression. In addition association analysis in breeds segregating for the two promoter SNPs and for which estimated breeding values for several conformational and performance traits are available could be useful to further evaluate the association of these polymorphic sites with phenotypic traits.

Table 4: Minor allele frequency (MAF), observed and expected heterozygosity (Het*), and haplotype (Hap§) frequencies of the two promoter SNPs of the MSTN gene in horses with different morphological types

Types#	Number of horses	MAF g.26C	MAF g.156C	Observed Het(s.d.)x	Expected Het (s.d.)x	Hap [T:T]	Hap [T:C]	Hap [C:T]
B	107	0.11	0.21	0.24 (0.09)	0.26 (0.10)	0.69	0.22	0.09
M	131	0.02	0.22	0.18 (0.20)	0.19 (0.22)	0.76	0.22	0.02
M-D	80	0.04	0.07	0.11 (0.03)	0.11 (0.03)	0.89	0.08	0.03
D	78	0.01	0.01	0.02 (0.01)	0.02 (0.01)	0.98	0.01	0.01
Total	396	0.05	0.15	0.15 (0.09)	0.17 (0.11)	0.81	0.15	0.04

*Means for the two loci and standard deviation, in parenthesis. x Haplotypes for the g.26T>C and g.156T>C polymorphisms. # Types: B= brachimorphic or heavy, M= mesomorphic, M-D= meso-dolichomorphic, D= dolichomorphic or light.

ACKNOWLEDGMENTS

The authors thank horse breeders, Italian Horse National Breeders Associations, Associazione Italiana Allevatori (A.I.A.), Istituto Sperimentale per la Zootecnia of Rome (Italy), and Association Rural de Uruguay for providing horse samples and genealogical information. They also thanks three anonymous reviewers for their comments that made it possible to improve the manuscript. This study was funded by the University of Bologna RFO.

REFERENCES

1. A. C. McPherron, A. M. Lawler, and S.-J. Lee, "Regulation of skeletal muscle mass in mice by a new TGF-β superfamily member," Nature, vol. 387, no. 6628, pp. 83–90, 1997.
2. A. C. McPherron and S.-J. Lee, "Double muscling in cattle due to mutations in the myostatin gene,"Proceedings of the National Academy of Sciences of the United States of America, vol. 94, no. 23, pp. 12457–12461, 1997.
3. D. Joulia-Ekaza and G. Cabello, "Myostatin regulation of muscle development: molecular basis, natural mutations, physiopathological aspects," Experimental Cell Research, vol. 312, no. 13, pp. 2401–2414, 2006.
4. N. F. Gonzalez-Cadavid, W. E. Taylor, and W. E. Taylor, "Organization of the human myostatin gene and expression in healthy men and HIV-infected men with muscle wasting," Proceedings of the National Academy of Sciences of the United States of America, vol. 95, no. 25, pp. 14938–14943, 1998.
5. A. Stratil and M. Kopecny, "Genomic organization, sequence and polymorphism of the porcinemyostatin (GDF8; MSTN) gene," Animal Genetics, vol. 30, no. 6, pp. 468–469, 1999.
6. F. Jeanplong, M. Sharma, W. G. Somers, J. J. Bass, and R. Kambadur, "Genomic organization and neonatal expression of the bovine myostatin gene," Molecular and Cellular Biochemistry, vol. 220, no. 1-2, pp. 31–37, 2001.
7. R. Du, Y.-F. Chen, and Y.-F. Chen, "Cloning and sequence analysis of myostatin promoter in sheep,"DNA Sequence, vol. 16, no. 6, pp. 412–417, 2005.

8. A. Stinckens, T. Luyten, and T. Luyten, "Characterization of the complete porcine MSTN gene and expression levels in pig breeds differing in muscularity," Animal Genetics, vol. 39, no. 6, pp. 586–596, 2008.
9. M. Schuelke, K. R. Wagner, and K. R. Wagner, "Myostatin mutation associated with gross muscle hypertrophy in a child," New England Journal of Medicine, vol. 350, no. 26, pp. 2682–2688, 2004.
10. R. Kambadur, M. Sharma, T. P. L. Smith, and J. J. Bass, "Mutations in myostatin (GDF8) in double-muscled Belgian Blue and Piedmontese cattle," Genome Research, vol. 7, no. 9, pp. 910–916, 1997.
11. L. Grobet, L. J. R. Martin, and L. J. R. Martin, "A deletion in the bovine myostatin gene causes the double-muscled phenotype in cattle," Nature Genetics, vol. 17, no. 1, pp. 71–74, 1997.
12. L. Grobet, D. Poncelet, and D. Poncelet, "Molecular definition of an allelic series of mutations disrupting the myostatin function and causing double-muscling in cattle," Mammalian Genome, vol. 9, no. 3, pp. 210–213, 1998.
13. C. Marchitelli, M. C. Savarese, A. Crisà, A. Nardone, P. A. Marsan, and A. Valentini, "Double muscling in Marchigiana beef breed is caused by a stop codon in the third exon of myostatin gene,"Mammalian Genome, vol. 14, no. 6, pp. 392–395, 2003.
14. A. Clop, F. Marcq, and F. Marcq, "A mutation creating a potential illegitimate microRNA target site in the myostatin gene affects muscularity in sheep," Nature Genetics, vol. 38, no. 7, pp. 813–818, 2006.
15. I. A. Boman, G. Klemetsdal, T. Blichfeldt, O. Nafstad, and D. I. Våge, "A frameshift mutation in the coding region of the myostatin gene (MSTN) affects carcass conformation and fatness in Norwegian White Sheep (Ovis aries)," Animal Genetics, vol. 40, no. 4, pp. 418–422, 2009.
16. I. A. Boman and D. I. Våge, "An insertion in the coding region of the myostatin (MSTN) gene affects carcass conformation and fatness in the Norwegian Spælsau (Ovis aries)," BMC Research Notes, vol. 2, article 98, 2009.

17. D. S. Mosher, P. Quignon, C. D. Bustamante, N. B. Sutter, C. S. Mellersh, H. G. Parker, and E. A. Ostrander, "A mutation in the myostatin gene increases muscle mass and enhances racing performance in heterozygote dogs," PLoS Genetics, vol. 3, no. 5, pp. 779–786, 2007.
18. R. H. S. Bellinge, D. A. Liberles, S. P. A. Iaschi, P. A. O›Brien, and G. K. Tay, "Myostatin and its implications on animal breeding: a review," Animal Genetics, vol. 36, no. 1, pp. 1–6, 2005.
19. J. L. Gill, S. C. Bishop, C. McCorquodale, J. L. Williams, and P. Wiener, "Associations between the 11-bp deletion in the myostatin gene and carcass quality in Angus-sired cattle," Animal Genetics, vol. 40, no. 1, pp. 97–100, 2009.
20. S. E. F. Guimaraes, C. H. Stahl, S. M. Lonergan, B. Geiger, and M. F. Rothschild, "Myostatin promoter analysis and expression pattern in pigs," Livestock Science, vol. 112, no. 1-2, pp. 143–150, 2007.
21. L. Yu, H. Tang, and H. Tang, "Polymorphisms in the 5′ regulatory region of myostatin gene are associated with early growth traits in Yorkshire pigs," Science in China C, vol. 50, no. 5, pp. 642–647, 2007.
22. T. Hosoyama, S. Kawada, and S. Kawada, "Molecular cloning of equine (thoroughbred) myostatincDNA and detection of myostatin precursor proteins in the serum," Journal of Reproduction and Development, vol. 48, no. 4, pp. 335–342, 2002.
23. A. R. Caetano, D. Pomp, J. D. Murray, and A. T. Bowling, "Comparative mapping of 18 equine type I genes assigned by somatic cell hybrid analysis," Mammalian Genome, vol. 10, no. 3, pp. 271–276, 1999.
24. E. W. Hill, J. Gu, and J. Gu, "A sequence polymorphism in MSTN predicts sprinting ability and racing stamina in thoroughbred horses," PLoS ONE, vol. 5, no. 1, article e8645, 2010.
25. A. T. Bowling and A. Ruvinsky, "Genetic aspect of domestication, breeds and their origins," in The Genetics of the Horse, A. T. Bowling and A. Ruvinsky, Eds., CAB International, Oxfordshire, UK, 2000.
26. G. Aparicio, "Zootecnia especial. Etnologia compendiada," Deposito Legal, vol. 16, pp. 25–27, 1960.

27. A. Falaschini, S. Rizzi, and M. Pasquini, "Morphological evolution of the Haflinger horse," Italian Journal of Animal Science, vol. 2, no. 1, pp. 595–597, 2003.
28. A. Sabbioni, V. Beretti, A. Zanon, G. P. Pagani, S. Filippini, P. Superchi, and A. L. Catalano, "Morphological evolution of Bardigiano horse," Italian Journal of Animal Science, vol. 4, no. 2, pp. 412–414, 2005.
29. C. Dario, D. Carnicella, M. Dario, and G. Bufano, "Morphological evolution and heritability estimates for some biometric traits in the Murgese horse breed," Genetics and Molecular Research, vol. 5, no. 2, pp. 309–314, 2006.
30. A. Falaschini and C. Gallinelli, "Morphological evolution of the Throroughbred reared in Italy,"Annual Meeting of the Italian Society for Veterinary Sciences, vol. 60, pp. 497–498, 2006.
31. F. C. Yeh, R. Yang, and T. Boyle, "POPGENE Version 1.31. Microsoft Windows-based freeware for population genetic analysis," 1999, .
32. M. Stephens, N. J. Smith, and P. Donnelly, "A new statistical method for haplotype reconstruction from population data," American Journal of Human Genetics, vol. 68, no. 4, pp. 978–989, 2001.
33. M. P. Spiller, R. Kambadur, F. Jeanplong, M. Thomas, J. K. Martyn, J. J. Bass, and M. Sharma, "Themyostatin gene is a downstream target gene of basic helix-loop-helix transcription factor MyoD,"Molecular and Cellular Biology, vol. 22, no. 20, pp. 7066–7082, 2002.
34. B. Langley, M. Thomas, A. Bishop, M. Sharma, S. Gilmour, and R. Kambadur, "Myostatin inhibits myoblast differentiation by down-regulating MyoD expression," Journal of Biological Chemistry, vol. 277, no. 51, pp. 49831–49840, 2002.
35. X. Jin, J.-G. Kim, and J.-G. Kim, "Opposite roles of MRF4 and MyoD in cell proliferation and myogenic differentiation," Biochemical and Biophysical Research Communications, vol. 364, no. 3, pp. 476–482, 2007.
36. K. Ma, C. Mallidis, J. Artaza, W. Taylor, N. Gonzalez-Cadavid, and S. Bhasin, "Characterization of 5′-regulatory region of human myostatin gene: regulation by dexamethasone in vitro," American Journal of Physiology, vol. 281, no. 6, pp. E1128–E1136, 2001.

37. D. L. Allen and T. G. Unterman, "Regulation of myostatin expression and myoblast differentiation by FoxO and SMAD transcription factors," American Journal of Physiology, vol. 292, no. 1, pp. C188–C199, 2007.
38. D. L. Allen and M. Du, "Comparative functional analysis of the cow and mouse myostatin genes reveals novel regulatory elements in their upstream promoter regions," Comparative Biochemistry and Physiology, vol. 150, no. 4, pp. 432–439, 2008.
39. L. Di Stasio, G. Perrotta, M. Blasi, and C. Lisa, "Genetic characterization of the Bardigiano horse using microsatellite markers," Italian Journal of Animal Science, vol. 7, no. 2, pp. 243–250, 2008.

Chapter 2

A 15-Year Survey of Reproductive Efficiency of Standardbred and Finnhorse Trotters in Finland - Descriptive Results

Terttu Katila[1], Tiina Reilas[2], Kaisa Nivola[3], Terttu Peltonen[4], and Anna-Maija Virtala[5]

[1]Department of Production Animal Medicine, University of Helsinki, Paroninkuja 20,

04920 Saarentaus, Finland

[2]MTT Agrifood Research Finland, Opistontie 10, 32100 Ypäjä, Finland

[3]Kallelan oriasema, Isonummentie 212, 23600 Kalanti, Finland

[4]Suomen Hippos, Tulkinkuja 3, 02650 Espoo, Finland

[5]Department of Veterinary Biosciences, University of Helsinki, P.O. Box 66, 00014 Helsinki, Finland

ABSTRACT

Background

The major horse breeds in Finland are the Finnhorse (FH) and the American Standardbred (SB). The foaling rates of the FH have consistently been lower than those of the SB. During the last years, a decreasing trend in foaling rates of both breeds has been observed. The purpose of this study was to describe and compare the structure of these two mare populations for age, reproductive history and mating type. In addition, changes over the years were studied that could explain the decline in foaling rates.

Methods

In Finland, the mating statistics and foaling rates per stallion are published yearly by Suomen Hippos, which is the Finnish trotting and breeding association authorized by the EU. The studied material was the electronic breeding data of Suomen Hippos in 1991-2005 which contained 69 180 cases (one mare bred in one year with one stallion), 20 168 mares, 2 230 stallions and 5 397 stud managers. The effect of mare age and type, mating type and changes during the study period were examined separately for FH and SB using SAS 9.1 for descriptive statistical analyses (frequencies, percentages, means, standard deviations and confidence intervals). The outcome of the last mating per season (foal or not) was used in the calculation of the foaling rates.

Results

The FH mares were on average one year older and belonged to the older age groups more often than the SB mares. Ageing decreased foaling rates and even more in FH; the foaling rates were the following: young FH 68.6 and SB 72.1%, middle-aged FH 66.1 and SB 71.9%, ageing FH 61.2 and SB 68.4%, and very old FH 52.8 and SB 61.8%. The foaled mares were more frequent in the SB (45%) than in the FH (37%), but the barren and rested mares were more common in the FH. Natural mating was more commonly practiced in the FH as compared to the SB. The foaling rates decreased from 1991 to 2005 in SB from 75.1 to 65.9% and in FH from 66.5 to 60.8%. For both breeds, the proportion of young mares decreased and the proportion of very old mares increased over the years. Similarly, the proportion of foaled mares in both breeds decreased and the proportion of barren mares increased during the study period. In both breeds, insemination (AI) by transported cooled semen increased, diminishing the on-site AI in the SB and the natural mating in the FH.

Conclusions

The results of this study suggest that mare age and type and mating type all affect foaling rates and that the structural differences in the mare populations can explain differences in the foaling rates between the horse breeds and between the time periods.

BACKGROUND

Profitable horse breeding requires general information about the reproductive traits of horses, which horse breeders can then utilize in decision making. However, most research in equine reproduction has focused on individual animals, physiology and pathology. Only one epidemiological study based on a large number of horses (535 746 matings) has been published [1]. This French study comprised several breeds: the Thoroughbred (TB), Anglo-Arab, Selle Francais, French Trotter and the cold-blooded French breeds. An Australian study compared the reproductive efficiency of the TB and the Standardbred (SB) horses [2]. Whereas several reports on TB farms have been published [3-12], less has been published on other breeds: Hannoverians[13], Icelandic horses [14], feral horses [15] and different horse breeds in the USA [16] and in Finland [17].

In Finland, the mating statistics and foaling rates per stallion are published yearly by Suomen Hippos, which is the Finnish trotting and breeding association authorized by the EU. During the recent years, a decreasing trend in foaling rates has been suspected.

Finland has its own horse breed, the Finnish cold blood, the Finnhorse (FH). This breed is of universal type and is mostly used for sports. The average height at withers is 156 cm and the weight is 550 kg. The present population is 19 500 horses from which 200 are breeding stallions and 2 300 brood mares. Furthermore, approximately 1 300 foals are born yearly [18].

Annual reports of Suomen Hippos show higher foaling rates for the SB than for the FH.

The total population of the SB in Finland is about 25 000 making it the largest horse breed in Finland. According to the data base of Suomen Hippos, 64% of the SB mares were born in Finland and 36% were imported. Annually, 90 stallions and 2 600 mares are used for breeding and 1 600 foals are born. In addition, semen from approx. 50 foreign stallions is imported both as cooled and frozen, mainly from Sweden, Italy, Germany and USA. The use of imported semen has increased from 50 to approximately 500 mares per year; half of the mares are inseminated with frozen semen.

The Finnish studbooks and horse registers are kept and administered by Suomen Hippos. To maintain these records, the stallion managers have to report all matings of the breeding season to one of the sixteen local horse breeding associations by the end of October. If the mating has not been reported, the foals are not registered and they are not allowed to race. As a consequence, one can assume that practically all the matings of the trotter mares and births of the foals are reported. Moreover, since 1990, local breeding associations submit the mating records in digital form to the central database of Suomen Hippos.

The objective of this study was to examine the Finnish horse breeding data for possible differences between the two breeds and for changes in the foaling rates through the years. The frequency distributions and foaling rates are reported for each breed, year, time period, age, mare type and mating type. The aim was to seek for any structural changes and differences in the mare populations or mating methods that could explain the possible differences between the breeds and years.

METHODS

The data originates from all the reported inseminations of the FH and SB trotter mares in Finland during the years 1991-2005. For this project, the records in the database of Suomen Hippos were imported to Excel®.

One case was defined as one mare bred in one year with one stallion. Only the outcome of the last mating per season (foal or not) was used. The original data consisted of 70 238 cases; 1 002 cases were excluded from the data because the mare type could not be defined. These excluded mares had entered the database in the first years of the digital registration and their foaling history was unknown. Mares over 25 years old (n = 28) were all excluded owing to the small likelihood of their conceiving at this advanced age. One-year-old mares were also excluded (n = 25) because their mating was not planned but accidental, and therefore, only mares which foaled had been reported. Another group excluded from this study was the only three FH mares artificially inseminated (AI) with frozen semen. After these exclusions, the final number of cases was 69 180. It is important to note that the same mares, stallions and stallion managers occur several times because the data covers 15 years.

Definitions

Foaling rate was used as the measure of reproductive efficiency. In the horse breeding literature, the foaling rate is used for the proportion of mares (%) that have foaled the following year of all mares mated. The Finnish database also includes matings per cycle, but since they had not been consistently reported, the foaling rate was considered to be a more reliable measure.

In the database of Suomen Hippos, the result of the breeding is divided into seven categories. In this study, the categories filly, colt, dead foal and foal died after birth were assigned the value 1 (foaled), and the categories barren, aborted and mare died pregnant were given the value 0 (not foaled).

The change in foaling rates through the years was studied both from year to year and in longer time periods. The 15 years in the study were divided in four time periods (TP): TP1 = 1991 - 1994, TP2 = 1995 - 1998, TP3 = 1999 - 2002 and TP4 = 2003 - 2005.

Mares were divided into four age groups: young (2 - 9 years), middle-aged (10 - 13 years), ageing (14 - 16 years), and very old (17 - 25 years). The different mare types in the data were 1) maiden (never mated), 2) barren (mated earlier, but aborted or did not conceive), 3) rested (not mated after the last foaling), and 4) foaled (mare with a live or dead foal).

The type of breeding was categorised as 1) on-site AI (mare inseminated with fresh semen at the same station where the stallion was resident), 2) AI using transported semen (mare inseminated with cooled semen transported to another station or home stable), 3) AI using frozen semen (only in SB), and 4) natural mating.

Statistics

After the data had been checked for possible mistakes, typing errors and outliers, they were transported to the SAS 9.1 statistical package (SAS Institute Inc.) for descriptive statistical analyses. The data were described using frequencies, percentages, means, and standard deviations. The 95% binomial confidence intervals for the percentages were calculated using the FREQ procedure.

RESULTS

There were altogether 69 180 breeding cases and 102 615 cycles, out of which 33 699 breeding cases/49 339 cycles were for the FH mares and 35 481 cases/53 276 cycles for the SB mares. The data included 20 143 mares: 9 633 FH and 10 510 SB. About 30% of the mares appeared in the data more than once. The same FH mare appeared in the data a maximum of 24 times and the same SB mare 18 times. About 3% of the mares (594 mares) had more than 10 breeding seasons.

There were altogether 2 230 stallions (1 201 FH and 1029 SB) and 5 397 stallion managers. Stallion managers were divided according to the breed of the stallion: 3 472 stallion managers had FH stallions and 2 190 SB stallions.

Mares

The young mares were the largest age group, but whereas they comprised 47% of the SB mare population, they represented only 37% of the FH mares. Correspondingly, the FH occurred more frequently in the very old mare group than the SB (13 versus 8%). The proportions of middle-aged mares were 33% in FH and 32% in SB and the proportions of ageing mares 17 and 13%, respectively. The median ages were 11 years for the FH and 10 years for the SB.

Foaled mares were the largest mare type in both breeds, but more frequent in the SB (45%) than in the FH (37%). On the other hand, barren and rested mares were more common in the FH (26 and 15%) than in the SB (21 and 12%). The proportions of maiden mares were 21% in FH and 22% in SB.

When the age within the mare types was considered, the young SB mares were more frequent in the categories of maiden, barren and foaled mares than the FH; no difference was detected in the rested mares (Table 1). In the middle-aged and ageing groups, the maiden FH mares were more common than the SB mares.

Table 1: Proportions (% and 95% CI) of different mare age groups in different mare types for Finnhorses (FH) and Standardbreds (SB) in years 1991 – 2005

	Maiden		Barren		Rested		Foaled	
	%	95% CI	%	95% CI	%	95% CI	%	95% CI
Young								
FH	83.2	82.3 - 84.1	25.0	24.1 - 25.9	26.3	25.1 - 27.5	23.8	23.0 - 24.5
SB	90.5	89.8 - 91.1	35.9	34.8 - 37.0	25.6	24.3 - 26.9	37.0	36.3 - 37.8
Middle-aged								
FH	14.7	13.9 - 15.5	34.9	33.9 - 35.9	39.2	37.8 - 40.5	38.8	37.9 - 39.6
SB	8.2	7.6 - 8.8	36.7	35.6 - 37.8	43.4	42.0 - 44.9	39.3	38.5 - 40.0
Ageing								
FH	1.7	1.4 - 2.0	21.7	20.9 - 22.6	20.3	19.2 - 21.4	22.0	21.2 - 22.7
SB	1.1	0.8 - 1.3	15.9	15.1 - 16.7	18.7	17.5 - 19.8	15.1	14.6 - 15.7
Very old								
FH	0.3	0.2 - 0.5	18.3	17.5 - 19.1	14.3	13.4 - 15.3	15.5	14.8 - 16.1
SB	0.3	0.2 - 0.4	11.6	10.8 - 12.3	12.3	11.3 - 13.3	8.6	8.2 - 9.0

n FH	6987	8870	5236	12606
n SB	7869	7401	4355	15856

Age groups: Young = 2 - 9 years, Middle-aged = 10 - 13 years, Ageing = 14 - 16 years, Very old = 17 - 25 years.

Katila et al. Acta Veterinaria Scandinavica 2010 52:40, doi: 10.1186/1751-0147-52-40

In the whole material, half of the FH were naturally mated, whereas only one quarter of the SB mares were. In the SB, the on-site AI was the most common mating type (41%), as compared to 28% of the FH mares; natural mating was most common for the FH population. Transported semen was used more frequently to the foaled mares as compared to the other mare types (Table 2).

Table 2: Proportions (% and 95% CI) of different mating types in different mare types for Finnhorses (FH) and Standardbreds (SB) in years 1991 - 2005

	Maiden		Barren		Rested		Foaled	
	%	95% CI	%	95% CI	%	95% CI	%	95% CI
On-site AI								
FH	29.3	28.2 - 30.3	28.1	27.1 - 29.0	27.8	26.6 - 29.0	27.4	26.6 - 28.2
SB	42.4	41.3 - 43.5	44.2	43.1 - 45.3	40.5	39.0 - 41.9	39.8	39.0 - 40.6
Transported semen								
FH	19.5	18.5 - 20.4	18.0	17.2 - 18.8	19.9	18.8 - 21.0	27.1	26.3 - 27.9
SB	25.5	24.6 - 26.5	24.9	23.9 - 25.9	26.8	25.5 - 28.2	32.9	32.1 -- 33.6
Frozen semen								
SB	5.3	4.8 - 5.8	4.8	4.3 - 5.3	3.7	3.2 - 4.3	5.5	5.1 - 5.9
Natural cover								

FH	51.3	50.1 - 52.5	53.9	52.9 - 55.0	52.3	50.9 - 53.6	45.5	44.7 -- 46.4
SB	26.8	25.8 - 27.8	26.1	25.1 - 27.1	29.0	27.6 - 30.3	21.8	21.2 - 22.5
n FH	6987		8870		5236		12606	
n SB	7869		7401		4355		15856	

Katila *et al. Acta Veterinaria Scandinavica* 2010 52:40, doi: 10.1186/1751-0147-52-40

Changes over the Study Period

The structure of the Finnish broodmare population changed during the study period. For instance, the proportion of young mares decreased over the years in both breeds (Table 3); the proportion of young mares in the FH group fell from 40 to 30% between 1991 and 2005 and those in the SB group fell from 54 to 41% during the same period. In addition, during the same years, the proportion of the very old mares changed from 11 to 16% in the FH and from 6 to 11% in the SB.

Table 3: Proportions (% and 95% CI) of different mare age groups in different time periods for Finnhorses (FH) and Standardbreds (SB)

	1991-1994		1995-1998		1999-2002		2003-2005	
	%	95% CI	%	95% CI	%	95% CI	%	95% CI
Young								
FH	39.9	38.9 - 41.0	41.3	40.3 - 42.2	33.8	32.8 - 34.8	30.3	29.2 - 31.4
SB	53.9	52.8 - 54.9	50.6	49.6 - 51.6	42.8	41.8 - 43.8	40.8	39.7 - 41.9
Middle-aged								
FH	31.0	30.0 - 32.0	32.3	31.4 - 33.2	34.5	33.5 - 35.5	33.7	32.6 - 34.8

SB	29.8	28.8 - 30.7	31.6	30.6 - 32.5	34.6	33.6 - 35.5	33.6	32.6 - 34.7
Ageing								
FH	18.3	17.5 - 19.1	14.4	13.7 - 15.1	17.9	17.1 - 18.7	20.3	19.4 - 21.3
SB	10.7	10.1 - 11.4	11.1	10.5 - 11.8	14.3	13.6 - 15.0	14.5	13.7 - 15.3
Very old								
FH	10.8	10.1 - 11.4	12.0	11.4 - 12.7	13.8	13.1 - 14.5	15.7	14.8 - 16.6
SB	5.7	5.2 - 6.1	6.7	6.2 - 7.2	8.3	7.8 - 8.9	11.1	10.4 - 11.8
n FH	8313		9917		8791		6678	
n SB	8971		9401		9434		7675	

Age groups: Young = 2 - 9 years, Middle-aged = 10 - 13 years, Ageing = 14 - 16 years, Very old = 17 - 25 years.

Katila et al. Acta Veterinaria Scandinavica 2010 52:40, doi: 10.1186/1751-0147-52-40

Another finding is that over the years, the proportion of foaled mares decreased from 46 to 30% in the FH and from 53 to 39% in the SB. The proportion of barren mares increased in both breeds, but no changes were observed in the maiden mares (Table 4).

Table 4: Proportions (% and 95% CI) of different mare types in different time periods for Finnhorses (FH) and Standardbreds (SB)

	1991-1994		1995-1998		1999-2002		2003-2005	
	%	95% CI	%	95% CI	%	95% CI	%	95% CI
Maiden								
FH	20.1	19.3 - 21.0	21.8	21.0 - 22.6	19.1	18.3 - 19.9	22.1	21.1 - 23.1
SB	20.3	19.5 - 21.2	25.1	24.2 - 25.9	20.5	19.7 - 21.4	22.8	21.9 - 23.8

Barren								
FH	24.7	23.8 - 25.6	24.7	23.8 - 25.5	27.3	26.4 - 28.3	29.5	28.4 - 30.6
SB	18.5	17.7 - 19.3	18.9	18.1 - 19.7	22.2	21.3 - 23.0	24.4	23.5 - 25.4
Rested								
FH	9.6	9.0 - 10.3	16.0	15.3 - 16.7	18.3	17.4 - 19.1	18.6	17.7 - 19.5
SB	8.1	7.6 - 8.7	13.0	12.3 - 13.6	14.2	13.5 - 14.9	13.9	13.1 - 14.7
Foaled								
FH	45.6	44.5 - 46.6	37.5	36.6 - 38.5	35.3	34.3 - 36.3	29.8	28.7 - 30.9
SB	53.0	52.0 - 54.1	43.1	42.1 - 44.1	43.1	42.1 - 44.1	38.8	37.7 - 39.9
n FH	8313		9917		8791		6678	
n SB	8971		9401		9434		7675	

Katila *et al. Acta Veterinaria Scandinavica* 2010 52:40, doi: 10.1186/1751-0147-52-40

In mating types, the change in favour of insemination with transported semen was quite marked in both breeds (FH from 14 to 31% and SB from 15 to 36%) (Table 5). On-site AI decreased in SB (from 50 to 36%) but stayed the same in FH. The use of natural mating became less popular in both breeds: from 55 to 40% in FH and from 31 to 20% in SB. The use of frozen semen increased slightly (from 4 to 8%) in SB.

Table 5: Proportions (% and 95% CI) of different mating types in different time periods for Finnhorses (FH) and Standardbreds (SB)

	1991-1994		1995-1998		1999-2002		2003-2005	
	%	95% CI	%	95% CI	%	95% CI	%	95% CI
On-site AI								

FH	30.8	29.8 - 31.8	25.7	24.8 - 26.6	27.2	26.2 - 28.1	29.2	28.1 - 30.3
SB	50.1	49.0 - 51.1	42.6	41.6 - 43.6	36.5	35.5 - 37.5	35.7	34.6 - 36.8
Transported semen								
FH	14.0	13.2 - 14.7	19.8	19.0 - 20.6	25.4	24.5 - 26.3	30.7	29.6 - 31.8
SB	15.4	14.7 - 16.2	26.4	25.5 - 27.3	38.1	37.1 - 39.1	36.1	35.1 - 37.2
Frozen semen								
SB	3.9	3.5 - 4.3	4.7	4.3 - 5.1	4.4	4.0 - 4.8	7.8	7.2 - 8.4
Natural cover								
FH	55.2	54.2 - 56.3	54.5	53.5 - 55.5	47.4	46.4 - 48.5	40.1	39.0 - 41.3
SB	30.7	29.7 - 31.6	26.3	25.4 - 27.2	21.0	20.1 - 21.8	20.3	19.4 - 21.2
n FH	8313		9917		8791		6678	
n SB	8971		9401		9434		7675	

Katila *et al. Acta Veterinaria Scandinavica* 2010 52:40, doi: 10.1186/1751-0147-52-40

Foaling Rate

The foaling rate in the whole material was 68%: 64% in the FH and 71% in the SB. There was a lowering trend in the foaling rates from 71% (66% in FH and 75% in SB) in 1991 to 63% (61% in FH and 66% in SB) in 2005 (Figure 1). Foaling rates declined with increasing age in both breeds (Figure 2). Barren mares displayed the lowest foaling rates (Figure 3). In both breeds, the rested and foaled mares in young and middle-aged groups were the most fertile while the very old maidens were the least fertile (Table 6). Moreover, the very old and ageing barren and the ageing maiden FH mares showed low foaling rates.

Table 6: Foaling rates in different mare types and age groups for Finnhorses (FH) and Standardbreds (SB) in years 1991 – 2005

	FH			SB		
	n	foaling rate%	95% CI	n	foaling rate %	95% CI
Young	12405			16756		
Maiden		67.9	66.7 - 69.1		71.7	70.6 - 72.7
Barren		63.9	61.9 - 65.9		69.4	67.7 - 71.2
Rested		71.9	69.6 - 74.3		76.4	73.9 -78.9
Foaled		72.1	70.5 - 73.8		72.9	71.8 - 74.1
Middle-aged	11066			11479		
Maiden		59.9	56.9 - 62.9		67.9	64.3 - 71.5
Barren		59.1	57.4 - 60.1		68.7	67.0 - 70.5
Rested		68.9	66.9 - 70.9		73.8	71.9 - 75.8
Foaled		70.7	69.4 - 72.0		73.1	72.0 - 74.2
Ageing	5880			4470		
Maiden		39.7	30.9 - 48.4		63.9	53.5 - 74.2
Barren		54.4	52.2 - 56.6		66.2	63.4 - 68.9
Rested		67.9	65.1 - 70.7		69.8	66.6 - 72.9
Foaled		64.4	62.6 - 66.1		69.3	67.4 - 71.1
Very old	4348			2776		
Maiden		37.5	18.1 - 56.9		52.2	31.8 - 72.6
Barren		47.8	45.4 - 50.2		58.8	55.5 - 62.1

Rested		53	49.4 - 56.6		65.4	61.4 - 69.5
Foaled		57	54.8 - 59.2		62.4	59.8 - 65.0

Age groups: Young = 2 - 9 years, Middle-aged = 10 - 13 years, Ageing = 14 - 16 years, Very old = 17 - 25 years.

Katila et al. Acta Veterinaria Scandinavica 2010 52:40, doi: 10.1186/1751-0147-52-40

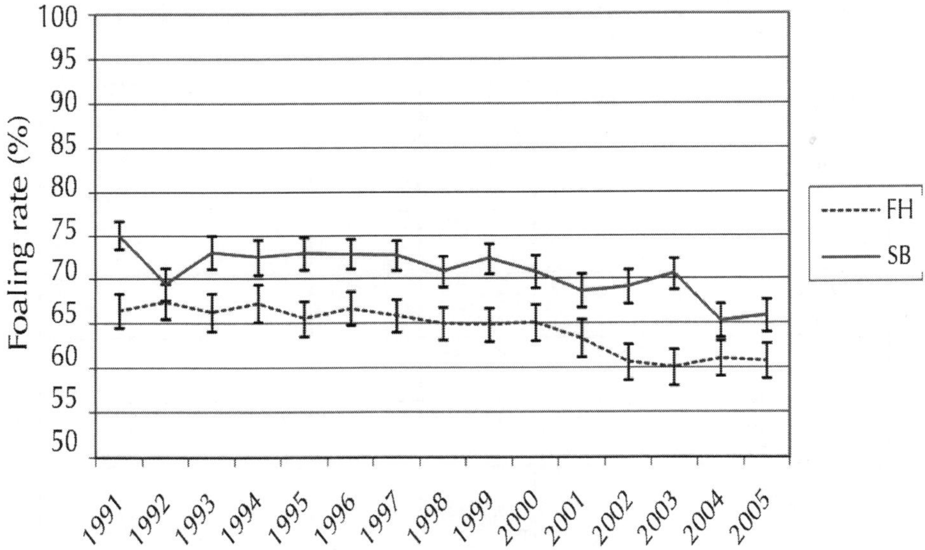

Figure 1: Foaling rates (mean with 95% confidence interval) in the different years for the Finnhorses (FH) and Standardbreds (SB).

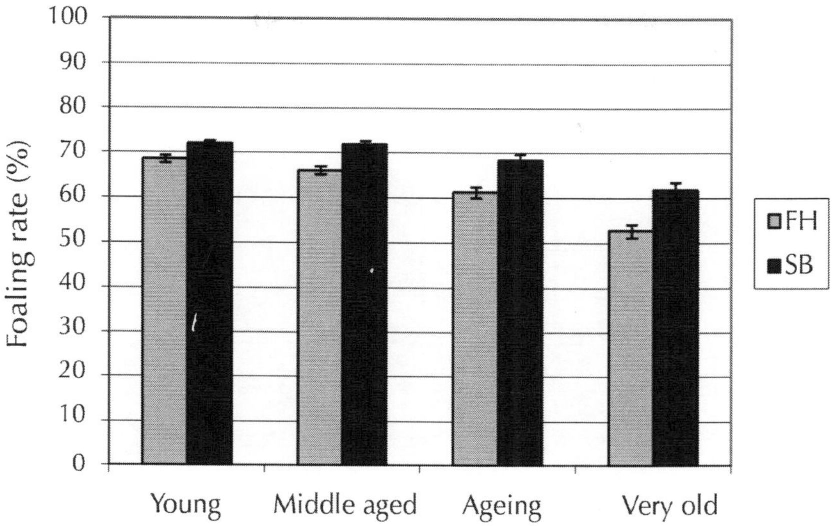

Figure 2: Foaling rates (mean with 95% confidence interval) in the different age groups for the Finnhorses (FH) and Standardbreds (SB) in the years 1991 - 2005. Age groups: Young = 2 - 9 years, Middle-aged = 10 - 13 years, Ageing = 14 - 16 years, Very old = 17 - 25 years.

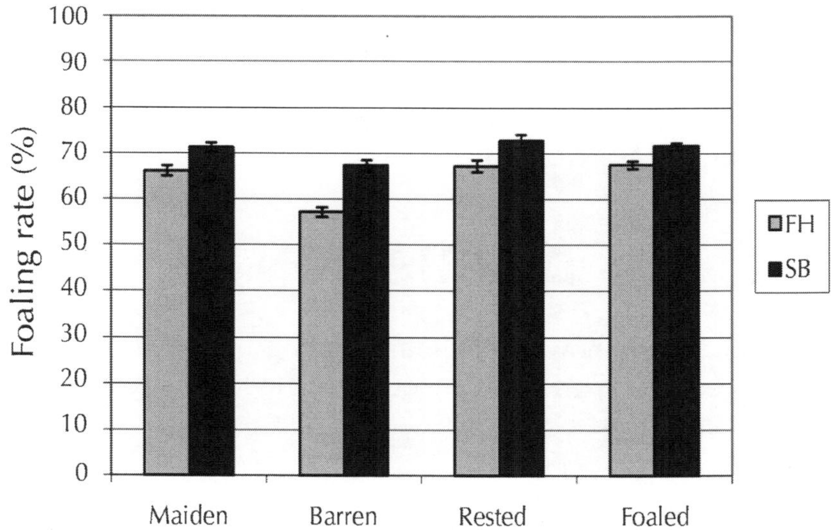

Figure 3: Foaling rates (mean with 95% confidence interval) in the different mare types for the Finnhorses (FH) and Standardbreds (SB) in the years 1991 - 2005.

The least successful mating type of the FH was natural mating and the most successful was the on-site AI. For the SB, the lowest foaling rate was found in the frozen semen group and the highest rate in the on-site AI group (Figure 4).

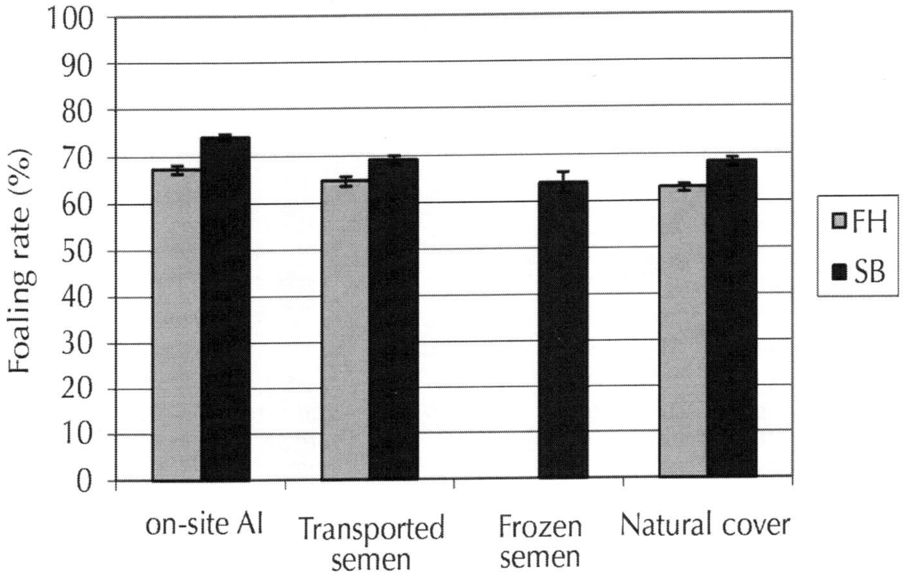

Figure 4: Foaling rates (mean with 95% confidence interval) in the different mating types for the Finnhorses (FH) and Standardbreds (SB) in the years 1991 - 2005.

DISCUSSION

The data analysed showed declining foaling rates during the study period. Moreover, it was very obvious that the foaling rates of the FH were lower than those of the SB.

Differences between FB and SB

The FH exhibited lower foaling rates than the SB. It is possible that the FH has genetically inferior fertility as compared to the SB, but the differences in the management of the mares and stallions, in both the age structure of the horses and in the proportions of the different mare types, may also explain the difference in foaling rates. Langlois and Blouin [1] reported lower fertility for cold-blooded horses, but pointed out that this may be related to the differences in reporting foals. Management plays an important role: the intensively and professionally managed TB mares have very high pregnancy and foaling rates [9]. In contrast, the FH owners may represent a more traditional horse owner because natural mating was more commonly practiced for the FH than for the SB. Foaling rates after natural mating were lower than after on-site AI which was more common in the SB. The FH mares are probably more often owned and handled by amateurs who might not even sell their foals. The breeding and foal fees are lower for the FH which may also exert an effect on the efforts to get a foal.

The FH mares were on average one year older than the SB mares, which is likely to cause some difference in the foaling outcome. Many studies report the negative effect of ageing of mares on the rates of pregnancy and foaling and on the pregnancy loss [1,3,6,8-12,16,19-21]. It is well established that fertility starts to decrease in middle age: according to Allen et al. > 9 years [11], Laing and Leech > 10 years [3], Hutton and Meacham > 12 years [16], Hemberg et al. > 13 years[10], Morris and Allen, Sanderson and Allen, and Bosh et al. ≥ 14 years [6,9,12], and Hearn et al. > 15 years [8]. In our data, the FH were overrepresented by about 10 percentage points in the two older age classes as compared to the SB. Moreover, the foaling rates in these two higher age groups were lower than in the two younger age groups for both breeds. The FH had foaling rates that were 4-5 percentage points lower than the SB in all age groups, except in the very old mare group where the difference was 9 percentage points higher. Since the FH have lower foaling rates at all ages, age alone may not explain the difference between the breeds, although the higher mean age of the FH certainly contributes to the difference.

Factors that affect a mare's chance of foaling are the age and the reproductive history of the mare. There were less foaled mares in the FH than in the SB. Correspondingly, the barren mare group was larger in the FH than in the SB. Foaled mares are the most fertile group [9], with the exception of the mares bred in foal heat which have lower pregnancy rates [5,9] and higher pregnancy loss rates [9,19] than the mares mated in subsequent heats. Maiden mares are also highly fertile [8,9,11,12]. In contrast, barren mares have the lowest pregnancy rates and the highest pregnancy loss rates [6,8,11,12,19]. In all mare types, the FH had 4-5 percentage points lower foaling rates than the SB, but for barren mares, the difference was 10 percentage points. Although mare type alone may not explain the difference between the FH and SB, it may be a contributing factor to the difference, since the distribution of mares into mare types was less favourable in the FH than in the SB.

The interaction of age and mare type has to be considered as well. Particularly in the maiden mare group, the FH mares were older than those of the SB. Moreover, the old maiden mares have been shown to be the least fertile of all when inseminated with frozen semen [22]. The FH mares seemed to enter the barren mare category at a younger age than the SB mares. In all, the FH mare population differed from the SB population both in terms of age and mare type and age within the mare type. All these differences were unfavourable to the FH and can at least partly explain the lower foaling rates of the FH mares.

Decreasing Foaling Rates

The foaling rates showed a decline over the years, which was particularly noticeable since 2000. The decrease in the foaling rate from 1991 to 2005 was over 10 percentage points for the SB, which was greater than for the FH. In fact, the foaling rate difference between the breeds has diminished from the initial 10% to 5%. The foaling rates (for live foal) in TB breeding increased from 1983 to 1998 by 5 percentage points [9] but decreased from 1998 to 2002 by 3 percentage points [9,11]. During the decade 1989-1999 in France, foaling rates increased in all breeds, but more so for the cold-blooded horses, which were less productive to start with; the TB breed progressed very little [1]. However, these studies are from a different time period as the present study and therefore cannot be directly compared. Finland has seen the same trend, with the foaling rates increasing in the 1980 s because of the new reproductive technology, the on-site AI and ultrasonography.

During the follow-up time, the proportion of young mares decreased both in the FH and the SB, and correspondingly the proportions of other age classes increased. Thus, the development in the mares' age has been unfavourable and may contribute to the decline in foaling rates. Furthermore, the proportion of foaled mares diminished (16 percentage points for FH and 14 for SB) and the proportion of barren mares increased in both breeds (5 percentage points for FH and 6 for SB). During this time, the proportion of the rested FH mares doubled and the proportion of these increased in the SB mares by almost 5 percentage points. These represent major changes from the most fertile mare groups to the less fertile mare types.

The structure of the brood mare population for age and reproductive history has not been studied in other breeds with the exception of the TB. Allen and his coworkers published three studies about reproductive efficiency in TB in Newmarket area. These publications contain pregnancy and foaling rates and their analysis from mating seasons 1982-3, 1998 and 2002 [6,9,11]. This allows also us to look at changes over the years and compare the distributions of ages (Table 7) and mare types (Table 8) between TB, SB, and FH. The division of mares into age categories in the English studies was slightly different from ours but the results are still comparable. The time periods were not exactly the same, since the first English study was carried out 10 years earlier than our first time period.

Table 7: Age distribution of Thoroughbreds (TB), Standardbreds (SB) and Finnhorses (FH)

Mating seasons	Young (%)	Middle-aged (%)	Ageing (%)	Very old (%)
TB				
1982-3	51.8	30.0	14.6	3.6
1998	53.5	29.7	14.0	2.8
2002	45.1	32.8	17.0	4.3
SB				
1991-4	53.9	29.8	10.7	5.7
1995-8	50.6	31.6	11.1	6.7
1999-2002	42.8	34.6	14.3	8.3
FH				
1991-4	39.9	31.0	18.3	10.8
1995-8	41.3	32.3	14.4	12.0
1999-2002	33.8	34.5	17.9	13.8

Young = 3-8 y for TB and 2-9 y for SB and FH; middle-aged = 9-13 y for TB and 10-13 y for SB and FH; ageing = 14-18 y for TB and 14-16 y for SB and FH; very old = > 18 for TB and 17-25 for SB and FH.

TB data 1982-3 from Sanderson and Allen (1987), 1998 from Morris and Allen (2002), and 2002 from Allen et al. (2007) [6,9,11].

Katila et al. Acta Veterinaria Scandinavica 2010 52:40, doi:10.1186/1751-0147-52-40

Table 8: Distribution of different mare types in Thoroughbreds (TB), Standardbreds (SB) and Finnhorses (FH)

Mating seasons	Maiden (%)	Barren (%)	Foaling (%)	Rested (%)
TB				
1982-3	11.9	24.7	63.4	N.R.
1998	16.2	16.8	65.5	1.5
2002	17.7	24.7	57.6	N.R.
SB				
1991-4	20.3	18.5	55.0	8.1
1995-8	25.1	18.9	43.1	13.0
1999-2002	20.5	22.2	43.1	14.2
FH				
1991-4	20.1	24.7	45.6	9.6
1995-8	21.8	24.7	37.5	16.0
1999-2002	19.1	27.3	35.3	18.3

Barren mare category includes also aborted mares. N.R. = not reported.

TB data 1982-3 from Sanderson and Allen (1987), 1998 from Morris and Allen (2002), and 2002 from Allen et al. (2007) [6, 9, 11].

Katila et al. Acta Veterinaria Scandinavica 2010 52:40, doi: 10.1186/1751-0147-52-40

The age structure of TB and SB was similar, but FH were much older. While the mares in our material became older, the TB population was younger in 1998 than earlier or later. Maybe this is also the reason for the higher pregnancy and foaling rates reported for the season 1998 as compared to 1982-3 and 2002. However, a clear ageing of the TB mare population from 1982-3 to 2002 was evident similar to our observations.

The proportion of foaling mares throughout these years was approximately 10 percentage points higher in TB than in SB and 20 percentage points higher than in FH (Table 8). The maiden mare population was smaller in TB than in our trotters but the barren mare group was similar in size. It is unclear, why rested mares were lacking in the TB studies from 1982-3 and 2002, but since they comprised only 1.5% in 1998, it can be concluded that they did not represent a large group. This group was much higher in the SB and FH trotters. This may reflect the professionalism in TB breeding: once the mare has started as a brood mare, it is consistently bred each year. In Finland, many breeders have one or two mares which they breed only for their own purposes, not for sale. Economical constraints may also play a role; in Finland the foal prices and selling prospects have sometimes been so low that it is better not to breed the mare again for a year or two.

During the first half of the 1980 s natural mating gave way to the on-site AI in Finland. In the second half of the 1980 s, transported semen started to replace the on-site AI. This development - a decrease in natural mating and in the on-site AI and an increase in transported semen - continued during the study period of 1991-2005. In the FH, the proportion of the on-site AI did not change much, but while the proportion of transported semen doubled, the proportion of natural mating decreased by 15.1 percentage points. Moreover, the proportion of transported semen doubled in the SB, but both the on-site AI (-14 percentage points) and natural mating (-10 percentage points) decreased. In addition, the use of frozen semen increased by 4 percentage points. Almost 44% of the SB mares are inseminated using techniques where the individual stallion differences in the sperm survival during storage can result in a large variation in the foaling rates.

Natural cover - which is the only allowed mating method for the TB - results in very high rates of pregnancy and foaling in the TB industry [9-12], but in other breeds where the AI is allowed and used, higher pregnancy rates have usually been reported for the AI than for the natural mating. For instance, Langlois and Blouin [1] demonstrated the highest foaling rates for the on-site AI. The next best method was free pasture mating (not practiced in Finland); similar results were yielded for transported semen, frozen semen and in-hand natural mating. For both breeds in Finland, the on-site AI was the best method; foaling rates after the use of natural mating and transported semen were similar, but lower as compared to the on-site AI, and frozen semen resulted in the lowest foaling rate. The differences in foaling rates between the on-site AI and the transported semen were almost 3 percentage points for the FH and 5 percentage points for the SB.

The high pregnancy and foaling rates of the TB as a result of natural cover are in conflict with the results achieved in other breeds. Probably the high value of the breeding stock and foals creates pressures, but also offers opportunities for veterinarians and stud managers to intensively manage, control and treat mares. The AI as such may not be any better than natural mating, but its use requires the use of a veterinarian and as a result, the mares are carefully controlled and examined.

Foaling rate vs. Pregnancy rates

Unfortunately, the original goal to use the pregnancy rate per cycle as the fertility measure was not possible because of frequent missing data. Pregnancy rate per cycle reflects the true fertility of the mare and stallion, whereas the seasonal pregnancy rate can be greatly improved by persistent trying, hard work and good management. Foaling rate, on the other hand, includes the effect of the pregnancy losses. Although this does not necessarily reflect innate fertility, it is the best economical measure. One example for the difference between the fertility measures can be taken from the study of Morris and Allen [9]: the pregnancy rates per cycle were 55.3% for barren mares and 61.4% for foaling mares, the respective seasonal pregnancy rates were 92.4 and 85.6%, and foaling rates 88.8 and 81.2%. The barren mares may be valuable problem mares which get more attention and benefit from veterinary treatments, but also have a risk to lose the pregnancy. In an Australian study, the pregnancy rate per cycle was significantly higher in TB than in SB, but the seasonal pregnancy rates were the same, which was explained by the longer breeding season in SB industry [2]. One can speculate whether the low foaling rates of barren and old mares in Finnish trotters, particularly FH, as compared with those of TB could be explained by deficient veterinary care and reluctance of owners to invest money in the treatments. In the intensive and professional TB industry, veterinarians are an integral part of the business, but in Finland this is not as self-explanatory.

Another example can be taken from the use of frozen semen. There per cycle pregnancy rates are typically low (20-50%), but the seasonal pregnancy rates are close to fresh semen AI (60-90%)[23]. In our data, the foaling rate after frozen semen AI was 64%, which was 6 percentage points lower than for transported semen, but presumably the pregnancy rates per cycle would have differed more. Pregnancy rate per cycle is a more sensitive indicator when the efficiency and economy of breeding is evaluated.

Sources of Error

Our results are prone to some errors due to several steps and several people handling the data starting from the level of accuracy among the stallion holders providing the first information.

It is also possible that some stallion owners purposely left some of the non-pregnant mares out of the book in an attempt to get better pregnancy results for their stallion. Moreover, not all breedings are necessarily reported, because stallion managers might not be aware of the purpose of reporting matings in all heats, not just the last heat of the season.

CONCLUSIONS

For the future, it is very important that the data collection is precise, reliable and as inclusive as possible. This means that all matings in all cycles should be recorded. As the foaling rate is not a very sensitive indicator for fertility and the pregnancy rate per cycle or per first mating would be much better, their use should be made possible. Furthermore, the stud farms should give the breeding reports in real time or at least once a month to avoid the possibility of leaving out data on the non-successful matings.

Precise, accurate and timely breeding data are necessary to detect the possible changes in fertility and breeding efficiency. For this reason, the horse breeding industry needs to be informed in good time about the possible threats to the efficiency of horse breeding.

The descriptive results of this study suggest that factors such as age and type of the mare as well as mating type all have important effects on foaling rates. Moreover, structural differences exist between the two horse breed populations which may explain the differences in foaling rates. Structural differences in the mare populations have taken place during the study period and they are likely to explain the declining foaling rates. A more in-depth statistical multivariable analysis of the data considering the hierarchy of the breeding structure would reveal the relative significance of the different variables.

AUTHORS' CONTRIBUTIONS

KN imported, checked, corrected and analysed the material and drafted the figures. A-M V instructed and supervised the description and statistical analysis of the data and participated in the revision of the manuscript. TR actively participated in the revision and writing of the manuscript. TP represented the organisation that owned the data and was actively involved in the planning of the research and made comments to the text. TK was the initiator and leader of the project and had the major responsibility for writing and finalizing the manuscript. All authors read and approved the final manuscript.

ACKNOWLEDGEMENTS

The authors wish to thank the Ministry of Agriculture and Forestry for funding this study, the Suomen Hippos for generously providing the data, and statistician Tero Vahlberg for his work.

REFERENCES

1. Langlois B, Blouin C: Statistical analysis of some factors affecting the number of horse births in France. *Reprod Nutr Dev* 2004, 44:583-595.
2. Reproductive efficiency of horses in Australia[http://www.gvequine.com.au/breeding_efficiency.htm] *webcite* 9.1.2009.
3. Laing JA, Leech FB: The frequency of infertility in Thoroughbred mares. *J Reprod Fertil* 1975, (Suppl 23):307-310.
4. Osborne VE: Factors influencing foaled percentages in Australian mares. *J Reprod Fertil* 1975, (Suppl 23):477-483.

5. Sullivan JJ, Turner PC, Self LC, Gutteridge HB, Bartlett DE: Survey of reproductive efficiency in the Quarter-horse and Thoroughbred. *J Reprod Fertil* 1975, (Suppl 23):315-318.
6. Sanderson MW, Allen WR: *Reproductive efficiency of Thoroughbred mares in the United Kingdom*. 9th edition. Edited by Huntigton T. Proc Bain Fallon Memorial Lectures, AEVA, Sydney; 31-41.
7. Brück I, Anderson GA, Hyland JH: Reproductive performance of thoroughbred mares on six commercial stud farms. *Aust Vet J* 1993, 70:299-303.
8. Hearn P, Bonnett B, Samper J: Factors influencing pregnancy and pregnancy loss on one thoroughbred farm.*39th Ann Conv Am Assoc Equine Pract* 1993, 161-163.
9. Morris LHA, Allen WR: Reproductive efficiency of intensively managed Thoroughbred mares in Newmarket. *Equine Vet J* 2002, 34:51-60.
10. Hemberg E, Lundeheim N, Einarsson S: Reproductive performance of Thoroughbred mares in Sweden. *Reprod Dom Anim* 2004, 39:81-85.
11. Allen WR, Brown L, Wright M, Wilsher S: Reproductive efficiency of Flatrace and National Hunt Thoroughbred mares and stallions in England. *Equine vet J* 2007, 39:438-445.
12. Bosh KA, Powell D, Shelton B, Zent W: Reproductive performance measures among Thoroughbred mares in central Kentucky, during the 2004 mating season. *Equine vet J* 2009, 41:883-888.
13. Merkt H, Jacobs K-O, Klug E, Aukes E: An analysis of stallion fertility rates (foals born alive) from the breeding documents of the Landgestüt Celle over a 158-year period. *J Reprod Fertil* 1979, (Suppl 27):73-77.
14. Davies Morel MCG, Gunnarson V: A survey of the fertility of Icelandic stallions. *Anim Reprod Sci* 2000, 64:49-64.
15. Keiper R, Houpt K: Reproduction in feral horses: An eight-year study. *Am J Vet Res* 1984, 45:991-995.
16. Hutton CA, Meacham TN: Reproductive efficiency on fourteen horse farms. *J Anim Sci* 1968, 27:434-438.
17. Katila T: Effects of hormone treatments, season, age and type of mares on ovulation, twinning and pregnancy rates of mares

inseminated with fresh and frozen semen. *Pferdeheilkunde* 2003, 19:619-624.

18. Jalostustilastot[http://www.hippos.fi/hippos/jalostus_ja_kasvatus/Jalostustilastot.php]*webcite Suomen Hippos* 2008. 24.4.2009
19. Chevalier-Clément F: Pregnancy loss in the mare. *Anim Reprod Sci* 1989, 20:231-244.
20. Carnevale EM, Ginther OJ: Relationship of age to uterine function and reproductive efficiency in the mare. *Theriogenology* 1992, 37:231-246.
21. McDowell KJ, Powell DG, Baker CB: Effect of book size and age of mare and stallion on foaling rates in thoroughbred mares. *J Equine Vet Sci* 1992, 1:364-367.
22. Samper JC: Management and fertility of mares bred with frozen semen. *Anim Reprod Sci* 2001, 68:219-228.
23. Barbacini S, Marchi V, Zavaglia G: Equine frozen semen: results obtained in Italy during the 1994-1997 period. *Equine vet Educ* 1999, 11:109-112.

Chapter 3

Stallion Mate Choice and Mare Sexual Behaviour in a Herd of Sorraia Horses (Equus caballus)

Filipa Paiva Brandão Deslandes Heitor and Luís António Matos Vicente

Centro de Biologia Ambiental, Faculdade de Ciências, Universidade de Lisboa, Campo Grande, Edifício C2, 1749-016 Lisboa, Portugal

ABSTRACT

We examined the relationship between male mate choice, female sexual behaviour, and individual factors in a managed group of Sorraia horses. The herd comprised 9–11 adult mares and their foals. Two stallions were introduced into the mare group in different years for pasture breeding. Mare receptivity during oestrus was poorly correlated with individual factors. Stallions did not prefer to mate with mares that showed the greatest behavioural receptivity during oestrus. The older and more experienced stallion preferred to mate with the older, higher-ranking, or barren oestrous mares. The younger stallion preferred to mate with the more genetically related mares and showed higher oestrus discrimination of mares to who he kept proximity during oestrus. Mate choice was not associated with probability of foaling in the following year. The differential influence of individual factors on mate choice between the stallions could stem from differences in breeding experience and familiarity with the mares.

INTRODUCTION

The Sorraia horse is a Portuguese autochthonous breed which is believed to be a direct descendant from the primitive South Iberian horse [1]. The population currently includes less than 200 individuals, which are mainly located in Portugal and Germany and presents high inbreeding levels [1]. Due to its small effective number, that includes less than 100 brood mares, the Sorraia horse is considered to be at critical-maintained risk status by FAO [2]. A breeding management plan is necessary to minimize inbreeding and preserve genetic variation of the population [1]. In order to implement such breeding management plan and increase the effective number of the Sorraia horse population, it is important to know the factors that affect sexual behaviour and its impact on reproductive success.

Feral band stallions defend the mare group and their mating opportunities from other males year round, as is typical of female defence polygyny [3–6]. Unlike feral stallions, Sorraia stallions are kept in managed mare groups at pasture during the reproductive season and cannot choose group members. However, Sorraia stallions can choose who to mate with, and opportunity for mate choice arises when more than one female is in oestrus.

Mares are seasonally polyestrous, cyclically showing periods of oestrus and dioestrus during spring and summer, and experiencing a prolonged anoestrus during fall and winter [7]. Stallions may not mate with all mares when they come into oestrus simultaneously [8] and show preference for certain females with whom they mate repeatedly

[9–11]. Factors such as mare coat colour, size, days from ovulation, lactation status, age, and dominance rank are known to affect sexual preferences [7, 10].

The stallion may use cues such as age, rank, or reproductive state to assess a mare's future ability to raise a foal. Mare age is an important factor for foal survival because older mothers target their investment better due to experience and are more successful at raising offspring [12]. Higher-ranking mares may benefit from higher quality diets, produce faster growing offspring [13], and their foals may be more protected against aggression [14, 15]. Maternal care entails costs in terms of immediate loss of body condition which translates into decreased conception rates and costs to future reproduction [12, 16]. Therefore, mares that foal on a given year may have lower probability of conceiving or reduced ability to invest in offspring in the following year.

Female sexual behaviour and receptivity during oestrus are also related to individual factors. As mares get older, sexual experience increases and residual reproductive value decreases [12]. Older and more experienced mares are usually more receptive [17]. The dominance status of females relative to the stallion may also be relevant, as Przewalski's stallions are sometimes rejected by mares dominant to them and fail to breed them [18]. Barren mares may show greater receptivity than mares with foals [11].

Mares avoid mating with familiar males, who are usually close relatives, and prefer to join bands with unfamiliar males after natal dispersal, which functions to prevent inbreeding [19–21]. Therefore, stallions could prefer to mate with mares that are less genetically related to him, and mares that are more genetically related to the stallion could be less receptive to his mating attempts.

Male mate choice could also be aimed at reducing mating effort (e.g., time, energy, and risk of injury). Mares play an important role in sexual stimulation and timing of copulation [22, 23]. Therefore, females that solicit the stallion during oestrus more often or more overtly may be preferred mating partners [8, 9] because mating with them requires lower effort and oestrus detection is improved.

We conducted behavioural observations on one of the largest Sorraia horse subpopulations in Portugal, to test the following specific hypotheses: (1) oestrous mares that are older, less genetically related to the stallion, subordinate, or barren display greater sexual activity towards the stallion; (2) the stallion chooses to mate with the oldest, highest-ranking, least genetically related, subordinate or barren mares among oestrous females; (3) the stallion chooses to mate with mares that show greatest sexual activity towards him among oestrous females; (4) male mate choice is associated with probability of foaling in the following year.

METHODS

Subjects and Study Site

Observations were conducted on a pastured group of Sorraia horses kept at Alter studfarm (39°11′N, 7°39′W), Portugal, in 2003 and 2005. The herd comprised 9–11 adult mares and their foals. Mares ranged in age from 4 to 22 years and had known each other since birth. Each year, a different stallion was introduced into the mare group in February, and remained there until June for pasture breeding. In 2003, the stallion was 11 years old and had been used for reproduction in this herd since 2001. In 2005, a 5-year-old stallion was used for the first time and therefore was unacquainted with the mares when he entered the group. Both stallions and mares were experienced in pasture breeding, which was implemented since 1998. Six foals were born in 2003 and seven foals were born in 2005, but three died within few hours or days after birth in each year. Shortly after the beginning of observations in 2005, a mare died a few weeks after a miscarriage and was excluded from analysis. Foals were weaned and removed from the herd at approximately nine months of age.

The herd occupied two 5.5 and 17.2 ha pastures enclosed by 1.5-m high wire fences and walls and fed mainly on grasses. Horses had access to supplemental feed in summer and veterinary care. Water was available from temporary water lines, watering ponds and canals connected to reservoirs. Animals were taken to a paddock a few times per year for pregnancy detection, foal removal, branding, tail and mane shearing, and collection of blood samples for paternity analyses.

Data Collection

Behavioural observations were conducted on foot, 3–10 m from the horses, between 06:30 and 18:30 h solar time. We collected data on social interactions during a series of 25-min focal samples [24] randomly assigned to the subjects. For every interaction, the type of behaviour, initiator, and receiver(s), reaction of the receiver(s), and context were noted. Sexual interactions consisted of courting behaviours (approach, follow, and body contacts), presenting to the stallion, mounting, and copulation. Copulation was recorded when the stallion gained intromission, performed several pelvic thrusts, remained stationary on the mare for a short period of time and finally dismounted with loss of erection [22]. Agonistic-related interactions included displacements, mild threats, bite threats, bites, kick threats, kicks, chases, attacks, and herding (descriptions are presented elsewhere [25]). In 2005, we recorded approaches across one body-length distance, the identity of the focal animal's nearest neighbour (relative to the closest body part) and of its associates (horses within one body-length) by instantaneous sampling at 5-min intervals [24].

This study was part of a broader research project on social relationships of Sorraia horses. We conducted 206 h of focal sampling on both stallion and mares over 316 h of observation in 2003, and 42 h of focal sampling on the stallion over 188 h of observation in 2005. The difference between observation time and focal sampling time corresponds to ad libitum sampling. As sexual behaviours occurred at low frequencies, ad libitum data collected throughout the project in 2003 and 2005 were also included in statistical analyses. Mare body condition was estimated in 2005, according to a scale which varies from 0 (very thin) to 5 (obese), with half point gradations [26].

Data Analysis

Observation days when each female was in oestrus or dioestrus were determined according to her reproductive state (pregnant mares were not in oestrus [27]) and estimated conception date (obtained by subtracting the average gestation period of 336 days to foal birth date in the following year [17]), in conjunction with criteria adapted from Asa et al. [28] and Waring [7] described below. A mare was classified as being in oestrus on a given day if at least one of the following signs of oestrus were recorded: (1) she initiated sexual behaviours at least once; (2) when receiving sexual behaviours from the stallion, she remained calm, with raised tail and one of the following components: (i) straddled hind legs, (ii) clitoral winking, (iii) voiding small amounts of urine; (3) copulation. If no copulation was recorded and the mare directed agonistic interactions or moved away from the stallion when sexually approached by him, we concluded she was not in oestrus. Intervals of 1–3 days with missing data between oestrus days, as assessed by the previous criteria, were also considered to be oestrus days.

Sexual behaviours were analysed at the level of the "mating attempt", which was defined as a behavioural sequence that includes one or more sexual behaviours. We considered the following categories of mare reactions to mating attempts:

- positive: raised tail, straddled hind legs, clitoral winking, voiding small amounts of urine, or affiliative interactions;
- negative: avoid, withdraw or agonistic interactions;
- ambivalent: showing behaviours included both in the positive and negative categories;
- neutral: includes all other reactions (e.g., look at the stallion, vocalizations).

We computed the following measures of female sexual activity: proximity to the stallion during oestrus (only in 2005), receptivity and frequency of sexual behaviours initiated by the mare. Proximity of mares to the stallion during oestrus periods was measured by the time spent as associate and nearest neighbour to him (i.e., estimated by the percentage of instantaneous samples as associate or nearest neighbour) and by the frequency of approaches given to the stallion and received from the stallion by mares. Receptivity was measured as the percentage of positive reactions to mating attempts received from the stallion during oestrus.

We examined three parameters of sexual behaviour associated with male mate choice: frequency of mating attempts, mating success, and oestrus discrimination. We computed the frequency of mating attempts directed to oestrous mares, during total oestrus time and during days when several mares were in oestrus simultaneously. Mating success was measured as the percentage of mating attempts with copulation, during oestrus and during the whole study (i.e., total success). We attributed the cause of the lack of success of a mating attempt to combinations of the following observed reactions: avoidance (mare moves away from the stallion), aggression (mare directs agonistic interactions to the stallion), interference (another mare directs an interaction to the stallion and/or the mare), and quit (termination by the stallion). Oestrus discrimination was computed as the number of mating attempts directed to a mare during oestrus, divided by the total number of mating attempts directed by the stallion to that mare over the whole study. Frequencies of mating attempts were computed from focal sampling data. Receptivity, mating success, oestrus discrimination scores, and cause of unsuccessful mating attempts were estimated from the complete data set (focal and ad libitum data).

Dominance relationships were determined on the basis of agonistic-related interactions. We excluded kicks and kick threats due to their defensive function [29, 30]. Herding was also excluded because it was performed only by the stallion. The dominant individual within a dyad was the one that initiated the majority of agonistic-related interactions that caused a submissive response from the other animal. We measured linearity of mare dominance relationships by Kendall's coefficient of consistence K, based on the number of circular triads, d [31, 32]. Linearity was significant in both years (2003: $K = 0.85$, $d = 6$, $N = 10$, $P < .02$; 2005: $K = 0.93$, $d = 3$, $N = 10$, $P < .03$) and therefore mares were ordered in a linear hierarchy by the "I and SI" method [33]. An ordinal dominance rank, which increased from the bottom to the top of the hierarchy, was then assigned to each female.

Kinship coefficient between the stallion and the mares was computed from pedigree data up to the founder animals.

Spearman's rank correlation coefficient was used to assess the relationship between sexual behaviour patterns and mare individual factors: age, rank, and kinship relative to the stallion. Frequency of mating attempts directed to the oldest, highest-ranking, or least genetically related mare among those in oestrous was compared with the mean frequency directed to other simultaneous oestrous mares by means of Wilcoxon paired-sample tests. We tested for differences in sexual behaviours patterns between dominants and subordinates to the stallion and between mares that were in different reproductive states (foaled versus barren) by means of Mann-Whitney U-test. Mares whose foals died soon after birth were treated as barren.

All statistical tests were one-tailed and the significance level was set at 0.05. Standard statistical tests were performed on Statistica 5.1 StatSoft, Inc.

RESULTS

The stallion in 2003 was dominant over two mares, which occupied ranks 2 and 6 in the mare dominance hierarchy. The stallion in 2005 was dominant over three mares: the oldest, a 13-year-old, and the youngest female (ranks 5, 4, and 1, resp.).

Barren mares were all in better body condition (range: 2.5–3) than mares with foals (range: 1–1.5) in 2005. Every mare came into oestrus during the study period, except the third highest-ranking female in 2003. There was at least one female in oestrus during 35 of the 60 (58.3%) observation days in 2003, and during 31 of the 57 (54.4%) observation days in 2005. Two or more mares were simultaneously in oestrus in 19 (54.3%) of the 35 oestrus days in 2003 (mean 2.16, maximum 3 mares per day), and in 11 (35.5%) of the 31 oestrus days in 2005 (mean 2.36, maximum 4 mares per day). Therefore, the two stallions had similar opportunities for mate choice.

The stallion in 2003 copulated with seven out of nine mares (77.8%) and the stallion in 2005 was observed copulating with five out of 10 mares (50%). Five copulations were recorded during focal samples in 2003 (49 copulations in the complete data set) and four copulations in 2005 (25 copulations in the complete data set). Copulation frequency (mean ± S.D.) was 0.013 ± 0.017 h–1 per mare in 2003 (0.090 ± 0.100 h–1 per mare during oestrus time) and 0.010 ± 0.024 h–1 per mare in 2005 (0.061 ± 0.130 h–1 per mare during oestrus time). The main cause of unsuccess (Table 1) was "interference" in 2003 (33.8%) and "quit" in 2005 (44.5%). The stallions had similar oestrus discrimination scores and frequencies of mating attempts, but the stallion in 2003 had higher mating success (Table 2). Frequency of mating attempts during oestrus was not significantly correlated with mating success during oestrus in either year (2003: s= 0 . 2 4, = 8, > . 0 5; 2005: s= – 0 . 3 2, = 1 0, > . 0 5).

Table 1: Cause of unsuccess of mating attempts

Cause of unsuccess (%)	2003	2005
Avoidance	6.8	4.2
Aggression	23.6	12.6
Interference	33.8	20.2
Quit	26.2	44.5
Avoidance + aggression	2.1	4.2
Avoidance + interference	3.8	7.6
Aggression + interference	3.0	4.2
Quit + interference	0	0.8
Avoidance + aggression + interference	0.8	1.7
Total number of mating attempts	237	119

Table 2: Influence of dominance status and reproductive state on male mate choice and female receptivity, as measured by the Mann-Whitney U-test

	Mean ± S.D.	Dominance			Reproductive state		
		D	S	U	B	F	U
2003							
Simultaneous oestrus frequency (h–1)	0.91 ± 0.65	6	2	10	5	3	15*
Total oestrus frequency (h–1)	0.72 ± 0.45	6	2	10	5	3	15*
Total success (%)	14.9 ± 11.7	7	2	6	6	3	11.5
Success in oestrus (%)	27.8 ± 17.1	6	2	7	5	3	5
Oestrus discrimination (%)	74.3 ± 17.3	6	2	0	5	3	3
Receptivity (%)	55.3 ± 23.0	6	2	10	5	3	8
2005							
Simultaneous oestrus frequency (h–1)	0.86 ± 0.57	6	3	7	6	3	4
Total oestrus frequency (h–1)	0.87 ± 0.61	7	3	7.5	6	4	10
Total success (%)	10.6 ± 12.9	7	3	10	6	4	10
Success in oestrus (%)	17.2 ± 20.4	7	3	8	6	4	9
Oestrus discrimination (%)	72.9 ± 18.0	7	3	21*	6	4	22*

Receptivity (%)	57.9 ± 23.0	7	3	8	6	4	17

Number of mares: *N*D: dominants, *N*S: subordinates, *N*B: barren and *N*F: with foals; $*P < .05$.

Influence of Individual Factors on Female Sexual Activity

Oestrous subordinate mares spent more time as the stallion nearest neighbour than oestrous dominant mares, as predicted (Table 3). However, this difference was probably due to stallion behaviour rather than mare behaviour, because the stallion approached subordinates significantly more often than he approached dominants (Table 3). Barren mares made a greater effort to keep proximity to the stallion during oestrus than mares that foaled (Table 3). Contrary to our predictions, younger mares spent more time as the stallion's associates and approached him more frequently than older mares during oestrus periods (Table 4). Moreover, mares that were more genetically related to the stallion spent more time as his associates during oestrus than the less related mares (Table 4).

Table 3: Influence of dominance status and reproductive state on proximity of mares to the stallion during oestrus, as measured by the Mann-Whitney U-test

	Mean ± S.D.	Dominance			Reproductive state		
		D	S	U	B	F	U
Associate	0.10 ± 0.12	7	3	13	6	4	21*
Nearest neighbour	0.13 ± 0.10	7	3	19*	6	4	22*
Approaches r (h–1)	0.19 ± 0.33	7	3	21*	6	4	20
Approaches g (h–1)	1.01 ± 0.89	7	3	15	6	4	22*

Number of mares: *N*D: dominants,S: subordinates, *N*B: barren, and *N*F: with foals; r: received from the stallion, g: given to the stallion; $*P < .05$. Time as associate and as nearest neighbour are expressed as proportions. Frequencies of approaches is measured in number of occurrences per hour.

Table 4: Influence of mare age and kinship on proximity to the stallion during oestrus, as assessed by the Spearman's rank correlation coefficient (N = 1 0)

	Age	Kinship
Associate	–0.89	0.57
Nearest neighbour	–0.38	–0.09
Approaches r	0.02	–0.29
Approaches g	–0.77	0.43

r: received from the stallion, g: given to the stallion.

During oestrus periods in 2003, mares showed 55.3 ± 23.0% positive, 15.3 ± 19.7% negative, 14.9 ± 8.0% ambivalent, and 14.9 ± 8.0% neutral reactions (mean ± S.D.) to mating attempts. The stallion in 2005 received less negative reactions from oestrous mares than the stallion in 2003 (mean ± S.D.): 57.9 ± 23.0% positive, 5.8 ± 11.0% negative, 13.5 ± 15.8% ambivalent, and 22.9 ± 16.0% neutral. Subordinate and barren females were not more receptive during oestrus in either year (Table 2). Age, rank and kinship were also unrelated to receptivity (Table 5).

Table 5: Influence of mare age, rank, and kinship on sexual behaviour patterns, as assessed by the Spearman's rank correlation coefficient

	Simultaneous oestrus frequency	Total oestrus frequency	Total success	Success in oestrus	Oestrus discrimination	Receptivity
2003	= 8	= 8	= 9	= 8	= 8	= 8
Age	0.69*	0.52	–0.16	–0.07	0.24	–0.33
Rank	0.69*	0.52	–0.12	–0.07	0.24	–0.33
Kinship	0.16	0.06	–0.03	–0.29	0.17	–0.51
2005	= 9	= 1 0	= 1 0	= 1 0	= 1 0	= 1 0
Age	0.23	0.26	–0.32	–0.33	–0.13	–0.09
Rank	0.38	0.39	–0.14	–0.14	–0.53	–0.17
Kinship	0.19	0.41	0.46	0.39	–0.30	0.33

*P < . 0 5.

We could not analyse the influence of individual factors on the frequency of mating attempts initiated by mares, because mares initiated them only once each year during focal samples. Considering both focal and ad libitum data, eight attempts in 2003 and five attempts in 2005 were initiated by mares. Mare presentations to the stallion were observed only in 2005: five times in focal data and seven times in ad libitum data. The stallion responded sexually to mare presentations only twice in ad libitum data.

Influence of Individual Factors on Male Mate Choice

Dominance relationships with the stallion were not related to frequencies of mating attempts in either year (Table 2). The stallion in 2003 attempted to mate more frequently with oestrous barren mares than with oestrous mares with foals, both during the whole reproductive season and during simultaneous oestrous periods, but not the stallion in 2005 (Table 2). Contrary to our predictions, the stallion in 2003 showed greater oestrus discrimination of females dominant to him and reproductive state was not related to oestrus discrimination (Table 2). In 2005, the stallion made higher oestrus discrimination of subordinates and barren mares (Table 2). During simultaneous oestrus periods in 2003, frequency of mating attempts was significantly higher with the oldest and highest-ranking mares (Wilcoxon paired-sample test: $T = 7$, $N = 19$ days, $P < .005$; Table 5) but not with the less genetically related mares ($T = 51.5$, $N = 18$ days, $P > .05$; Table 5). The stallion in 2005 did not show sexual preference for the oldest, highest-ranking, or least genetically related mares (Wilcoxon paired-sample test: age: $T = 22$, $N = 11$ days, $P > .05$; rank: $T = 20$, $N = 11$ days, $P > .05$; kinship: $T = 5.5$, $N = 11$ days, $P > .05$; Table 5). Contrary to our predictions, this stallion directed lower frequencies of mating attempts to the less related mare among those in oestrus. Mating success was not related to individual factors in either year (Tables 2 and 5).

Influence of Female Sexual Activity on Male Mate Choice

In 2005, oestrus discrimination was significantly higher for mares that the stallion approached more frequently and that spent more time as his nearest neighbour, but frequency of mating attempts and mating success were not related to proximity during oestrus (Table 6).

Table 6: Influence of proximity of mares to the stallion during oestrus on male mate choice, as assessed by the Spearman's rank correlation coefficient

	Simultaneous oestrus frequency	Total oestrus frequency	Total success	Success in oestrus	Oestrus discrimination
	= 9	= 1 0	= 1 0	= 1 0	= 1 0
Associate	−0.48	−0.28	0.28	0.26	0.34
Neighbour	−0.56	−0.63	0.14	0.15	0.82*
Approaches r	−0.29	−0.19	−0.07	−0.25	0.88*
Approaches g	−0.31	−0.30	0.19	0.20	0.44

r: received from the stallion, g: given to the stallion; *$P < .05$.

Mare receptivity was not significantly correlated with oestrus discrimination, frequency of mating attempts, or mating success, neither in 2003 (frequency simultaneous oestrus: $rs= 0.05$, $N = 8$, $P > .05$; frequency total oestrus: $rs= 0.26$, $N = 8$, $P > .05$; success in oestrus: $rs= 0.40$, $N = 8$, $P > .05$; oestrus discrimination: $rs= -0.29$, $N = 8$, $P > .05$) nor in 2005 (frequency simultaneous oestrus: $rs= -0.19$, $N = 9$, $P > .05$; frequency total oestrus: $rs= 0.18$, $N = 10$, $P > .05$; success in oestrus: $rs= -0.07$, $N = 10$, $P > .05$; oestrus discrimination: $rs= 0.08$, $N = 10$, $P > .05$).

Male Mate Choice and Probability of Foaling

Six of the nine mares in 2003 (66.7%) and two of the 10 mares in 2005 (20%) foaled in the following year. Mares that foaled had not been involved in higher frequencies of mating attempts during oestrus, with higher mating success or higher oestrus discrimination than mares that did not foal in the year following 2003 (Mann-Whitney U-test: frequency simultaneous oestrus: $U = 8$; frequency total oestrus: $U = 6$; success in oestrus: $U = 0$; oestrus discrimination: $U = 2$; $NB= 2$, $NF= 6$, $P > .05$) and 2005 (Mann-Whitney U-test: frequency total oestrus: $U = 4$; success in oestrus: $U = 12$; oestrus discrimination: $U = 5$; $NB= 8$, $NF= 2$, $P > .05$). Only one of the two mares that foaled in the year following 2005 had been in oestrus simultaneously with other mares, which precluded statistical tests. The mare that received the highest percentage of copulations in each year (2003: 30.6% of 49 copulations; 2005: 52% of 25 copulations) did not foal in the following year. Moreover, mares that foaled in the following year had not received a higher total number of copulations than those that did not foal (2003: $U = 9.5$, $NB = 3$, $NF = 6$, $P > .05$; 2005: $U = 11$, $NB = 8$, $NF = 2$, $P > .05$).

DISCUSSION

This study examined four main hypotheses on the relationship between male mate choice, female sexual behaviour, and individual factors in a managed herd of Sorraia horses. The results regarding each hypothesis are discussed below.

Influence of Individual Factors on Female Sexual Activity

Contrary to our predictions, younger mares and mares that were more genetically related to the younger stallion spent more time in proximity to him during oestrus periods than older and less related mares. Subordinates did not make a greater effort to keep proximity to the stallion than did dominants during oestrus. Nevertheless, the stallion made a greater effort to keep proximity to subordinate females than to dominants during their oestrus periods, possibly because the risk of receiving agonistic interactions from subordinates is lower [25]. As predicted, barren mares spent more time as associates to the stallion and approached him more often during oestrus periods than mares with foals. Barren mares may invest more in future reproduction, whilst mares with foals invest more in current reproduction, which entails greater social isolation after foaling [34]. These findings suggest that proximity during oestrus could reflect affiliative and agonistic relationships between the stallion and mares, as well as female sexual activity.

Although mares kept proximity to the stallion during oestrus, sexual behaviours were mostly initiated by the stallion and not by the mares. In contrast, Tyler [3] and McDonnell [23] stated that mares play an active role in initiation of sexual behaviours.

Receptivity was not related to any of the individual factors tested. Consistent with other studies on horses [7,22, 23, 28], some oestrous mares displayed aggressive or ambivalent reactions to mating attempts and minimal behavioural signs of oestrus. Aggressive behaviours during oestrus could be a mechanism used by dispersing mares in feral populations to test quality of a stallion before joining his band. Resistance behaviours could then function to promote female mate choice [35, 36]. In managed conditions, although mares cannot choose the stallions that will breed them, resistance behaviours may also be used to assess mate quality.

Influence of Individual Factors on Male Mate Choice

The two males in our study had similar oestrus discrimination scores and frequencies of mating attempts, but the older stallion had higher mating success than the younger male. Copulation frequency was similar to that reported by Cunha [11] in a previous study of this herd with a different stallion (0.012 copulations h^{-1} per mare). The younger stallion interrupted almost half his mating attempts for no apparent reason, even when he was not receiving aggression from the mares ("quit"), and despite receiving fewer negative reactions and more neutral reactions from mares than the older stallion did. Perhaps because the younger stallion had less breeding experience and was unacquainted with the mares, he needed to tease them repeatedly to assess oestrus state and attempted to mount a female only when she was clearly receptive. In contrast, the main cause of unsuccess in mating attempts initiated by the older stallion was interference by other mares. Interference behaviours consisted mostly of agonistic interactions directed to the stallion and caused disruption of the sexual behaviour in which he was involved. The functions of sexual interference behaviours are discussed elsewhere by Heitor et al. [37].

The older stallion in this study tried to mate more often with older, higher-ranking, and barren mares, as predicted. Consistent with these findings, Cunha [11] observed that the stallion in a former study of this Sorraia horse herd copulated only with older females and Waring [7] referred that stallions show greater sexual interest in older mares. Asa et al. [28] reported that stallions select the higher-ranking oestrous mare for copulation when more than one oestrous female was present, but Bristol [22] found no such preference. A 15-year-old stallion observed by Steinbjörnsson [8] mated exclusively with barren mares. However, contrary to our predictions, the older stallion showed greater oestrus discrimination of dominant than subordinate females. By targeting better his mating attempts to oestrus periods of dominants, the older stallion could avoid receiving aggression from them.

The younger stallion showed higher oestrus discrimination of subordinate and barren mares, as predicted, but female age and rank did not seem to affect mate choice. Female age and rank were not related to frequency of mating attempts of either stallion in their first year as breeders at Alter studfarm both in the present study and in a previous one [38]. Breeding experience is known to affect stallion sexual behaviour [39]. Therefore, the greater general breeding experience and familiarity with the mares of the older stallion before being introduced into the group may have promoted the development of sexual preferences based on mare age, rank, and reproductive state. Future studies should assess whether stallions use these factors as cues to assess female quality or ability to raise foals.

The younger stallion in our study seemed to prefer the most genetically related mares among those in oestrus. Such preference is contrary to our predictions, but it is consistent with sexual patterns of the older stallion in his first year as a breeder in this herd [38]. Cunha [11] found no evidence that a Sorraia stallion avoided copulating with close relatives via the mother (half-sisters). Feral horses do not to avoid mating with close kinper se but with familiar individuals of their natal band, which are usually close relatives [19–21]. In our study, the stallion was unfamiliar with the mares, and he may have chosen the most genetically related mares because they spent more time as his associates during oestrus. However, because both the number of mares that were simultaneously in oestrus per day and the number of days in which there was more than one oestrous female both in the present study and that of Heitor et al. [38] were small, this finding may reflect a spurious relationship and deserves further study.

Contrary to Przewalski's stallions [18], mating success of Sorraia stallions was not lower with dominant females than with subordinates. Therefore, the fact that both stallions were subordinate to the majority of mares did not seem to affect mating success.

Influence of Female Sexual Activity on Male Mate Choice

We found little evidence that male mate choice is aimed at reducing mating effort. Maintaining proximity to the stallion during oestrus did not seem to afford mares with higher frequency of mating attempts or higher mating success. Maintaining proximity to the stallion could have a larger effect on frequency of mating attempts in groups where a higher number of mares are simultaneously in oestrus. Bristol [22] reported that the stallion usually attempted to mate with the mare that was closest to him in a group of 20 pastured mares in synchronized oestrus. In contrast, only 2–4 Sorraia mares were simultaneously in oestrus per day.

Consistent with our predictions, the younger stallion made greater oestrus discrimination of mares to whom he kept proximity during oestrus. Oestrus discrimination provides an inverse estimate of the level of sexual harassment received by mares when they are not in oestrus. This finding suggests that proximity could reduce the costs associated with sexual harassment (e.g., disruption of other activities, risk of injury).

We did not find a preference in Sorraia stallions for mating with mares that showed the greatest receptivity. In contrast, Ginther [9] observed that stallions copulated repeatedly with the same mares, who were usually the most sexually active. Our study focused on behavioural receptivity, which in some cases does not match ovarian activity [7, 17, 28]. Olfactory cues also play an important role in sexual stimulation of the stallion during courtship [7, 17, 39]. Although there is no evidence that stallions can detect the oestrus condition of a mare based on olfactory investigation, stallions exhibit the flehmen response to mare urine, which promotes coordination between male and female sexual behaviour [40]. Therefore, stallions probably responded sexually to perceived chemical signs of physiological oestrus, as well as to behavioural signs of oestrus.

Male Mate Choice and Probability of Foaling

Mate choice was not related to the probability of foaling in the following year. This finding may have several, not mutually exclusive, explanations. The occasional absence of tail flagging at the end of copulations and the occurrence of intervals shorter than the average postejaculatory refractory period of 20-min [28] between copulations suggest that ejaculation was not always achieved by Sorraia stallions. Anovulatory oestrus periods may also have occurred, which are behaviourally undistinguishable from ovulatory oestrus periods [7, 17,

28]. Moreover, there may have been differences in the frequency of copulation around the time of ovulation, which is the period when mares have the highest probability of conception and occurs within the last two days of oestrus [28]. It has been suggested that stallions may be able to detect the timing of mare ovulation [8], although no evidence that stallions preferred to mate with mares that were closest to ovulation was found [9]. Finally, some mares may have conceived and suffered abortion at an early gestation phase, due to the high inbreeding levels in this herd of Sorraia horses [38]. Future studies on sexual behaviour of Sorraia horses should complement behavioural data with an assessment of physiological variables (e.g., hormone levels) and ovarian activity (e.g., ultrasonography), to measure the extent to which behavioural signs and physiological oestrus match each other and to assess their relative influence on stallion mate choice.

Final Remarks

In sum, Sorraia stallions do not seem to display similar and consistent patterns of mate choice. The two stallions in this study may have adopted different reproductive strategies: the older stallion may have based mate choice on female quality or ability to raise offspring, whereas the younger stallion may have based mate choice on reduction of mating effort. Moreover, the older stallion had shown different patterns of mate choice in a previous study when compared to the present one. These differences could be related to differences in breeding experience and familiarity with the mares. However, the observed patterns of mate choice could simply be related to particular characteristics and sexual preferences of the two stallions. The low effective number of the Sorraia population and the low number of breeding groups kept at pasture precluded the collection of data on a higher number of stallions in this study. Therefore, more data should be collected on different stallions before conclusions can be drawn regarding the factors that affect stallion mate choice in Sorraia horses.

Mare receptivity during oestrus was poorly correlated with the individual factors tested in this study. Other factors such as individual temperament or physiological variables could have a greater influence on behavioural receptivity and deserve further study. In addition, behavioural receptivity did not seem to affect male mate choice. Stallions could rely more on chemical signs of oestrus than behavioural signs because there is large variability in behavioural receptivity during oestrus among mares. In addition, we did not find evidence that mate choice affected the probability of foaling in the following year. Future studies should address the influence of physiological variables and ovarian activity on male mate choice as well as long-term effects of mate choice on female reproductive success.

ACKNOWLEDGMENTS

The authors thank Dr. João Costa Ferreira for permission to conduct this study at Alter studfarm and Dr. Maria do Mar Oom for providing the kinship data. Sónia Emídio participated in data collection. F. Heitor was supported by a Doctoral Fellowship granted by the Fundação para a Ciência e a Tecnologia (SFRH/BD/8792/2002).

REFERENCES

1. C. Luís, The Sorraia horse, a case study of a small and closed population: contribution of molecular markers to the genetic conservation and management of an endangered breed, Ph.D. thesis, University of Lisbon, Lisbon, Portugal, 2006.
2. B. D. Scherf, World Watch List for Domestic Animal Diversity, Food and Agriculture Organization of the United Nations, Rome, Italy, 3rd edition, 2000.
3. S. J. Tyler, "The behaviour and social organization of the new forest ponies," Animal Behaviour, vol. 5, no. 2, pp. 87–196, 1972.
4. R. E. Salter and R. J. Hudson, "Social organization of feral horses in western Canada," Applied Animal Ethology, vol. 8, no. 3, pp. 207–223, 1982.
5. Y. Kaseda, A. M. Khalil, and H. Ogawa, "Harem stability and reproductive success of Misaki feral mares," Equine Veterinary Journal, vol. 27, no. 5, pp. 368–372, 1995.
6. W. L. Linklater, E. Z. Cameron, E. O. Minot, and K. J. Stafford, "Stallion harassment and the mating system of horses," Animal Behaviour, vol. 58, no. 2, pp. 295–306, 1999.

7. G. H. Waring, Horse Behavior: The Behavioral Traits and Adaptations of Domestic and Wild Horses, Including Ponies, Noyes Publications, Park Ridge, NJ, USA, 1983.
8. B. Steinbjörnsson, "Sexual behavior in herds of Icelandic horses," in Horse Behavior and Welfare. A Dorothy Russell Havemeyer Foundation Workshop, S. McDonnell and D. Mills, Eds., pp. 47–50, Hólar, Iceland, 2002.
9. O. J. Ginther, "Sexual behaviour following introduction of a stallion into a group of mares,"Theriogenology, vol. 19, no. 6, pp. 877–886, 1983.
10. S. M. McDonnell, "Stallion sexual behavior," in Equine Breeding Management and Artificial Insemination, J. C. Samper, Ed., pp. 53–61, W. B. Saunders, Philadelphia, Pa, USA, 2000.
11. M. B. Cunha, Comportamento social do Cavalo do Sorraia em regime extensivo, M.S. thesis, Instituto Superior de Psicologia Aplicada, Lisbon, Portugal, 2004.
12. E. Z. Cameron, W. L. Linklater, K. J. Stafford, and E. O. Minot, "Aging and improving reproductive success in horses: declining residual reproductive value or just older and wiser?" Behavioral Ecology and Sociobiology, vol. 47, no. 4, pp. 243–249, 2000.
13. P. Duncan, Horses and Grasses: The Nutritional Ecology of Equids and Their Impact on the Camargue, Springer, New York, NY, USA, 1992.
14. A. T. Rutberg and S. A. Greenberg, "Dominance, aggression frequencies and modes of aggressive competition in feral pony mares," Animal Behaviour, vol. 40, no. 2, pp. 322–331, 1990.
15. J. W. Weeks, S. L. Crowell-Davis, A. B. Caudle, and G. L. Heusner, "Aggression and social spacing in light horse (Equus caballus) mares and foals," Applied Animal Behaviour Science, vol. 68, no. 4, pp. 319–337, 2000.
16. D. R. Henneke, G. D. Potter, J. L. Kreider, and B. F. Yeates, "Relationship between condition score, physical measurements and body fat percentage in mares," Equine Veterinary Journal, vol. 15, no. 4, pp. 371–372, 1983.
17. A. F. Fraser, The Behaviour of the Horse, CAB International, Wallingford, UK, 1992.

18. L. E. Boyd, "The behaviour of Przewalski's horses and its importance to their management," Applied Animal Behaviour Science, vol. 29, no. 1–4, pp. 301–318, 1991.
19. P. Duncan, C. Feh, J. C. Gleize, P. Malkas, and A. M. Scott, "Reduction of inbreeding in a natural herd of horses," Animal Behaviour, vol. 32, no. 2, pp. 520–527, 1984.
20. A. M. Monard and P. Duncan, "Consequences of natal dispersal in female horses," Animal Behaviour, vol. 52, no. 3, pp. 565–579, 1996.
21. A. M. Monard, P. Duncan, andV. Boy, "The proximate mechanisms of natal dispersal in female horses,"Behaviour, vol. 133, no. 13-14, pp. 1095–1124, 1996.
22. F. Bristol, "Breeding behaviour of a stallion at pasture with 20 mares in synchronized oestrus," Journal of Reproduction and Fertility, vol. 32, supplement, pp. 71–77, 1982.
23. S. M. McDonnell, "Reproductive behavior of stallions and mares: comparison of free-running and domestic in-hand breeding," Animal Reproduction Science, vol. 60-61, pp. 211–219, 2000.
24. J. Altmann, "Observational study of behavior: sampling methods," Behaviour, vol. 49, no. 3-4, pp. 227–267, 1974.
25. F. Heitor, M. M. Oom, and L. Vicente, "Social relationships in a herd of Sorraia horses. Part I. Correlates of social dominance and contexts of aggression," Behavioural Processes, vol. 73, no. 2, pp. 170–177, 2006.
26. C. L. Carroll and P. J. Huntington, "Body condition scoring and weight estimation of horses," Equine Veterinary Journal, vol. 20, no. 1, pp. 41–45, 1988.
27. C. S. Asa, D. A. Goldfoot, and O. J. Ginther, "Assessment of the sexual behavior of pregnant mares,"Hormones and Behavior, vol. 17, no. 4, pp. 405–413, 1983.
28. C. S. Asa, D. A. Goldfoot, and O. J. Ginther, "Socio-sexual behavior and the ovulatory cycle of ponies (Equus caballus) observed in harem groups," Hormones and Behavior, vol. 13, no. 1, pp. 49–65, 1979.
29. S. M. Wells and B. von Goldschmidt-Rothschild, "Social behaviour and relationships in a herd of Camargue horses," Zeitschrift für Tierpsychologie, vol. 49, no. 4, pp. 363–380, 1979.

30. M. C. van Dierendonck, H. de Vries, and M. B. Schilder, "An analysis of dominance, its behavioural parameters and possible determinants in a herd of icelandic horses in captivity," Netherlands Journal of Zoology, vol. 45, no. 3-4, pp. 362–385, 1995.
31. M. C. Appleby, "The probability of linearity in hierarchies," Animal Behaviour, vol. 31, no. 2, pp. 600–608, 1983.
32. H. de Vries, "An improved test of linearity in dominance hierarchies containing unknown or tied relationships," Animal Behaviour, vol. 50, no. 5, pp. 1375–1389, 1995.
33. H. de Vries, "Finding a dominance order most consistent with a linear hierarchy: a new procedure and review," Animal Behaviour, vol. 55, no. 4, pp. 827–843, 1998.
34. F. Heitor and L. Vicente, "Affiliative relationships among Sorraia mares: influence of age, dominance, kinship and reproductive state," Journal of Ethology, vol. 28, no. 1, pp. 133–140, 2009.
35. E. J. A. Cunningham and T. R. Birkhead, "Sex roles and sexual selection," Animal Behaviour, vol. 56, no. 6, pp. 1311–1321, 1998.
36. T. Chapman, G. Arnqvist, J. Bangham, and L. Rowe, "Sexual conflict," Trends in Ecology and Evolution, vol. 18, no. 1, pp. 41–47, 2003.
37. F. Heitor, S. Emídio, and L. Vicente, "Sexual interference behaviour by Sorraia mares (Equus caballus)," in Horses: Biology, Domestication, and Human Interactions, J. E. Leffhalm, Ed., pp. 65–84, Nova Science Publishers, New York, NY, USA, 2011.
38. F. Heitor, M. M. Oom, and L. Vicente, "Social relationships in a herd of Sorraia horses. Part II. Factors affecting affiliative relationships and sexual behaviours," Behavioural Processes, vol. 73, no. 3, pp. 231–239, 2006.
39. S. McDonnell, "Reproductive behavior of the stallion," The Veterinary Clinics of North America. Equine Practice, vol. 2, no. 3, pp. 535–555, 1986.
40. C. C. Stahlbaum and K. A. Houpt, "The role of the Flehmen response in the behavioral repertoire of the stallion," Physiology and Behavior, vol. 45, no. 6, pp. 1207–1214, 1989.

Chapter 4

Effect of Cholesterol and Equex-STM Addition to an Egg Yolk Extender on Pure Spanish Stallion Cryopreserved Sperm

Lidia Gil[1], Iván Galindo-Cardiel[2], C. Malo[1], N. González[1], and C. Álvarez[3]

[1]Reproduction and Obstetrics Area, Department of Animal Pathology, Faculty of Veterinary, University of Zaragoza, Spain

[2]WorldPathol Ltd. Co., Zaragoza, Spain

[3]Equine Reproduction Center, Torre Abejar, Garrapinillos, Zaragoza, Spain

ABSTRACT

Cholesterol and Equex-STM are frequently added to different commercial and experimental extenders improving postthawing sperm quality. Doses of 125–150 mM of cholesterol from pig liver and 0.5–0.7% of Equex-STM were evaluated in a standard eggyolk extender (Martin et al., 1979). Six ejaculates per stallion from six pure Spanish stallions (6–8 years old) were collected in Martin's extender (B) and different mixtures of 125 mM-0.5% (I), 125 mM-0.7% (II), 150 mM-0.5% (III), and 150 mM-0.7% (IV) were added to original Martin's extender. Samples were frozen in 0.5 mL straws (100×10^6 spermatozoa) and thawed (21 s ,37°C water bath). After thawing the following parameters were evaluated: viability (V), motility (computer assisted sperm analysis, CASA; % nonprogressive NP; % progressive MP), hipoosmotic swelling test (HOST), acrosome integrity (A), fluorescence test (FL), and resistance test (RT). Sperm quality was significantly affected by stallion (in the parameters V, VI, NP, MP, HOST, A, FL, and RT), extraction (VI, NP, MP, HOST, A, and FL), and the different combinations of Equex-STM-cholesterol (FL). We concluded that 0.5% of Equex-STM mixed with 125 mM of cholesterol has obtained better sperm quality results than those of original Martin›s extender, showing a simple and economic improvement of this home-made practical seminal extender.

INTRODUCTION

Artificial insemination remains as one of the most important assisted reproductive technologies. It is a simple, economical and successful method for animal reproduction [1]. Freezing/thawing sperm techniques are a widely used method to manage equine breeds and maintain genetic stallion pool [2]. Different sperm cryopreserving methods have been developed for a lot of species, such as Sea Urchin (Evechinus chloroticus) [3], Carp (Cyprinus carpio) [4], Pacific oyster (Crassostrea gigas) [5], Red Deer (Cervus elaphus) [6], Human (Homo sapiens sapiens) [7], and practically all domestic and farmer species (reviewed by [8, 9]). Seminal cryopreservation techniques should be performed taking into account physiological individual stallion-depending sperm variation and the specific cooling, freezing, and thawing rates, such as the necessary equipment [10–14].

Frozen/thawed sperm protocols have been described as an improving reproductive tool related to a better breed management and reproductive potential stallion optimization due to its ability to preserve fertile inseminating doses [15, 16]. Cryopreservation extends the availability of sperm for fertilization; however, the fertilizing potential of the frozen-thawed sperm is compromised because of alterations in the structure and physiology of the sperm cell [17–19]. Sperm capacitation-like alterations are present in the motile population and decrease sperm life span, interaction with female tract, and its fertilizing ability [20]. The etiology of such alterations may represent a combination of factors, such as inherited fragility of the sperm cell to withstand the cryopreservation process and the semen dilution. Sperm membrane cholesterol, reactive oxygen species, and seminal plasma have been related as mediators of cryopreservation effects on sperm functions, just as capacitation process [8, 9, 21–23].

Several articles have been carried out to analyze the effect of the cholesterol added as cryoprotective agent, using different techniques such as cyclodextrin incubation, liposomes, or low density lipoproteins, getting different results which will be discussed [24–26]. The addition of Equex-STM has been tested to yield high cryopreservation results, mainly in the dog [27–32], stallion [33], lama (Lama glama) [34], boar [35, 36], gazelle [36], rat, and sheep [28, 32, 37, 38]. As for other lauryl sulphate derivatives, the positive effects of these compounds are thought to be brought about by two combined mechanisms: interaction between the egg yolk in the extender and Equex-STM, modifying the protein structure of lipoproteins [35, 39] and improving the stability of plasma membrane lipids [27] by adding cholesterol.

The goal of the present study was to evaluate plasmatic sperm membrane protection and sperm quality parameters improvement in pure Spanish stallion sperm stored in conventional frozen straws, after thawing process, related to the addition of four different combinations of cholesterol (cholesterol of liver of pig 99%, SIGMA) and Equex-STM (Nova Chemical Sales, Scituate, MA, USA) in a lactose-EDTA-egg yolk home-made extender.

MATERIALS AND METHODS

Semen was collected from six pure Spanish stallions aged 6 to 8 years belonging to a reproduction center in NE Spain (Equine Reproduction Center Torre Abejar, Garrapinillos, Zaragoza, Spain). Six ejaculates per stallion were collected from January to May 2004. Minimum quality was required to be frozen according to previous studies [2, 40, 41] (Table 1).

Table 1: Means and minimum sperm quality parameters for ejaculates

Statistics	Concentration (Spr/mL)	Motility (%)	Viability (%)	Intact acrosome (%)	HOS test (%)
N	36	36	36	36	36
Mean	266,86	74,44	65,69	62,36	58,22
SD	8890,18	73,96	235,18	85,15	168,92
CV	94,28	8,60	15,33	9,227	12,99
Minimum required	>200	>60%	>50%	>50%	>50%

Spr/mL: millions of spermatozoa per milliliter. %: percentage of positive evaluated spermatozoa. N: observation data. SD: standard variation. CV: coefficient of variation. HOS test: hyperosmotic test.

Semen was collected by artificial vagina, keeping the sample at 37.5°C in a double boiler immediately. Each ejaculate was diluted immediately after collection in glucose-EDTA extender [42] (1 : 1) and centrifuged to 400 g for 10 minutes to remove seminal plasma and possible gross contamination. The extender used for freezing/thawing semen consisted of lactose-EDTA-egg yolk [42] with cholesterol from pig spleen (Sigma C 3137–56) (125–150 mM) and Equex-STM (Paste 30 mg, Minitüb) (0.5–0.7%) added. Mixtures of 125 mM, 0.5% (I), 125 mM, 0.7% (II), 150 mM, 0.5% (III), and 150 mM, 0.7% (IV) were added to original Martin's extender (0 mM, 0.5%) (W) (Table 2).

Table 2: Composition of the Equex-STM-cholesterol mixtures tested

Mixture	Cholesterol (mM)	Equex-STM (%)
White	0	0.5
I	125	0.5
II	125	0.7
III	150	0.5
IV	150	0.7

m/M: millimolar. %: percentage in total volume.

After definitive dilution, samples were refrigerated at 5°C in a keeper box in the laboratory (Obstetric and Reproduction Area, Animal Pathology Department, Faculty of Veterinarian Sciences, University of Zaragoza, Spain). Then, equilibrated mixture was packed in 0.5 mL straws (100×10^6 spz/mL). The straws were held at 4 cm above liquid nitrogen level for 10 minutes and then plunged into liquid nitrogen. Frozen samples were thawed by placing the straws at 37°C water bath for 21 seconds [43]. Three straws per treatment and boar were performed.

Sperm Evaluation

Total motility was measured by means of a computer-assisted semen analysis (CASA) system [44–46]. The following parameters were analysed: total motility (M), progressive motility (MP), and nonprogressive motility (NP). Sperm viability was evaluated by using eosin-nigrosin stain as described in [47]. A semen sample was diluted 1 : 1 with stain solution (5% eosin, 10% nigrosin in a citrate solution) and smeared. Live spermatozoa remained unstained. The percentage of live spermatozoa was expressed as viability. In addition, acrosomal integrity was evaluated under a phase contrast microscope after a 1 : 1 dilution in buffered 8% glutaraldehyde solution [48]. The percentage of spermatozoa with intact acrosome was determined. Membrane functional integrity was further assessed by the hypoosmotic swelling test (HOST) [49]. The technique consisted of incubating

30 μL of diluted semen with 100 μL of BTS hypoosmotic solution (100 mOsm/Kg) at 37°C for 15 min. The samples were then fixed in 8% glutaraldehyde buffered solution. The proportion of spermatozoa with swollen or coiled tails was considered as HOST positive as well as the integrity of acrosome after hypoosmotic incubation to determine the osmotic resistance (ORT). To evaluate spermatozoa capacitation state, chlortetracycline (CTC) fluorescence assay was performed [50]. Sperm samples were thawed at 37°C for 21 s and resuspended in PBS. Sperm-PBS was mixed with CTC solution (1 : 1), incubated at 37°C for 30 seconds, and subsequently fixed with glutaraldehyde (1 : 2). Briefly, the CTC solution was composed of 5 μL CTC, 5 μL cysteine, and 40 μL buffer (20 mmol/L TRIS-HCl and 130 mmol/L NaCl), kept at 37°C, and incubated for 30 min. One hundred cells were assessed for each preparation under a differential interference microscope equipped with epifluorescence (excitation 450490 nm: B2-A filter, 400x). Capacitated sperm (FL) consisted of low fluorescence in the postacrosomal and relatively bright fluorescence in the intact acrosome, almost no fluorescence over the entire head except a thin band of fluorescence in the equatorial segment, or low fluorescence in the postacrosomal and relatively bright fluorescence in the disintegrated acrosome.

Statistical Analysis

An analysis of factorial variance was applied (ANOVA) for the analysis, following the equation below, where the independent factors applied are stallion, ejaculate, and the different combinations of Equex-STM (percentage) and cholesterol (concentration) added to the different mixtures (called EQCOL factor) and the dependent variables are M, MP, NP, A, HOST, V, FL, and RT:

$$\delta = \text{Stallion}_i + \text{Ejaculate}_j + \text{Equex} - \text{STM} - \text{cholesterol}_k + e_{ijklm} \quad (1)$$

An interval of confidence of the 0.05% was applied in the model. Ejaculates for freezing/thawing fulfilling certain conditions were chosen (Table 1). Ejaculates data have been incorporated into the ANOVA in order to compare the variations of the factors implied (stallion, extraction, and the EQCOL) in respect of sperm quality. All the factors tested were independent of each other. Variables have been consistent with respect to the presence or absence of missing values. Tukey's Studentized Range (HSD) test has been used in order to establish significant mean comparisons between the mixtures of EQCOL. Statistical analysis was performed using the SPSS 11.0 Windows Package.

RESULTS

We identified interactions between extender and stallion in all the parameters analysed (M, MP, NP, HOST, V, FL, and RT), indicating the importance of individual factor and ejaculate. Interactions of the extender with the fixed factor extraction in M, MP, NP, HOST, and A were obtained.

No interactions between the extender and the fixed factor EQCOL in any dependent variables, indicating that there is not different behavior of the extender combinations depending on the different combinations of Equex-STM (percentage) and cholesterol (concentration) added (Table 3). However, closed proximity to significance observed for FL in this fixed factor motivated us to analyse the different implications of each extender combination in this apparently annoying result (by Tukey's Studentized Range test). That is the reason why significant differences in the mean comparison of the extender combinations were identified for A (IV > II > I), HOST (IV > I), and FL (I > II > IV; W > II) (Table 4) after thawing process.

Table 3: General linear model procedure for independent variable (t)

Dependent variable	n	R2	CV	Root MSE	Mean	Independent variable (Pr > F)		
						Stallion	Ejaculate	EQCOL
M	396	0.68	28.57	13.72	48.03	<0.0001	<0.0001	0.9850
MP	210	0.49	94.53	14.66	15.51	<0.0001	<0.0001	0.5153
NP	210	0.20	136.4	16.87	12.37	0.0009	0.0006	0.1798
A	396	0.45	26.63	12.49	46.89	<0.0001	<0.0001	0.1691
HOST	396	0.38	27.30	11.67	42.76	<0.0001	<0.0001	0.0811
V	384	0.56	28.50	13.97	49.02	<0.0001	0.2194	0.3268
FL	61	0.47	68.23	8.01	11.74	0.0009	0.0413	0.0160
RT	121	0.35	38.57	8.80	22.81	<0.0001	0.0772	0.6244

M: individual motility; MP: progressive motility; NP: nonprogressive motility; A: acrosome integrity; HOST: hypoosmotic swelling test; FL: fluorescence test;

RT: resistance test; n: observation data; R^2 : regression coefficient; CV: coefficient of variation; Root MSE: root of mean standard error; EQCOL: tested Equex-STM-cholesterol mixtures.

Table 4: Tukey's Studentized Range (HSD) test for EQCOL

EQCOL comparison		Difference between means	95% confidence limits	
Acrosome integrity				
IV	I	4.125	0.033	8.217
IV	II	4.722	0.639	8.814
HOS test				
IV	I	4.972	1.146	8.798
Fluorescence				
I	IV	8.026	1.583	14.468
I	II	11.083	4.513	17.653
W	II	7.333	0.763	13.093

Means with nonsignificant comparisons have not been added into the table (Alpha = 0.05). W: 0–0.5; I: 125–0.5; II: 125–0.7; III: 150–0.5; IV: 150–0.7 (cholesterol mM-Equex-STM%). HOS: hypoosmotic swelling test.

DISCUSSION

Cryopreservation and thawing of equine sperm led to a significant decrease in the number of CASA-measured motile sperms to 11.3 ± 5.8% in May [45], which does not exactly correspond with the obtained results (6.78 ± 10.319). Moreover, CASA-measured objective motility and sperm survival rate after thawing process showed a marked lack of significant effect related to the different combinations of Equex-STM-cholesterol. However, sperm subjective motion capacity (analyzed by researchers) was modified by the different combinations of Equex-STM-cholesterol (data not shown), which indicates that it is not a good sperm quality parameter to check in other related experiments, such as was observed by different authors reviews, [8, 9, 14, 16].

As far as the authors know, first descriptive results in the literature of seminal quality of postthawed pure Spanish breed sperm are showed (Table 5).

Table 5: Descriptive statistics for sperm quality parameters after thawing

Statistics	M	MP	NP	A	HOST	FL	RT
N	180	100	100	180	180	60	120
Mean	28.139	6.7800	10.670	36.600	35.628	11.733	22.750
SD	13.496	10.319	20.142	13.648	12.302	9.9930	10.348
CV	47.961	152.19	188.78	37.290	34.529	85.168	45.485

M: individual motility; MP: progressive motility; NP: nonprogressive motility; A: acrosome integrity; HOST: hypoosmotic swelling test; FL: fluorescence test; RT: resistance test; N: observation data; SD: standard variation; CV: coefficient of variation.

Stallions were selected for this study following the criteria of the different authors reviews which found bad cryosurvival sperm results in those that failed in diverse seminal cooling studies [43, 44, 52]. This preliminary cooling sperm study was made by Gil et al. (2005, data not published), discarding those stallions which presented sperm quality deficiencies in the cooling process such as recommend Aurich [16]. The obtained results have demonstrated the significance of individual (M, MP, NP, HOST, V, FL, and RT) and extraction (M, MP, NP, HOST, and A), indicating the different behavior of the extender combinations depending on the horse employed or collection moment, as observed by other authors [19, 45, 51, 53–56].

Low density lipoproteins extracted from hen egg yolk have been also tested as cryoprotective media with an optimum extender concentration of 8%, in order to protect the spermatozoa against cold shock due to its protective effect in membranes [26]. On the other hand, it has been suggested that a close relationship among cold susceptibility, lipid phase transition, and lipids profile (polyunsaturated/saturated fatty acids) in gametes of ram, fowl, and bee spermatozoa exists [57] but no studies are carried out in stallions. We identified no interactions of the extender with the fixed factor EQCOL in any dependent variables, indicating that there is no different behaviors of the extender combinations depending on the laboratory technique used. However, significant differences in the mean comparison of the extender combinations were identified for A (IV > II > I), HOST (IV > I), and FL (I > II > IV; W > II) (Table 4) after thawing process in a posterior statistical analysis (Turkey's Studentized Range test). This result confirms that the combination of Equex-STM (0.5%) mixed with cholesterol (125 mM) has obtained better sperm quality results than those of original Martin's extender, possibly due to better balance on lipids membrane profile and its positive relationships with oxidative stress caused by ROS.

The function of the Equex-STM is related to outer cleaning of the sperm plasmatic membrane, at the time of the separation of the plasmatic and spermatic fractions of the ejaculate [38, 58]. Different authors reviews [38, 40, 43, 59] have found significant differences by using different percentages of Equex which contradicts the results obtained in this study, with no significant differences in sperm quality in neither of the two percentages used. We hypothesize that all the effects observed in the results were related to cholesterol adding (125 mM), independently of Equex adding (0.5 or 0.7%).

After analysing by fluorescence trials, we have concluded that the extender composed of 0.5% of Equex-STM and 125 mM of cholesterol has improved stallion semen quality after thawing than original Martin's extender.

ACKNOWLEDGMENTS

The authors would like to thank specially the deceased Publio Rodriguez (Vet Captain of the Spanish Army Forces, DVM, Ph.D.), who was the principal interested person in straighting forward with this work. This paper is dedicated to his memory.

REFERENCES

1. R. Vishwanath, "Artificial insemination: the state of the art," Theriogenology, vol. 59, no. 2, pp. 571–584, 2003.
2. T. L. Blanchard, D. D. Varner, et al., Manual of Equine Reproduction, C.V. Mosby, 2002.

3. S. L. Adams, P. A. Hessian, and P. V. Mladenov, "Cryopreservation of sea urchin (Evechinus chloroticus) sperm," Cryo-Letters, vol. 25, no. 4, pp. 287–299, 2004. View at Scopus
4. S. I. Drokin, H. Stein, and T. P. Govorukha, "Ultrastructure of carp Cyprinus carpio spermatozoa after cooling, dilution and freeze-thawing," Cryo-Letters, vol. 24, no. 1, pp. 49–55, 2003.
5. J.-C. Gwo, C.-Y. Wu, W.-S. P. Chang, and H.-Y. Cheng, "Evaluation of damage in Pacific oyster (Crassostrea gigas) spermatozoa before and after cryopreservation using comet assay," Cryo-Letters, vol. 24, no. 3, pp. 171–180, 2003.
6. M. R. Fernández-Santos, M. C. Esteso, A. J. Soler, V. Montoro, and J. J. Garde, "The effects of different cryoprotectants and the temperature of addition on the survival of red deer epididymal spermatozoa," Cryo-Letters, vol. 26, no. 1, pp. 25–32, 2005.
7. V. I. Grischenko, A. V. Dunaevskaya, and V. I. Babenko, "Cryopreservation of human sperm using rapid cooling rates," Cryo-Letters, vol. 24, no. 2, pp. 67–76, 2003.
8. A. S. L. Medeiros, G. M. Gomes, M. T. Carmo, F. O. Papa, and M. A. Alvarenga, "Cryopreservation of stallion sperm using different amides," Theriogenology, vol. 58, no. 2–4, pp. 273–276, 2002.
9. C. M. O. Medeiros, F. Forell, A. T. D. Oliveira, and J. L. Rodrigues, "Current status of sperm cryopreservation: why isn't it better?" Theriogenology, vol. 57, no. 1, pp. 327–344, 2002.
10. K. F. Weitze and R. Petzoldt, "Preservation of semen," Animal Reproduction Science, vol. 28, no. 1-4, pp. 229–235, 1992.
11. J. C. Samper and C. A. Morris, "Current methods for stallion semen cryopreservation: a survey,"Theriogenology, vol. 49, no. 5, pp. 895–903, 1998.
12. J. C. Samper, "Management and fertility of mares bred with frozen semen," Animal Reproduction Science, vol. 68, no. 3-4, pp. 219–228, 2001.
13. J. Saragusty, H. Gacitua, M. T. Pettit, and A. Arav, "Directional freezing of equine semen in large volumes," Reproduction in Domestic Animals, vol. 42, no. 6, pp. 610–615, 2007.
14. J. R. Clulow, L. J. Mansfield, L. H. A. Morris, G. Evans, and W. M. C. Maxwell, "A comparison between freezing methods for the

cryopreservation of stallion spermatozoa," Animal Reproduction Science, vol. 108, no. 3-4, pp. 298–308, 2008.

15. H. Sieme, G. Martinsson, H. Rauterberg et al., "Application of techniques for sperm selection in fresh and frozen-thawed stallion semen," Reproduction in Domestic Animals, vol. 38, no. 2, pp. 134–140, 2003.
16. C. Aurich, "Recent advances in cooled-semen technology," Animal Reproduction Science, vol. 107, no. 3-4, pp. 268–275, 2008.
17. M. H. T. Troedsson, I. K. M. Liu, and B. G. Crabo, "Sperm transport and survival in the mare,"Theriogenology, vol. 49, no. 5, pp. 905–915, 1998.
18. H. Sieme, R. A. P. Harrison, and A. M. Petrunkina, "Cryobiological determinants of frozen semen quality, with special reference to stallion," Animal Reproduction Science, vol. 107, no. 3-4, pp. 276–292, 2008.
19. P. R. Loomis and J. K. Graham, "Commercial semen freezing: individual male variation in cryosurvival and the response of stallion sperm to customized freezing protocols," Animal Reproduction Science, vol. 105, no. 1-2, pp. 119–128, 2008.
20. S. J. Bedford, D. D. Varner, et al., "Cryopreservation induces capacitation-like changes in acrosomal status of stallion spermatozoa.," 1998.
21. J. Baumber, B. A. Ball, C. G. Gravance, V. Medina, and M. C. G. Davies-Morel, "The effect of reactive oxygen species on equine sperm motility, viability, acrosomal integrity, mitochondrial membrane potential, and membrane lipid peroxidation," Journal of Andrology, vol. 21, no. 6, pp. 895–902, 2000.
22. G. B. Combes, D. D. Varner, F. Schroeder, R. C. Burghardt, and T. L. Blanchard, "Effect of cholesterol on the motility and plasma membrane integrity of frozen equine spermatozoa after thawing," Journal of Reproduction and Fertility. Supplement, no. 56, pp. 127–132, 2000.
23. D. M. Neild, B. M. Gadella, M. G. Chaves, M. H. Miragaya, B. Colenbrander, and A. Agüero, "Membrane changes during different stages of a freeze-thaw protocol for equine semen cryopreservation," Theriogenology, vol. 59, no. 8, pp. 1693–1705, 2003.

24. A. Heitland, "Motility and fertility of stallion spermatozoa cooled and frozen in a modified skim milk extender containing egg yolk and liposome," in Equine Reproduction VI, Biology of Reproduction Monograph Series 1, pp. 753–759, 1995.
25. F. S. Zahn, F. O. Papa, and J. A. Dell' Aqua Jr., "Cholesterol incorporation on equine sperm membrane: effects on post-thaw sperm parameters and fertility," Theriogenology, vol. 58, no. 2–4, pp. 237–240, 2002.
26. M. Moussa, V. Martinet, A. Trimeche, D. Tainturier, and M. Anton, "Low density lipoproteins extracted from hen egg yolk by an easy method: cryoprotective effect on frozen-thawed bull semen,"Theriogenology, vol. 57, no. 6, pp. 1695–1706, 2002.
27. A. Peña and C. Linde-Forsberg, "Effects of equex, one- or two-step dilution, and two freezing and thawing rates on post-thaw survival of dog spermatozoa," Theriogenology, vol. 54, no. 6, pp. 859–875, 2000.
28. T. Tsutsui, M. Hase, T. Hori et al., "Effect of addition of Orvus ES paste to frozen canine semen extender on sperm acrosomes," Journal of Veterinary Medical Science, vol. 62, no. 5, pp. 537–538, 2000.
29. T. Tsutsui, M. Hase, A. Tanaka, N. Fujimura, T. Hori, and E. Kawakami, "Intrauterine and intravaginal insemination with frozen canine semen using an extender consisting of orvus ES paste-supplemented egg yolk tris-fructose citrate," Journal of Veterinary Medical Science, vol. 62, no. 6, pp. 603–606, 2000.
30. W. Nizański, A. Dubiel, W. Bielas, and G. J. Dejneka, "Effects of three cryopreservation methods and two semen extenders on the quality of dog semen after thawing," Journal of Reproduction and Fertility. Supplement, vol. 57, pp. 365–369, 2001.
31. A. I. Peña, L. López-Lugilde, M. Barrio, J. J. Becerra, L. A. Quintela, and P. G. Herradón, "Studies on the intracellular Ca^{2+} concentration of frozen-thawed dog spermatozoa: influence of equex from different sources, two thawing diluents and post-thaw incubation in capacitating conditions,"Reproduction in Domestic Animals, vol. 38, no. 1, pp. 27–35, 2003.
32. T. Tsutsui, M. Hase, T. Hori, T. Ito, and E. Kawakami, "Effects of orvus ES paste on canine spermatozoal longevity after freezing and thawing," Journal of Veterinary Medical Science, vol. 62, no. 5, pp. 533–535, 2000.

33. J. D. Cochran, Effects of Centrifugation, Glycerol Level, Cooling to 5°C, Freezing Rate on the Post-Thaw Motility of Equine Spermatozoa, Special Series 33, Animal Reproduction Laboratory, Colorado State University, 1984.
34. L. Von Baer and C. Helleman, "Cryopreservation of Llama (Lama glama) Semen," Reproduction in Domestic Animals, vol. 34, no. 2, pp. 95–96, 1999.
35. V. G. Pursel, L. L. Schulman, and L. A. Johnson, "Effect of Orvus ES Paste on acrosome morphology, motility and fertilizing capacity of frozen-thawed boar sperm," Journal of animal science, vol. 47, no. 1, pp. 198–202, 1978.
36. T. Abaigar, W. V. Holt, R. A. P. Harrison, and G. Del Barrio, "Sperm subpopulations in Boar (Sus scrofa) and Gazelle (Gazella dama mhorr) semen as revealed by pattern analysis of computer-assisted motility assessments," Biology of Reproduction, vol. 60, no. 1, pp. 32–41, 1999.
37. M. A. El-Alamy and R. H. Foote, "Freezability of spermatozoa from Finn and Dorset rams in multiple semen extenders," Animal Reproduction Science, vol. 65, no. 3-4, pp. 245–254, 2001.
38. A. Akourki, L. Gil, A. Echegaray et al., "Effect of the extender supplement Equex-STM on cryopreserved semen in the Assaf sheep," Cryo-Letters, vol. 25, no. 2, pp. 147–154, 2004.
39. P. G. A. Thomas, V. Surman, et al., "Addition of sodium dodecyl sulphate to tris-citrate extender improves motility and longevity of frozen-thawed canine spermatozoa," in Proceedings of the 12th International Congress on Animal Reproduction (ICAR '92), vol. 4, pp. 1823–1825, The Hague, The Netherlands, 1992.
40. R. P. Amann and B. W. Pickett, An Overview of Frozen Equine Semen: Procedures for Thawing and Insemination of Frozen Equine Spermatozoa, Special Series 33, Animal Reproduction Laboratory, Colorado State University, 1984.
41. J. Juhász, P. Nagy, M. Kulcsár, and G. Huszenicza, "Methods for semen and endocrinological evaluation of the stallion: a review," Acta Veterinaria Brno, vol. 69, no. 4, pp. 247–259, 2000.
42. J. C. Martin, E. Klug, and A. R. Günzel, "Centrifugation of stallion semen and its storage in large volume straws," Journal of Reproduction and Fertility. Supplement, no. 27, pp. 47–51, 1979.

43. R. P. Amann and B. W. Pickett, "Principles of cryopreservation and a review of cryopreservation of stallion spermatozoa," 1987.
44. J. Verstegen, M. Iguer-Ouada, and K. Onclin, "Computer assisted semen analyzers in andrology research and veterinary practice," Theriogenology, vol. 57, no. 1, pp. 149–179, 2002.
45. C. Warnke, A. Tuchscherer, H. Alm, W. Kanitz, S. Blottner, and H. Torner, "Characterisation of movement pattern and velocities of stallion spermatozoa depending on donor, season and cryopreservation," Acta Veterinaria Hungarica, vol. 51, no. 3, pp. 395–408, 2003.
46. J. E. Bruemmer, "Collection and freezing of epididymal stallion sperm," Veterinary Clinics of North America: Equine Practice, vol. 22, no. 3, pp. 677–682, 2006.
47. R. Eliasson and L. Treichl, "Supravital staining of human spermatozoa," Fertility and Sterility, vol. 22, no. 2, pp. 134–137, 1971.
48. V. G. Pursel and L. A. Johnson, "Glutaraldehyde fixation of boar spermatozoa for acrosome evaluation," Theriogenology, vol. 1, no. 2, pp. 63–68, 1974.
49. R. S. Jeyendran and L. J. Zaneveld, "Human sperm hypoosmotic swelling test," Fertility and Sterility, vol. 46, no. 1, pp. 151–152, 1986.
50. C. Dubé, M. Beaulieu, C. Reyes-Moreno, C. Guillemette, and J. L. Bailey, "Boar sperm storage capacity of BTS and Androhep Plus: viability, motility, capacitation, and tyrosine phosphorylatio n,"Theriogenology, vol. 62, no. 5, pp. 874–886, 2004.
51. E. S. Metcalf, "The efficient use of equine cryopreserved semen," Theriogenology, vol. 68, no. 3, pp. 423–428, 2007.
52. R. P. Arruda, B. A. Ball, C. G. Gravance, A. R. Garcia, and I. K. M. Liu, "Effects of extenders and cryoprotectants on stallion sperm head morphometry," Theriogenology, vol. 58, no. 2–4, pp. 253–256, 2002.
53. B. A. Ball, V. Medina, C. G. Gravance, and J. Baumber, "Effect of antioxidants on preservation of motility, viability and acrosomal integrity of equine spermatozoa during storage at 5∘C,"Theriogenology, vol. 56, no. 4, pp. 577–589, 2001.

54. L. M. Thurston, P. F. Watson, and W. V. Holt, "Semen cryopreservation: a genetic explanation for species and individual variation?" Cryo-Letters, vol. 23, no. 4, pp. 255–262, 2002.
55. P. R. Loomis, "Advanced Methods for Handling and Preparation of Stallion Semen," Veterinary Clinics of North America: Equine Practice, vol. 22, no. 3, pp. 663–676, 2006.
56. C. López-Fernández, F. Crespo, F. Arroyo et al., "Dynamics of sperm DNA fragmentation in domestic animals. II. The stallion," Theriogenology, vol. 68, no. 9, pp. 1240–1250, 2007.
57. A. Arav, M. Pearl, and Y. Zeron, "Does lipid profile explain chilling sensitivity and membrane lipid phase transition of spermatozoa and oocytes?" Cryo-Letters, vol. 21, no. 3, pp. 179–186, 2000.
58. M. Vidament, P. Vincent, J. M. Yvon, B. Bruneau, and F. X. Martin, "Glycerol in semen extender is a limiting factor in the fertility in asine and equine species," Animal Reproduction Science, vol. 89, no. 1-4, pp. 302–305, 2005.
59. M. Henry, P. P. N. Snoeck, and A. C. P. Cottorello, "Post-thaw spermatozoa plasma membrane integrity and motility of stallion semen frozen with different cryoprotectants," Theriogenology, vol. 58, no. 2–4, pp. 245–248, 2002.

Chapter 5

Nutraceuticals in Reproduction of Bulls and Stallions

Rubens Paes de Arruda[1], Daniela Franco da Silva[1], Maria Augusta Alonso[1], André Furugen Cesar de Andrade[1], Juliana Nascimento[1], Andres Mejia Gallego[1], Simone Maria Massami Kitamura Martins[1], and Thaís Marques Granato[1]

[1]Laboratory of Semen Biotechnology and Andrology, Department of Animal Reproduction, School of Veterinary Medicine and Animal Science, Universidade de São Paulo (USP), Pirassununga, SP, Brazil.

ABSTRACT

The industry has made available in the market a series of substances (nutraceuticals) which intent would be to optimize the use of nutrients in some metabolic paths, influencing positively reproductive performance in animals. However, the response to the use of nutraceuticals varies according to the animal. As the organism is highly complex and in order to achieve a perfect activity of the hypothalamic-pituitary-gonadal axis, an ideal interaction in molecular basis is needed, where the nutraceuticals can have their direct action. The aim of this study was to review the function and research results using the main nutraceuticals (β carotene, vitamin A, L-carnitine, omegas 3, 6 and 9 and Gamma-oryzanol) on reproductive characteristics of bulls and stallions.

INTRODUCTION

Functional foods and nutraceuticals commonly have been considered synonyms, however functional foods is any healthy or fictional food claimed to have health-promoting or disease preventing properties beyond the basic function of supplying nutrients, such as reduction of disease risk and maintenance of physical and menthal well-being and consumed as part of the diet. Biologically active substances encountered in functional foods can be classified in groups as: probiotics and prebiotics, sulfured and nitrogen foods, pigments and vitamins, phenolic compounds, polyunsaturated fatty acids and fibers. In the other hand, nutraceuticals are food or part of the food that have benefits to health, including prevention and/or disease treatment. They can include isolated nutrients, diet supplements, genetic engineered products, herbal products and processed food (Moraes & Colla, 2006).

Spermatogenesis, the processes of masculine gamete formation, which takes place within the testicles, more specifically in seminiferous tubules, demands a balanced function of all systems in the organism, knowing the sensitivity of the germinative epithelium. It is atablished that environmental factors can alter hormonal secretion and cellular differentiation in the testicles and maturation and transport in the epididymis. In face of adverse factors, especially nutritional, reproductive organs present degeneration and disturbances of different degrees and intensities, temporary or permanent, therefore determining a greater or lesser influence in the animal´s fertility.

In Central Brazil, testicular degeneration is considered the greatest cause of low fertility in *Bos taurus* bulls raised extensively (Vale Filho, 1974). No doubt, it can be affirmed that among other environmental factors, the occurrence of food shortage of diverse natures, mainly during the dry months of the year, significantly cause the low performance of the animals. Food shortage considered as a complex can be proteic, energetic, mineral or vitamin in its origin.

Unfortunately, there is a great individual variation among stallions in sperm viability maintenance during cooled semen storage. For some stallions, even with adequate care during the whole procedure, sperm that survive cooling are insufficient to provide a sufficient number of viable sperm for artificial insemination (Arruda et al., 2009).

Nowadays, athletic performance is required from a great part of the stallions, which have an intense training regimen associated with semen collection/live cover schedule, leading to an increase in nutritional requirements. Thus, a nutritional program becomes mandatory, aiming an optimization of performance as athletes and stallions (Franceschini, 2003).

Bulls raised under tropical conditions, such as in Brazil, can present quantitative and qualitative semen characteristics variations, promoted among other causes by thermal stress, management practices, nutritional status and, the specially the amount and quality of pastures (Aurélio, 2008).

β-Carotene and Vitamin A

In the literature, one can find that β-carotene, pro- vitamin A, acts beneficially in the organism in the same manner vitamin A does, although presenting specific physiological functions, being essential for the epithelial tissues functioning in reproductive organs (Arikan & Rodway, 2000). β-carotene is found in extremely high concentrations in the bovine corpus luteum (CL) (O›Fallon & Chew, 1984; Holt et al., 1995), causing the characteristic yellow color in the CL. Besides acting as a vitamin A precursor, there are evidences that β-carotene can be necessary for ideal steroid production, possibly acting as an antioxidant (Young et al., 1995). Moreover, several studies in dairy cattle couldn´t demonstrate the effect of β-carotene supplementation in steroid hormone levels (Folman et al., 1979; Wang et al., 1982).

Studies performed in laboratory demonstrated that β-carotene stimulates progesterone production in luteal cells cultivated *in vitro* and that β-carotene concentration in culture media lowers during incubation, being more abrupt when cells are stimulated with LH and/ or cAMP (Arikan & Rodway, 1997,1998), suggesting that β-carotene is metabolized during the steroidogenic process.

Weiss et al. (1979) investigated the influence of β-carotene on some sperm characteristics in young bulls under a food regimen with shortage of this substance, but supplemented with vitamin A. After 27 weeks of the experiment, results showed that β-carotene deficiency provoked a reduction in sperm progressive motility and an increase in morphological alteration percentage of the head and citoplasmatic droplet in middle piece, that indicate retarded spermatogenesis and spermatic maturation disturbances in the epididymis.

Erb et al. (1947) found that young dairy bulls that received food with low vitamin A content had, besides weight loss and vision alteration, seizures, spermatogenesis decrease and testicular atrophy. In adult bulls, no sterility cases were found, but vitamin A deficiency caused low fertilizing capacity, as a consequence of bad semen quality. Bratton et al. (1948) submitted 6 bulls to a deprived pro vitamin A food for 21 months. In the end of the experiment three bulls presented sperm motility decrease and increase in abnormal sperm shapes. Histologically, germinative epithelium of seminiferous tubules presented degeneration signs and few cells in the tubules lumen. Schmidt (1953) designed an experiment using white and red carrots in bulls feeding, maintaining basic food with normal carotenoids levels. After analyzing 124 seminal samples from 6 treated bulls, bulls supplemented with red carrots presented 7% higher values for volume, concentration and total sperm numbers compared with bulls receiving white carrots. The author attributed this superiority to β-carotene influence.

With the purpose of evaluating the effects of vitamin A deficiency on bull´s reproductive characteristics, Rode et al. (1995) delineated an experiment where Hereford bulls (16 months of age, 462 kg average body weight) were used. They were fed with a diet rich in concentrated with (+VIT) or without (-VIT) vitamin A supplement until hypovitaminosis A was apparent (28 and 32 weeks in years 1 and 2, respectively). Half of the bulls from each treatment were slaughtered and the remaining where re-fed with vitamin A. Retinol plasmatic concentration in -VIT bulls reached their lowest value in 25 weeks. In year 1, the proportion of sperm with progressive motility was lower in -VIT bulls after 17 weeks, but was similar to the +VIT bulls after receiving Vitamin A again. The proportion of sperm with primary morphological defects seemed higher in -VIT bulls compared with +VIT bulls in weeks 26 and 24 in year 1 and 2, respectively. The incidence of these defects decreased in -VIT bulls after being re-fed with Vitamin A in weeks 8 and 12. Vitamin A hypovitaminosis led to a decrease in testicles weight, daily sperm output, and epididymal sperm storage, but did not affect daily weight gain. Prolonged vitamin A diet deficiency was detrimental to sperm quality and production in the absence of other clinical signs. However, under practical feeding conditions, diets leading to marginal vitamin A deficiency or relative ingestion absence for a short period probably would have minimal effect on spermatogenesis.

L-Carnitine

In a very interesting introduction, Stradaioli et al. (2000) describe that among the factors that can affect semen quality and spermatozoa storage (Pickett, 1993; Bedford et al., 1995; Magistrini et al., 1996), seminal plasma constituents must be considered, which reflect changes in epididymis and accessory sexual gland secretions (Setchell et al., 1994). Stallion sexual gland markers include carnitine which has only been found in epididymal plasma (Magistrini et al., 1995a,b) and represents nearly all the carnitine available in seminal plasma, as observed in other mammals (Jeulin & Lewin, 1996). Carnitine is taken from the blood stream and then released in epididymal lumen by active epithelial pumps (Brooks, 1980), which are regulated by androgens in rat (Cooper et al., 1986a) and monkey (Cooper et al., 1986b). Carnitine is best acknowledged as a key compound in energy-producing processes since it modulates mitochondrial fatty acid oxidation. To accomplish this role, carnitine needs the concerted action of a discrete number of membrane-bound, carnitine-dependent, long-chain acyltransferases, also known as carnitine palmitoyltransferases (CPTI and CPTII), and acyl-carnitine translocase (Bieber, 1988).

Spermatozoa increase their carnitine content and progressive motility during passage through the epididymis where carnitine is esterified within sperm cells in acetylcarnitine (Casillas, 1973). Acetylated l-carnitine is the major form of acylcarnitine in mammal tissues (Bieber et al., 1982).

In this context, another important action of carnitine is to modulate the intramitochondrial acetyl-CoA/free CoA ratio via carnitine acetyltransferase (CAT) (Uziel et al., 1988; Abdel-Aleem et al., 1995), a mitochondrial enzyme able to catalyze the reversible transfer of the acetyl-unit from CoA to carnitine (Bieber et al., 1982).

Since elevated levels of mitochondrial acetyl-CoA cause the inhibition of a number of key enzymes of such oxidative pathways as pyruvate dehydrogenase and 3-keto-acyl-CoA thiolase, a reduction of acetyl-CoA by carnitine may relieve such an inhibitory effect (Wang et al., 1991; Abdel-Aleem et al., 1995; Jeulin an& Lewin, 1996). Both extra and intracellular acetylcarnitine provide readily available acetyl groups for spermatozoa motility (Milkowsky et al., 1976; Bruns & Casillas, 1990). In mature spermatozoa, high intracellular L-carnitine concentrations increase the utilization of pyruvate and lactate (Carter et al., 1980; Jones & Murdoch, 1996), thus holding the maximal "acetylation-state" of carnitine.

In human beings, seminal L-carnitine content is correlated with spermatozoa count and progressive motility (Menchini-Fabris et al., 1984; Borman et al., 1989) and a reduction of the acetylcarnitine/l-carnitine ratio has been observed in asthenospermic patients (Golan et al., 1984; Bartellini et al., 1987). Moreover, significant reduction of seminal carnitine concentrations has been reported in azoospermic patients affected by bilateral agenesis of the vas deferens and epididymal obstruction (Menchini-Fabris et al., 1984; Casano et al., 1987), as well as during severe testicular failures (Lewin et al., 1981). Recently, a reduction of seminal plasma carnitine has been reported in infertile men (Zöpfgen et al., 2000). The positive correlation observed among seminal parameters and seminal carnitine concentration allows proposing carnitine as a "good quality" semen marker (Menchini-Fabris et al., 1984).

L-carnitine is of major significance, because when administered in diet, acts on long chain fatty acid transport inside the mitochondria for beta oxidation and synthesis of phosphates rich in energy, optimizing energy and mitochondrial production, thus improving sperm motility and survival pre and post freezing (Franceschini, 2003).

The reproductive characteristics and seminal carnitine and acetylcarnitine content as well as carnitine acetyltransferase activity of young Maremmano stallions (*n* D 25) are reported (Stradaioli et al., 2000). The stallions were subjected to semen collections in November and January; in each trial two ejaculates were collected 1 h apart. The total motile morphologically normal spermatozoa (TMMNS) and the progressively motile spermatozoa at collection and during storage at +4°C were evaluated. Seminal L-carnitine (LC), acetylcarnitine (AC), pyruvate and lactate were measured using spectrophotometric methods, whereas carnitine acetyltransferase activity was measured by radioenzymatic methods. Significant differences ($P<0.001$) were observed between the first and second ejaculates for sperm count (0.249 ± 0.025 versus $0.133\pm0.014x10^9$/ml), total number spermatozoa by ejaculate (12.81 ± 1.23 versus $6.36\pm0.77x10^9$), progressively motile spermatozoa (48.6 ± 3.0 versus 52.6 ± 3.0%) and TMMNS (3.35 ± 0.50 versus $2.02\pm0.37x10^9$). In the raw semen the LC and AC were significantly higher in the first ejaculate than in the second ($P<0.001$), whereas, pyruvate and pyruvate/lactate ratio were higher in the second ejaculate ($P<0.05$). Seminal plasma AC and LC concentrations were higher in the first ejaculate ($P<0.001$). The pyruvate/lactate ratio was higher in the second ejaculate ($P<0.05$). Both raw semen and seminal plasma LC and AC concentrations were positively correlated with spermatozoa concentration ($P<0.01$); in raw semen AC was also correlated to TMMNS ($P<0.01$). Lactate levels of raw semen were correlated to progressively motile spermatozoa after storage ($P<0.01$). In the second ejaculate, significant correlations were also observed among AC/LC ratio in raw semen and progressively motile spermatozoa after 48 and 72 h of refrigeration. Furthermore, AC levels were correlated to lactate concentration. The positive correlation between LC, AC and spermatozoa concentration and between AC and TMMNS indicated carnitine as potential semen quality marker. Moreover, the correlation between AC/LC ratio and progressive spermatozoa motility after refrigeration, suggested that carnitine may contribute towards improving the maintenance of spermatozoa viability during in vitro storage.

To improve performance and reproductive indexes, a study was carried out to assess the effects of L-carnitine on reproductive parameters of pure Arabian horses (Rosas Filho et al., 2001). Horses were randomly divided into blocks by semen quality (good, medium, bad). After this, the blocks were divided in two groups. The first group was classified as control and the other one as treated. The second group received a diet containing 10 g of L-carnitine for a period of 90 days. Two weekly semen collections were performed to evaluate gel free volume, progressive motility, spermatic concentration, total sperm; spermatic morphology (major and minor defects) and once weekly testicular measurements were made. The results showed that there were no statistical differences ($P>0.05$) in the following semen parameters: gel free volume, progressive motility, spermatic concentration, total concentration, spermatic morphology (except minor defects, $P<0.05$) and testicular measurements.

Lima (2003) performed an experiment aiming to evaluate the influence of L-carnitine oral ingestion on stallion´s cryopreserved semen and its possible effect on total sperm per ejaculate, total and progressive motility, sperm velocity, membrane integrity and thermoresistance test (TRT). Means and standard deviations of progressive motility, linearity, path velocity, progressive velocity and curvilinear velocity were significantly higher for control group (TO) comparing with treated group (T1) before TRT was performed. After the TRT, means and standard deviations were significantly higher for TO for path velocity and progressive velocity; there was no significant difference among groups after TRT was conducted for progressive motility, linearity and curvilinear velocity. After TRT, there was an abrupt decrease in progressive motility, linearity, path velocity, progressive velocity and curvilinear velocity for the control group (TO) compared with the treated group (T1). According to the authors, results lead to the conclusion that L-carnitine can, in some circumstances, be an important therapeutic tool for stallion´s sperm quality improvement.

L-carnitine has an important role in diet administration and, among others, has the function of influencing the transport of long chain fatty acids inside mitochondria for beta oxidation and energy-rich phosphate, optimizing mitochondrial and energy production, thus improving motility and survival of spermatozoa pre and post freezing. Likewise, Franceschini (2003) designed and experiment to verify the effect of L-carnitine supplementation on stallion´s post freezing semen quality. Furthermore, evaluation of mitochondrial activity of sperm after freezing and thawing was performed. Results indicated that L-carnitine supplementation had a positive effect on mitochondrial activity, promoting reduction in the amount of sperm with inactive mitochondria. Besides causing an improvement in cryopreserved sperm total motility, possibly due to an optimization of their energy metabolism.

Omegas 3, 6 and 9

Differences in the ability of sperm from various animals to resist cold shock appear to be related to their sperm membrane lipid composition (Parks & Lynch, 1982; Brinsko et al., 2005). The lipid composition of sperm membranes not only influences the response of sperm to cooling and freezing, but also plays a major role in the physiologic changes leading to fertilization (Langlais & Roberts, 1985; Ladha, 1998).

Semen from all domestic species contains high levels of polyunsaturated fatty acids (PUFA), in particular, docosahexaenoic acid (DHA; 22:6 n-3, an omega-3 fatty acid) and docosapentaenoic acid (DPA; 22:5 n-6, an omega-6 fatty acid). The semen of boars has very high levels of DPA and the semen lipid profile of stallions is similar to that of the boar (Parks & Lynch, 1982). Studies in the boar have shown that a high DHA to DPA ratio in semen results in enhanced fertility, while higher levels of DPA relative to DHA results in reduced fertility (Penny et al., 2000; Maldjian et al., 2003; Brinsko et al., 2005). In asthenozoospermic men, the level of DHA in seminal plasma as well as the ratio of omega-3 to omega-6 fatty acids in sperm was found to be lower than in normozoospermic men (Conquer et al., 1999). Since animals are unable to synthesize PUFAs from saturated or monounsaturated fatty acids, they must acquire them from precursor PUFAs in their diet. The transfer of dietary PUFAs to sperm has been shown to be effective in a number of species (Drokin et al., 1999; Conquer et al., 2000; Penny et al., 2000). Unfortunately, most proprietary horse feeds are very high in precursors for omega-6 fatty acids while the precursors for omega-3 fatty acids, such as DHA, are very low. Brinsko et al. (2005) studied the effects of a DHA rich nutraceutical (omega 3) on fresh, cooled and frozen semen quality. Stallions were randomly assigned to one of two treatment groups (n=4 per group). Stallions were fed their normal diet (control) or their normal diet top-dressed with 250 g of a DHA-enriched nutraceutical. Feeding trials lasted for 14 week, after which a 14-week washout period was allowed and the treatment groups were reversed for another 14 week feeding trial. Feeding the nutraceutical resulted in a three-fold increase in semen DHA levels and 50% increase in the ratio of DHA to DPA in semen. Sperm motion characteristics in fresh semen were unaffected by treatment. After 24 h of cooled semen storage in an Equitainer™, total and progressive motility did not differ between treatment groups, but sperm from stallions fed the nutraceutical exhibited higher velocity and straighter projector ($P<0.05$). After 48 h of cooled storage, increases in the percentages of sperm exhibiting total motility ($P=0.07$), progressive motility ($P=0.06$) and rapid motility ($P=0.04$), were observed when stallions were being fed the nutraceutical. For a subset of four stallions, whose progressive sperm motility was <40% after 24 h of cooled storage when fed the control diet, feeding the nutraceutical resulted in improvements in mean progressive motility of sperm after 24 h ($P=0.10$) and 48 h ($P=0.03$) of storage. Feeding the nutraceutical resulted in similar improvements in motion characteristics being observed in frozen-thawed semen. While it appears that feeding the nutraceutical may improve the motion characteristics of cool-stored stallion semen, it may be most beneficial for stallions of marginal fertility whose sperm do not tolerate the rigors of cooling and storage. The nutraceutical also appeared to improve the freezability of semen. More dramatic improvements in semen quality may be observed if modifications in the main fat content of the diet are incorporated with the DHA supplement.

Elhordoy et al. (2008) investigated the action of the polyunsaturated fatty acids (PUFAs), in particular decosahexanoic acid (DHA; 22:6 n-3, omega-3 fatty acid), on the quality of fresh, cooled and frozen stallion semen. Six stallions were randomly assigned to two treatment groups ($n=3$ per group) and were kept under the same management conditions. Stallions of one group (group A) were fed 30 g of DHA per day for 80 days, while the others (group B) did not receive any supplementation. The treatment groups were then reversed, with the group B fed with 30 g of DHA and group A serving as a control. Both groups were subjected to a washout period before the second stage of this switch-back study. This period was established to allow DHA levels of treated stallions to return to pre-treatment levels. Preliminary results show that treated stallions experienced an increase in total spermatozoal number per ejaculate ($P<0.05$), motility ($P<0.05$), and a reduced percentage of dead and abnormal spermatozoa ($P<0.05$), especially in the acrosome and mid-piece abnormalities ($P<0.001$), in comparison with the control treatment. Mean percentage of progressively motile (PM) spermatozoa improved in some of the stallions after 48 h of cooled-semen storage and after semen cryopreservation. The greatest increase in these parameters was shown in PM of the stallions with initial poor quality semen. Moreover, the most significant morphological improvement was detected in the stallions with the poorest initial morphology, similarly to the stallions with the lowest PM following preservation. These data suggest that dietary DHA supplementation in stallions can increase daily spermatozoa output, and quality of cooled and cryopreserved semen, possibly due to an increase sperm plasma membrane DHA content. The effect was magnified in those stallions with initially poor-quality ejaculates. More research is needed to substantiate these findings in a larger group of stallions.

Gamma-Oryzanol

Gamma-oryzanol was discovered in rice oil in 1954 by Kaneco and Tsuchiya, in Japan (Gonzaga, 2008) and initially described as the only component, but later studies revealed that the substance is far from being simple, and the contrary, it is a variety of ferulate esters called α, β and γ-orizanol (Scavariello & Arellano, 1988). Gama-oryzanol has received most attention owing to health beneficial properties, such as plasmatic cholesterol reduction, platelet aggregation inhibition, reduction in hepatic cholesterol biosynthesis, reduction in cholesterol absorption and increase in fecal biliary salts excretion. It is used in pharmaceutical and cosmetic industry, as well as food additive due to antioxidant properties (Juliano et al., 2005; Gonzaga, 2008).

Gama-oryzanol components were isolated and identified by Xu & Godber (1999), as Δ-estigmastenol ferulate, estigmasterol ferulate, cycloarterol ferulate 24-metilen cicloarterol ferulate, Δ-campestenil ferulato, campesteril ferulato Δ-sitostenil ferulato, sitosteril ferulato, campestanil ferulato e sitostanil ferulato.

Fry et al. (1997) tested oral supplementaion efficiency (500 mg/day) of gamma-oryzanol in bodybuilder men. No significant differences were found in levels of circulating hormones (testosterone, cortisol, estradiol, GH, insulin, beta-endorphin), minerals (calcium and magnesium), albumin or blood lipids. Results showed that oral supplementation with 500mg/kg of gamma-oryzanol during 9 weeks did not interfere with physical performance or physiological parameters observed.

With the objective of evaluating the effects of dietary supplementation with Gamma-Oryzanol (GO) on seminal characteristics of stallions (Raphael et al., 2006), six light-horse stallions were split in two groups and supplemented for 60 days. The control group received 150 mL of soy oil, and the treatment group received 150 mL of rice oil containing

1,1% of GO (Gamahorse® 3).Volume, concentration and morphology were evaluated. Sperm membrane integrity was evaluated using the hypoosmotic swelling test (HOS). No effect of GO supplementation was detected on reproductive characteristics. In another study, Arlas et al. (2008) also evaluated the effects of supplementary feeding of stallions with commercial rice oil (gamma oryzanol) (Gama-Horse, HT Nutri®, Brazil) on sperm parameters. Four stallions with ages ranging between 6 and 30 years were used. Animals were similarly managed for 190 days during the trial. The experiment was divided in three periods: pre-treatment (PT)-30 days to stabilize sperm reserves; treatment (TR)-80 days of supplementation with 200 mL rice oil containing 34% linoleic acid, 1% linolenic acid, 1% gamma oryzanol and vitamin E; control (CN)-80 days without rice oil supplementation. Semen evaluations were performed immediately after collection: volume, concentration, total motility, hypo-osmotic test (HOST) evaluating functionality, carboxyfluorescein diacetate/propidium iodide (CFDA/PI) evaluating membrane integrity and total antioxidant potential (TRAP). A blood sample was obtained each 15 days to measure plasma testosterone and estradiol. The supplementation with rice oil increased concentration ($P<0.01$) (TR: 226×10^6 mL^{-1}; CN: 172×10^6 mL^{-1}), total motility ($P<0.01$) (TR: 59%; CN: 42%), HOST ($P<0.02$) (TR: 73%; CN: 69%) and TRAP ($P<0.01$) (TR: 1.9 nmol Trolox/mg of protein; CN: 0.98 nmol Trolox/mg of protein). No differences between periods of TR and CN were observed in volume, membrane integrity, testosterone or estradiol. The authors suggest that oral supplementation with the commercial rice oil containing PUFA and gamma-oryzanol increased the total antioxidant potential of the semen. In addition, higher membrane functionality and motility was detected, possibly due to antioxidant protection preventing lipid peroxidation of sperm membranes or attributable to improved membrane fluidity.

Commercial Nutraceuticals

With the purpose of investigating the effects of the commercial nutraceutical, Promater®, in body weight, semen, libido and hormones (testosterone and cortisol) in Nelore Bulls, Aurélio (2008) used two groups of ten Nelore bulls, aging between 30 and 36 months. Group 1 (G1) was control and Group 2 (G2) received 20 ml/animal/day of the product, during 70 days. Body weight, blood samples for testosterone and cortisol measurements and semen collection using eletroejaculation were obtained in days zero (D0), 35 (D35) and 70 (D70) in the two groups. Libido tests were conducted seven days before each collection (days -7, 28 and 63). There was difference (P<0.01) among collection days D70 = 33.28 cm, in relation to D0 = 32.30 cm and D35 = 32.18 cm in scrotal perimeter. There was difference in body weight (P<0.01) among days (0, 35 e 70) with means of 424, 30 kg, 480, 70 kg and 502, 60 kg, respectively. There was no difference among groups referring to libido, seminal aspects, cortisol and testosterone. The results demonstrated that nutraceutical supplementation did not lead to an improvement in evaluated parameters.

FINAL CONSIDERATIONS

The industry, in general, has made available in the market a series of substances (nutraceuticals) that would supposedly optimize the use of nutrients in some metabolic paths, influencing positively the animal´s athletic and reproductive performance.

However, the response to nutraceuticals use varies according to each individual, taking the breed, age, function, environmental and nutritional factors, etc in account. The organism is highly complex and, in order to possess a perfect functioning of hypothalamic pituitary gonadal axis, there is a need of perfect interactions in molecular basis. Nutraceuticals might be directly associated in these aspects. Therefore, the response to nutraceuticals utilization should be more efficient to one than other individual. Hence, a clinical and technical knowledge is essential for supplementing only when needed.

Further studies are needed to evaluate the real benefits from nutraceuticals supplementation as the experiments have small number of animals and results have low repeatability.

REFERENCES

1. ABDEL-ALEEM, S.; SAVED-AHMED, M.; NADA, M.A. et al. Stimulation of non-oxidative glucose utilization by l-carnitine in isolated myocytes. Journal of Molecular and Cellular Cardiology, v.27, p.2465-2472, 1995.

2. ARIKAN, S.; RODWAY, R.G. The effect of beta-carotene either in organic solvent or as HDL on progesterone production by bovine luteal cells. Journal of Reproduction and Fertility, v.19, p.64, 1997 (abstr.

3. ARIKAN, S.; RODWAY, R.G. Uptake and depletion of beta-carotene by bovine corpus luteum cells. In: BRITISH SOCIETY OF ANIMAL SCIENCE, 190., 1998, Ireland. Proceedings... Ireland: British Society of Animal Science., 1998. p.190.

4. ARIKAN, S; RODWAY, R.G. Effect of cyclodextrin-encapsulated β-carotene on progesterone production by bovine luteal cells. Animal Reproduction Science, v.64, p.149-160, 2000.

5. ARLAS, T.R.; PEDERZOLLI, C.D.; TERRACIANO, P.B. et al. Sperm quality is improved feeding stallions with a Rice oil supplement. Animal Reproduction Science, v.107, p.306, 2008.

6. ARRUDA, R.P.; ANDRADE, A.F.C.; CELEGHINI, E.C.C. et al. Manipulação e uso do sêmen transportado refrigerado de garanhões. In: SIMPÓSIO DE EQÜIDEOCULTURA - SIMEQ, 2., 2009, Viçosa, MG. Anais... Viçosa, MG: Universidade Federal de Viçosa, 2009. p.111-131.

7. AURÉLIO, P.T.F. Avaliação andrológica, libido e hormônios em touros nelore *Bos Taurus indicus*suplementados com nutracêutico. 2008. 76f. Dissertação (Mestrado em Ciência Animal) - Universidade do Oeste Paulista, Presidente Prudente.

8. BARTELLINI, M.; CANALE, D.; IZZO, P.L. et al. L-carnitine and acetylcarnitine in human sperm with normal and reduced motility. Acta Europaea Fertilitatis, v.18, p.29-31, 1987.

9. BEDFORD, S.J.; GRAHAM, J.K.; AMANN, R.P. et al. Use of two freezing extenders to cool stallion spermatozoa to 5°C with and without seminal plasma. Theriogenology, v.43, p.939-953, 1995.

10. BIEBER, L.L. Carnitine. Annual Review of Biochemistry, v.57, p.261-283, 1988.

11. BIEBER, L.L.; EMAUS, R.; VALKNER, K. et al. Possible functions of short-chain and medium-chain carnitine acyltransferases. Federation Proceedings, v.41, p.2858-2862, 1982.

12. BORMAN, M.S.; du TOIT, D.; OTTO, B. et al. Seminal carnitine, epididymal function and spermatozoal motility.South African Medical Journal, v.75, p.20-21, 1989.

13. BRATTON, R.W.; SALISBURY, G.W.; TANABE, T. et al. Breeding behavior, spermatogenesis, and semen production of mature dairy bulls fed rations low in carotene. Journal of Dairy Science, v.31, p.779-791, 1948.
14. BRINSKO, S.T.; VARNER, D.D.; LOVE, C.C. et al. Effect of feeding a DHA-enriched nutriceutical on the quality of fresh, cooled and frozen stallion semen. Theriogenology, v.63, p.1519-1527, 2005.
15. BROOKS, D.E. Carnitine in the male reproductive tract and its relation to the metabolism of the epididymis and spermatozoa. In: McGARRY, J.D.; FRENKEL, R.A. (Eds.) Carnitine biosynthesis metabolism and function. Academic Press: New York, 1980. p.219-235.
16. BRUNS, K.A.; CASILLAS, E.R. Partial purification and characterisation of an acetylcarnitine hydrolase from bovine epididymal spermatozoa. Archives of Biochemistry and Biophysics, v.277, p.1-7, 1990.
17. CARTER, A.L.; STRATMAN, F.W.; HUTSON, S.M.; LARDY, H.A. The role of carnitine and its esters in sperm metabolism. In: McGARRY, J.D.; FRENKEL, R.A. (Eds.) Carnitine biosynthesis metabolism and function. New York: Academic Press, 1980. p.251-269.
18. CASANO, R.; ORLANDO, C.; CALDINI, A.L. et al. Simultaneous measurement of seminal l-carnitine, a,1-4-glucosidase, and glycerylphophorylcholine in azoospermic and oligozoospermic patients. Fertility and Sterility, v.47, p.324-328, 1987.
19. CASILLAS, E.R. Accumulation of carnitine by bovine spermatozoa during maturation in the epididymis. Journal of Biological Chemistry, v.248, p.8227-8232, 1973.
20. CONQUER, J.A.; MARTIN, J.B.; TUMMON, I. et al. Fatty acid analysis of blood, serum, seminal plasma, and spermatozoa of normozoospermic vs. asthenozoospermic males. Lipids, v.34, p.793-799, 1999.
21. CONQUER, J.A.; MARTIN, J.B.; TUMMON, I. et al. Effect of DHA supplementation on DHA status and sperm motility in asthenozoospermic males. Lipids, v.35, p.149-154, 2000.
22. COOPER, T.G.; GUDERMANN, T.W.; YEUNG, C.H. Characteristics of the transport of carnitine into the cauda

epididymis of the rat as ascertained by luminal perfusion in vitro. International Journal of Andrology, v.9, p.348-358, 1986a.

23. COOPER, T.G.; YEUNG, C.H.; WEINBAUER, G.F. Transport of carnitine by the epididymis of the cynomolgus macaque (*Macaca fascicularis*). Journal of Reproduction and Fertility, v.77, p.297-301, 1986b.
24. DROKIN, S.I.; VAISBERG, T.N.; KOPEIKA, E.F. et al. Effect of cryopreservation on lipids and some physiological features of spermatozoa from rams pastured in highlands and in valleys. Cytobios, v.100, p.27-36, 1999.
25. ELHORDOY, D.M.; CAZALES, N.; COSTA, G. et al. Effect of dietary supplementation with DHA on the quality of fresh, cooled and frozen stallion semen. Animal Reproduction Science, v.107, p.319, 2008.
26. ERB, R.E.; ANDREWS, F.N.; HAUGE, S.M. et al. Observations on vitamin A deficiency in young dairy bulls. Journal of Dairy Science, v.30, p 687-702, 1947.
27. FOLMAN, Y.; ASCARELLI, L.; HERZ, Z. et al. Fertility of dairy heifers given a commercial diet free of β-carotene.British Journal of Nutrition, v.41, p.353-359, 1979.
28. FRANCESCHINI, G.C.S. Efeito da adição dietética de L-carnitina sobre a atividade mitocondrial dos espermatozóides criopreservados de garanhões. 2003. 58f. Dissertação (Mestrado em Medicina Veterinária) - Faculdade de Ciências Agrárias e Veterinárias/Universidade Estadual Paulista, Jaboticabal.
29. FRY, A.C.; BONNER, E.; LEWIS, D.L. et al. The effects of gamma-oryzanol supplementation during resistence exercise training. International Journal of Sport Nutrition, v.7, p.318-329, 1997.
30. GOLAN, R.; WEISSENBERG, R.; LEWIN, L.M. Carnitine and acetylcarnitine in motile and immotile human spermatozoa. International Journal of Andrology, v.7, p.484-494, 1984.
31. GONZAGA, I.V.F. Supplementation with rice bran oil semi-refined with high level of gamma-oryzanol in stallion´s diets. [Suplementação com óleo de farelo de arroz semi-refinado rico em gama-orizanol na dieta de garanhões]. 2008. 87f. Dissertação (Mestrado em Medicina Veterinária) - Faculdade de Medicina Veterinária e Zootecnia, Universidade de São Paulo, Pirassununga.

32. HOLT, A.J.; RODWAY, R.G.; FINDLAY, J.B.C. et al. Studies on β-carotene in bovine corpus luteum, Journal of Reproduction and Fertility, v.15, p.46-47, 1995 (abstr.

33. JEULIN, C.; LEWIN, L.M. Role of free l-carnitine and acetylcarnitine in postgonadal maturation of mammalian spermatozoa. Human Reproduction Update, v.2, p.87-102, 1996.

34. JONES, R.C.; MURDOCH, R.N. Regulation of the motility and metabolism of spermatozoa for storage in the epididymis of eutherian and marsupial mammals. Reproduction, Fertility and Development, v.8, p.553-568, 1996.

35. JULIANO, C.; COSSU, M.; ALAMANNI, M.C. et al. Antioxidant activity of gamma-oryzarol: mechanism of action and its effect on oxidative stability of pharmaceutical oil. International Journal of Pharmaceutics, v.299, p.146-154, 2005.

36. LADHA, S. Lipid heterogeneity and membrane fluidity in a highly polarized cell, the mammalian spermatozoon.Journal of Membrane Biology, v.165, p.1-10, 1998.

37. LANGLAIS, J.; ROBERTS, D. A molecular membrane model of capacitation and the acrosome reaction of mammalian spermatozoa. Gamete Research; v.12, p.183-224, 1985.

38. LEWIN, L.M.; PACE SHALEV, D.; WEISSENBERG, R. et al. Carnitine and acylcarnitines in semen from azoospermic patients. Fertility and Sterility, v.36, p.214-218, 1981.

39. LIMA, M.M. Influência da suplementação oral com L-carnitina na qualidade do sêmen criopreservado de garanhões. 2003. 61f. Dissertação (Mestrado em Medicina Veterinária) - Faculdade de Ciências Agrárias e Veterinárias/ Universidade Estadual Paulista, Jaboticabal.

40. MAGISTRINI, M.; SEGUIN, F.; BEAU, P. et al. 1H nuclear magnetic resonance analysis of stallion genital tract fluids and seminal plasma: contribution of the accessory sex glands to the ejaculate. Biology of Reproduction, v.1, p.599-607, 1995a (monograph).

41. MAGISTRINI, M.; McDONNEL, S.M.; SEGUIN, F. et al. Analysis of sex gland markers in equine seminal plasma of in copula and ex copula-induced ejaculates: quantification by magnetic resonance spectroscopy. In: INTERNATIONAL WORKSHOP ON ERECTION AND EJACULATION IN HORSES AND MEN, 2., 1995, Mount Joy. Proceedings... Mount Joy: 1995b, p.35-37.

42. MAGISTRINI, M.; VIDAMENT, M.; CLEMENT, F. et al. Fertility prediction in stallions. Animal Reproduction Science, v.42, p.181-188, 1996.
43. MALDJIAN, A.; PENNY, P.C.; NOBLE, R.C. Docosohexaenoic acid-rich marine oils and improved reproductive efficiency in pigs. In: De VRIESE, S.R.; CHRISTOPHE, A.B. (Eds.) Male fertility and lipid metabolism. Champaign: AOCS Press; 2003. p.60-72.
44. MENCHINI-FABRIS, G.F.; CANALE, D.; IZZO, P.L. et al. Free l-carnitine in human semen: its variability in different andrologic pathologies. Fertility and Sterility, v.42, p.263-267, 1984.
45. MILKOWSKY, A.L.; BABCOCK, D.F.; LARDY, H.A. Activation of bovine epididymal sperm respiration by caffeine: its transient nature and relationship to utilization of acetylcarnitine. Archives of Biochemistry and Biophysics, v.176, p.250-255, 1976.
46. MORAES, F.P.; COLLA, L.M. Alimentos funcionais e nutracêuticos: definições, legislação e benefícios à saúde.Revista Eletrônica de Farmácia, v.3, n.2, p.109-122, 2006.
47. O›FALLON, J.V.; CHEW, B.P. The subcellular distribution of β-carotene in bovine corpus luteum. In: PROCEEDINGS OF THE SOCIETY FOR EXPERIMENTAL BIOLOGY AND MEDICINE, 177., 1984, New York. Proceedings... New York: Society for Experimental Biology and Medicine, 1984. p.406-411.
48. PARKS, J.E.; LYNCH, D.V. Lipid composition and thermotrophic phase behavior of boar, bull, stallion, and rooster sperm membranes. Cryobiology, v.29, p.255-266, 1992.
49. PENNY, P.C.; MALDJIAN, A.; NOBLE, R.C. An enhancement of boar fertility and reproductive performance. In: INTERNATIONAL CONGRESS ON ANIMAL REPRODUCTION, 14., 2000, Stockolm. Proceedings... Stockolm: Organization International Committee for Animal Recording, 2000. p.109.
50. PICKETT, B.W. Factors affecting sperm production and sperm output. In: McKINNON, A.O.; VOSS, J.L. (Eds.)Equine reproduction. Philadelphia: Lea & Febiger, 1993. p.689-704.
51. RAPHAEL, C.F.; GOBESSO, A.A.O.; ANDRADE, A.F.C. et al. Effects of dietary supplementation with gamma-oryzanol on seminal characteristics of stallions. Animal Reproduction, v.3, p.253, 2006.

52. RODE, L.M.; COULTER, G.H.; KASTELIC, J.P. et al. Seminal quality and sperm production in beef bulls with chronic dietary Vitamin A deficiency and subsequent re-alimentation. Theriogenology, v.43, n.7, p.1269-1277, 1995.

53. ROSAS FILHO, A.C.; SPERS, A.; MAZZA P.H.R. et al. Effects of l-carnitin in alimentation of stallions arabian horse on reproductive parameters. Revista Brasileira de Reprodução Animal, v.25, n.3, p.369-371, 2001.

54. SCAVARIELLO, E.M.; ARELLANO, D.B. γ-oryzanol: um importante componente del aceite de salvado de arroz.Archivos Latinoamericanos de Nutricion, v.48, p.7-12, 1988.

55. SCHMIDT, K. Der Einfuâ der Fütterung mit weissen und roten Möhren auf die spermaproduktion des Zuchtbullen. 1. Mitteilung: Quantitative Undersuchung des Spermas. Monatshefte fur Veterinarmedizin, v.8, p.47-51, 1953.

56. SETCHELL, B.P.; MADDOCKS, S.; BROOKS, D.E. Anatomy, vasculature, innervation, and fluids of the male reproductive tract. In: KNOBIL, E.; NEILL, J.D. (Eds.) The physiology of reproduction. New York: Raven Press, 1994, v.1. p.1063-1175.

57. STRADAIOLI, G.; SYLLA, L.; ZELLI, R. et al. Seminal carnitine and acetylcarnitine content and carnitine acetyltransferase activity in young Maremmano stallions. Animal Reproduction Science, v.64, n.3-4, p.233-245, 2000.

58. UZIEL, G.; GARAVAGLIA, B.; Di DONATO, S. Carnitine stimulation of pyruvate dehydrogenase complex (PDHC) in isolated human skeletal muscle mitochondria. Muscle & Nerve, v.11, p.720-724, 1988.

59. VALE FILHO, V.R. Aspectos genéticos da subfertilidade e infertilidade dos touros. In: SIMPÓSIO NACIONAL DE REPRODUÇÃO ANIMAL, 1., 1974, Belo Horizonte. Anais... Belo Horizonte: Colégio Brasileiro de Reprodução Animal, 1974. p.67-76.

60. XU. Z.; GODBER, J.S. Purification and identification of components of γ-oryzanol in rice bran oil. Journal of Agricultural and Food Chemistry, v.47, p.2724-2728, 1999.

61. WANG, H.Y.; BAXTER Jr., C.F.; SCHULZ, H. Regulation of fatty acid beta-oxidation in rat heart mitochondria.Archives of Biochemistry and Biophysics, v.289, p.274-280, 1991.

62. WANG, J.Y.; LARSON, L.L.; OWEN, F.G. Effect of β-carotene supplementation on reproductive performance of dairy heifers. Theriogenology, v.18, p.461-473, 1982.

63. WEISS, R.R.; KLUG, E.; AHLSWEDE, L. Características do sêmen de touros jovens alimentados com carência de β-caroteno. Revista Brasileira de Reprodução Animal, v.3, p.7-16, 1979.

64. YOUNG, F.M.; LUDERER, W.B.; RODGERS, R.J. The antioxidant β-carotene prevents covalent cross-linking between cholesterol side-chain cleavage cytochrome P450 and its electron donor, adrenodoxin, in bovine luteal cells.Molecular and Cellular Endocrinology, v.109, p.113-118, 1995.

65. ZÖPFGEN, A.; PRIEM, F.; SUDHOFF, F. et al. Relationship between semen quality and the seminal plasma components carnitine, alpha-glucosidase, fructose, citrate and granulocyte elastase in infertile men compared with a normal population. Human Reproduction, v.15, p.840-845, 2000.

Chapter 6

Fertility of Frozen-Thawed Stallion Semen Cannot be predicted by the Currently Used Laboratory Methods

P Kuisma[1], M Andersson[1], E Koskinen[2], and T Katila[1]

of Clinical Veterinary Sciences, University of Helsinki, 04920 Saarentaus, Finland

[2]Department of Animal Sciences, University of Helsinki, PL 28, 00014 Helsingin yliopisto, Finland

ABSTRACT

The aim of the project was to use current simple and practical laboratory tests and compare results with the foaling rates of mares inseminated with commercially produced frozen semen. In Exp. 1, semen was tested from 27 and in Exp. 2 from 23 stallions; 19 stallions participated in both experiments. The mean number of mares per stallion in both experiments was 37 (min. 7, max. 121). Sperm morphology was assessed and bacterial culture performed once per stallion. In Exp. 1, progressive motility after 0, 1, 2, 3, and 4 h of incubation using light microscopy, motility characteristics measured with an automatic sperm analyzer, plasma membrane integrity using carboxyfluorescein diacetate/propidium iodide (CFDA/PI) staining and light microscopy, plasma membrane integrity using PI staining and a fluorometer, plasma membrane integrity using a resazurin reduction test, and sperm concentration were evaluated. In Exp. 2, the same tests as in Exp. 1 and a hypo-osmotic swelling test (HOST) using both light microscopy and a fluorometer were performed immediately after thawing and after a 3-h incubation. Statistical analysis was done separately to all stallions and to those having ≥ 20 mares; in addition, stallions with foaling rates < 60 or $\geq 60\%$ were compared. In Exp. 1, progressive motility for all stallions after a 2 – 4-h incubation correlated with the foaling rate (correlation coefficients 0.39 – 0.51), ($p < 0.05$). In stallions with > 20 mares, the artificial insemination dose showed a correlation coefficient of -0.58 ($p < 0.05$). In Exp. 2, the HOST immediately after thawing showed a negative correlation with foaling rate ($p < 0.05$). No single test was consistently reliable for predicting the fertilizing capacity of semen, since the 2 experiments yielded conflicting results, although the same stallions sometimes participated in both. This shows the difficulty of frozen semen quality control in commercially produced stallion semen, and on the other hand, the difficulty of conducting fertility trials in horses.

BACKGROUND

In many countries, artificial insemination (AI) has superseded natural mating as a breeding method for mares. Use of frozen semen, however, has not gained widespread use in horses, due to low pregnancy rates. In addition to semen quality, many other factors affect the outcome of AI, including the handling and freezing methods of semen, AI dose, timing of AI and management and fertility of the mares. There is considerable variation between individual stallions in how their semen survives freezing and thawing. Otherwise fertile stallions can produce semen that results in very poor post-thaw pregnancy rates. *Tischner* estimated that approx. 20% of stallions are "good freezers", another 20% are "bad freezers", and the majority of stallions, 60%, produce semen that is affected adversely, but may be freezable using certain techniques. Unlike bulls, stallions are not selected for breeding on the basis of fertility or semen freezability. Therefore, not much progress is to be expected in the use of frozen stallion semen. For prediction of fertility and for improving freezing methods, it is important to develop reliable techniques to assess the quality of semen *in vitro*. Many methods exist and are used, but not many studies have examined or showed the connection between laboratory test results and fertility of frozen-thawed stallion semen [4], [5]. The relationship between motility, the most frequently used test in horses, and fertility is far from clear [6], [7] and particularly for frozen semen it is not an exact measure of fertilizing potential [8]. In *Malmgren*'s review [9], conflicting correlations were reported between morphology – another commonly used test – and fertility of fresh stallion semen. It is often assumed that the condition of spermatozoa surviving after cryopreservation would be similar to the pre-freeze state. There is evidence that also the survivors have been affected [10]. Therefore, assessment and methods of examination applied for fresh semen may not be as useful for frozen semen.

Amann [11] stated that establishing a correlation between different attributes of semen and fertility is not sufficient. The goal is to develop laboratory tests that are predictive of fertility, which is not an easy task to achieve, particularly in horses. To determine if a laboratory test is correlated with fertility, one must have specific, precise, and accurate laboratory tests and precise and accurate fertility data from an adequate number of females. Tests of several independent parameters should be made [11-13,7]. *Graham* [14] listed several attributes that a sperm must possess to fertilize an oocyte, including motility, normal morphology, sufficient metabolism for energy production, and membrane integrity. Measurement of only a single attribute will fail to detect sperm defective in a different attribute and will overestimate the number of fertile sperm in the sample.

Obtaining good fertility data is difficult in horses. The number of mares and stallions used is too small, too few mares are inseminated at the appropriate time using adequate AI doses, too few semen samples are evaluated in an appropriate manner from each male, and the fertility data of mares is inaccurate [11].

Sperm membranes are particularly vulnerable during freezing [10]. This suggests that tests evaluating sperm membrane integrity should be used in the evaluation of frozen semen. On the other hand, spermatozoa that have survived freezing and thawing may be a selected subpopulation, which has unusually stable membranes. These membranes may also be unresponsive to physiological stimuli. If this is the case, then cryopreservation process may select viable, but relatively infertile sperm [10]. Membranes of cryopreserved spermatozoa are less able to withstand osmotic stress than fresh spermatozoa [15]. Velocity (curvilinear and mean path velocities) and linearity of cryopreserved spermatozoa are generally reduced [10]. A commonly used selection criterion in commercial stallion semen production is post-thaw progressive motility of ≥ 30–35%.

The aim of the present study was to use economically feasible and simple laboratory tests and correlate them with the foaling rates of mares. The pregnancy rates per cycle would have better reflected fertility [16], but they were not available from all mares. The aim of the study was also to analyze the overall quality of commercially produced semen doses.

MATERIALS AND METHODS

Results of frozen semen evaluation tests and foaling rates of mares were compared in 2 experiments. In the first experiment, semen of 27 stallions was tested and in the second experiment semen of 23 stallions; 19 stallions participated in both experiments. Only stallions having foaling data from at least 7 mares were included; the data were also analyzed separately for stallions having ≥ 20 mares.

Frozen Semen

First Experiment

Semen straws, frozen between 1988 and 1997, were available from 27 commercial stallions from Sweden (22), Finland (2), Italy (2), and the USA (1). Twelve of the stallions were American Standardbreds and 15 others represented various breeds of riding horses. Semen from one stallion was frozen in 5-mL straws, from 22 in 2.5-mL straws and from 4 stallions in 0.5-mL straws. The foaling data originated from Finland and

Sweden from 1989 to 1998. The mean number of mares per stallion was 37 (min. 7, max. 121). The average foaling rate was 56% (min. 0, max. 86%). Twelve stallions had foaling rates > 60% and 15 had foaling rates < 60%.

Second Experiment

Semen straws, frozen between 1988 and 1998, were available from 23 commercial stallions from Sweden (18), Finland (3), Italy (1) and Germany (1). Semen from 18 stallions was frozen in 2.5-mL straws and 5 in 0.5-mL straws. Seven stallions were American Standardbreds and 16 were various breeds of riding horses. The foaling data originated from Finland and Sweden from 1989 to 1999. The average number of mares per stallion was 37 (min. 7, max. 121). The mean foaling rate was 60% (min. 11%, max. 86%). Fourteen stallions had foaling rates of > 60% and nine < 60%.

Experiments

In the first experiment, the semen evaluations were performed once immediately after thawing, but motility assessment using light microscopy was continued for 4 h. Since the incubation appeared to differentiate sperm more readily than examination immediately after thawing, all tests were carried out 0 and 3 h after thawing in the second experiment. Bacterial culture was performed only in the first experiment and the hypo-osmotic swelling test (HOST) only in the second experiment. The HOST was included in the evaluation tools due to promising results in stallions [17,18]. The morphology was assessed from frozen-thawed spermatozoa once per stallion.

Thawing and Incubation

The 0.5-mL straws were thawed at 37°C for 30 sec, the 2.5-mL straws at 50°C for 40 and the 5-mL straws for 45 sec. The semen concentration was measured in a Bürker counting chamber, and the total number of spermatozoa per straw calculated. An insemination dose was one straw when the 2.5- or 5-mL straws were used and from 1 to 10 straws for the 0.5-mL straws. The semen was extended with a warm (+30°C) skim milk extender [19] to a concentration of 20–30 × 10^6spermatozoa/mL.

The sample for the longevity test was prepared by placing 0.5 mL of extended semen into a 3-mL vial enclosed with a cap. The sample was kept in a water bath at 37°C for 4 h (Exp. 1) or 3 h (Exp. 2). The total and progressive motility and velocity were evaluated by light microscope every hour (Exp. 1) or after 3 h (Exp. 2).

Motility

The post-thaw motility was evaluated with a light microscope for the percentage of progressively motile spermatozoa, total motility percentage and a velocity score (from 1 to 3). Motility parameters were measured with an automatic sperm analyzer (Hamilton Thorn Motility Analyzer, HTM-S, version 7.2, Hamilton Thorne Research, Beverly, MA, USA) using videotaping [20]. A 7-µL semen sample was placed into a Makler chamber at a temperature of 37.1°C; 2 chambers were prepared from the same sample. The chamber was placed on the thermostatically controlled stage of the motility analyzer and video recordings made as described by *Varner et al.* [20]. When the videotapes were analyzed the analyzer settings were: frames at frame rate 20 – 25/sec, minimum contrast 8, minimum size 6, low/high size gates 0.6 – 1.5, low/high intensity gates 0.6 – 1.5, motile head size 16, non- motile intensity 371, medium VAP (average path velocity) value 30, low VAP value 10, slow cells not motile, and threshold straightness 60. The videotapes were analyzed for the level of total (TMOT) and progressive motility (PROG), VAP and percentage of rapid sperm (RAP).

Plasma Membrane Integrity

Plasma membrane integrity was evaluated after thawing, using 3 methods in Exp. 1 and 5 methods in Exp. 2: 1) carboxyfluorescein diacetate/propidium iodide (CFDA/PI) staining and counting of cells with a fluorescence microscope, 2) PI staining and measurement with a fluorometer (Fluoroscan Ascent, Thermo Electron Inc., Milford, MA, USA), 3) resazurin reduction test with a fluorometer, 4) HOST and counting cells with a microscope (only in Exp. 2) and 5) HOST using a fluorometer (only in Exp. 2). In Exp. 1, the tests were performed once immediately after thawing, while in Exp. 2 they were repeated after a 3-h incubation.

For evaluation of plasma membrane integrity with CFDA/PI staining, the semen was extended with a skim milk extender [19] to a concentration of 50 × 10^6 spermatozoa/mL. Aliquots of 20 μL of CFDA stock solution consisting of 0.46 mg CFDA in 1 mL of DMSO (dimethylsulpfoxide) and 10 μl of PI stock solution (0.5 mg PI in 1 mL of 0.9% NaCl solution) were taken, mixed with 950 μl of semen, and incubated for 8 min at 30°C [21]. A 5-μL drop was placed on a slide and overlaid with a cover slip. The proportion of fluorescent cells was counted from 200 cells in a fluorescence microscope (Olympus BH2 with epifluorescence optics, Olympus Optical Co., Tokyo, Japan) using oil immersion and a fluorescein filter set.

The second plasma membrane viability test was performed using an automatic fluorometer (Fluoroscan Ascent, Thermo Electron Inc., Milford, MA, USA), which reads a 96-well microtitration tray and has an incubation compartment. The interference filter at the excitation path and that of the emission filter showed maximum transmission at 544 nm and 590 nm, respectively. For the fluorometric assay, 20 mg of PI was dissolved in 1 L of Beltsville Thawing Solution (BTS) (USDA, Beltsville, MD, USA) and dispensed in 3-mL aliquots. Equal aliquots (50 μL) of BTS diluted semen sample (80 × 10^6 spermatozoa/mL) and PI solution were dispensed into a well and shaken gently for 2 min. Spermatozoa from the same samples were killed by unprotected rapid freezing and slow thawing to obtain internal control samples consisting of only non- viable cells (100% fluorescence). The control sample was immersed in liquid nitrogen for 1 min and thereafter allowed to stand at room temperature for 30 sec and then 3 min in a water bath (37°C). Blanks containing 50 μl of diluted extender and 50 μl of PI were analyzed separately for every experiment in 4 replicates; the incubation time was 8 min. The percentage of fluorescence was calculated from the ratio of fluorescence intensities of the rapidly frozen control sample and the sample to be analyzed, after comparing with the blank values [22].

Resazurin Reduction Test

For the resazurin reduction test, 400 mg of resazurin was dissolved in 1 L of distilled water. One part of this solution and 9 parts of 0.9% NaCl were mixed [23]. An equal volume of this mixture and diluted sperm were combined and shaken for 2 min, then incubated for 30 min at

34°C and measured with the fluorometer, using the same fluorometer settings as in the plasma membrane viability test.

HOST

For the HOST, semen was extended to 4×10^6 spermatozoa/mL. The hypo-osmotic solution was prepared by dissolving 1.352 g fructose and 0.735 g Na-citrate to distilled water (150 mOsm, pH 7.2). An aliquot of 0.125 mL of sperm was added to 0.5 mL of solution and the mixture was incubated for 30–45 min at 37°C. A 5-μL drop was placed on a slide and overlaid with a cover slip. A total of 200 spermatozoa per sample were evaluated for the presence of bent tails in light microscopy [24] and also analyzed with an automatic fluorometer. For fluorometric determination of the HOST, 0.5 mL of the same hypo-osmotic solution (100 mOsmol/kg) were mixed with 0.125 mL of skim milk-extended semen (concentration 100×10^6 spermatozoa/mL). The fluorometric method was the same as for PI-stained semen. The mixture was incubated at 37°C and analyzed again after 3 h.

Morphology and Bacteriology

The frozen-thawed semen smears were air-dried and stained with Giemsa according to *Watson* [25]. A total of 100 spermatozoa were evaluated with light microscopy, magnification × 1250, for major abnormalities (underdevelopment, acrosomal granules, other major acrosomal defects, diadem effects, tails bent under the head, dag effects, mid piece defects, and proximal droplets) and minor abnormalities (bent tail, twisted tail, loose normal heads, large heads, loose acrosomes, and mild acrosomal abnormalities) according to *Blom* [26].

The bacterial culture was performed by spreading a drop of each sample onto half a blood agar plate, using a 10-μL sterile loop. After incubation for 24 and 48 h at 37°C, colony forming units (CFUs) were counted and bacterial species recognized. If more than 100 CFUs were detected per sample, the number was not calculated further.

Statistical Methods

Pearson and Spearm an correlation coefficients were used to study the association between the parameters. The results were accounted for, if both correlation coefficients were congruent. P-values < 0.05 were considered significant. The results were expressed as mean ± the standard error of the mean (s.e.m.). The stallions were divided into 2 groups: foaling rate of mares < 60% or > 60%. The independent sample t-test was used to test differences in the laboratory test parameters between the 2 groups of stallions. Statistical analysis was also performed separately from the material restricted to those stallions having > 20 mares (19 stallions in Exp. 1 and 16 in Exp. 2).

RESULTS

Experiment 1

The percentage of normal spermatozoa varied from 51% to 89%. Major abnormalities accounted for 9.5%, including head abnormalities in 4.1% (1–12%), tail bent under the head 2.5% (0–6%), and mid piece defects 2.4% (0–7%); minor abnormalities comprised 10.7% (3–31%) including mainly bent tails 6.9% (1–29%), normal loose heads 1.4% (0–7%), and loose acrosomes 2% (0–5%). There was no association between morphological findings and foaling rate.

A total of 52% of the samples showed no microbial growth, in 41% < 100 CFUs per plate were detected, and in 7% > 100 CFUs per plate. The microbes were mainly coagulase-negative staphylococci or belonged to the families Enterococcus, Enterobacteriaceae, or*Corynebacteriaceae*. There was no association between bacteriological findings and foaling rate.

Average CASA motility and s.e.m. were as follows: TMOT 37.0 ± 3.3, PROG 27.6 ± 2.7, and VAP 58.7 ± 2.0; these values did not correlate with fertility. Average progressive motility evaluated in light microscopy showed following changes during incubation: 0 h 40.2 ± 1.7 (min 10, max 60), 1 h 35.0 ± 1.4 (5, 50), 2 h 29.0 ± 1.6 (10, 40), 3 h 24.9 ± 1.7 (10–40), and 4 h 21.0 ± 1.7 (5–40). Progressive motility correlated significantly with foaling rate after 2–4 h of incubation (correlation coefficients 0.39 – 0.51; $p < 0.05$). Stallions (> 7 mares) with foaling rates of > 60% appeared to retain sperm motility slightly better than stallions with foaling rates of < 60%, although the difference was not statistically significant (Fig. 1). Similarly, semen resulting in foaling rates of > 60% showed higher plasma membrane integrity percentages measured with fluorometer than semen resulting in foaling rates of < 60%, but the differences were not statistically significant (Fig.2).

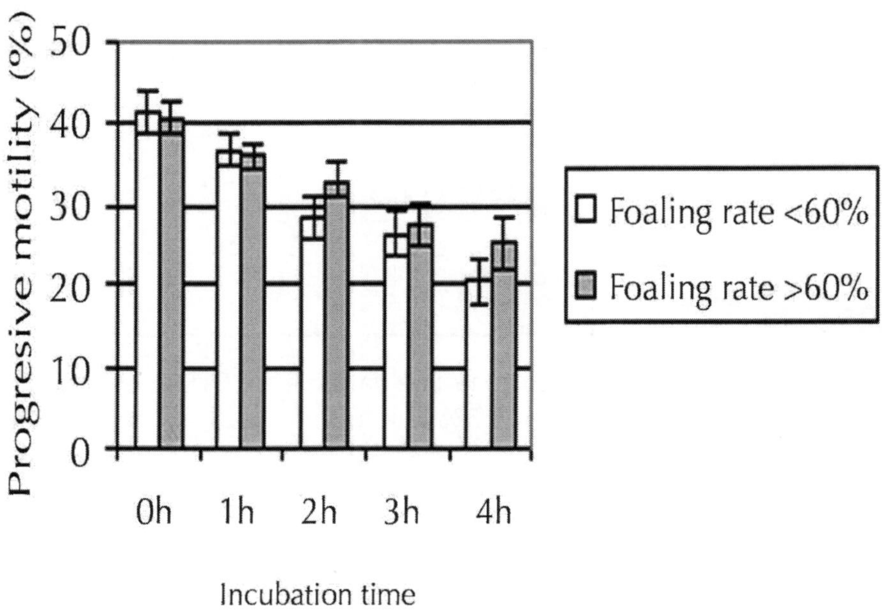

Figure 1: (Exp. 1) Mean (± s.e.m.) progressive motility in light microscopy during 4-h incubation in stallion groups with foaling rates of < 60% or > 60%. Number of mares per stallion was > 7.

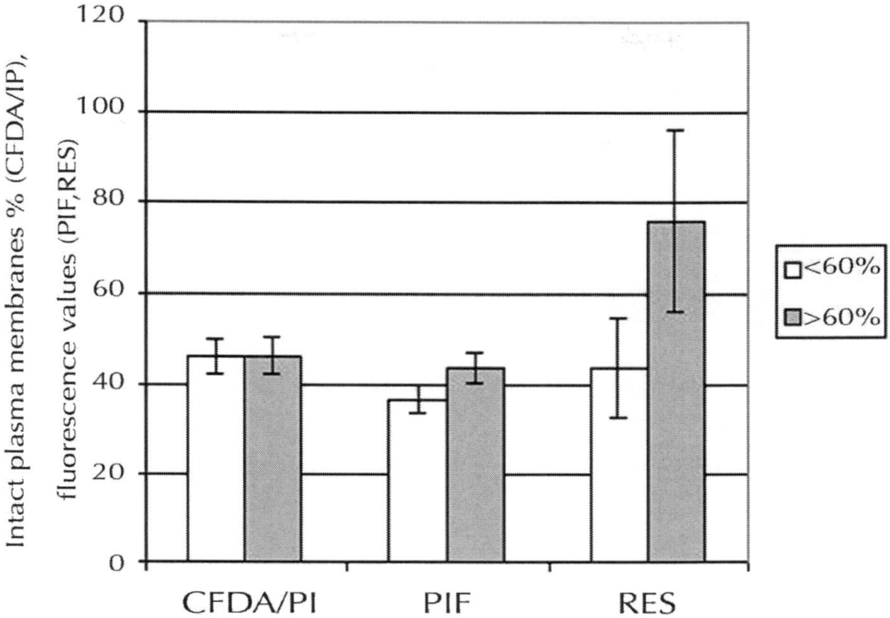

Figure 2: (Exp. 1) Mean (± s.e.m.) plasma membrane integrity parameters in stallion groups with foaling rates of < 60% or > 60%. Number of mares per stallion was > 7. CFDA/PI = plasma membrane integrity using light microscopy; PIF = plasma membrane integrity with PI staining using a fluorometer; RES = plasma membrane integrity with resazurin reduction test using a fluorometer.

Sperm concentration and the total number of sperm in an AI dose showed huge variation: the average concentration ± s.e.m. 383.2 ± 48.6, min 45, max 1593, and the average number of sperm/AI dose 713.2 ± 47.2, min 302, max 1777. When stallions having > 20 mares were analyzed, the total number of sperm in an AI dose showed a significant negative correlation of 0.58 with foaling rate ($p < 0.05$). The total number of sperm/AI dose and sperm concentration for stallion groups having foaling rates < 60% or > 60% are shown in Fig. 3, the difference being significant ($p < 0.05$). For all other parameters correlation coefficients with fertility were low and non-significant.

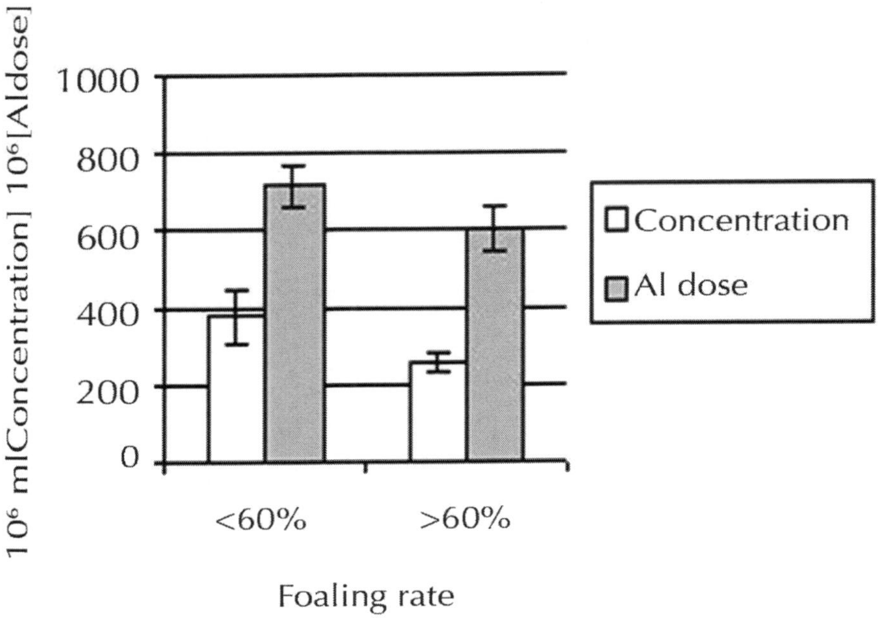

Figure 3: (Exp. 1) Mean (± s.e.m.) sperm concentration and total number of sperm in an AI dose in stallion groups with foaling rates of < 60% or > 60%. Number of mares per stallion was > 7.

When the various parameters were compared with each other, all motility parameters correlated significantly with each other (correlation coefficients varied from 0.44 to 0.81), similarly the plasma membrane integrity tests showed significant correlations between each other (0.37 – 0.83). CFDA/PI staining with light microscopy and with a fluorometer correlated significantly also with progressive motility before incubation. The total number of sperm/AI dose showed a significant negative correlation with the other parameters, except with progressive motility during incubation (3–4 h) and CFDA/PI with light microscopy.

Experiment 2

The average HOST-values were 30.1 ± 1.6 (18–49) before incubation and 21.7 ± 1.6 (9–46) after 3 h of incubation. A significant correlation coefficient of -0.50 with foaling rate ($p < 0.05$) was demonstrated before incubation. The average CFDA-values obtained in microscopy were 42.9 ± 2.4 (14–66) before incubation and 33.0 ± 1.8 (12–48) after the 3-h incubation. When stallions having > 20 mares were analyzed, CFDA/PI staining with light microscopy at 0-h incubation and HOST with fluorometer after a 3-h incubation showed correlation coefficients of 0.5 with foaling rate ($p > 0.05$). The HOST results in 2 stallion groups divided by their foaling rates are shown in Fig. 4. For other tests, correlation coefficients with foaling rate were low and non-significant. The TMOT and PROG values for stallions with foaling rates < 60% and > 60% are shown in Fig. 5.

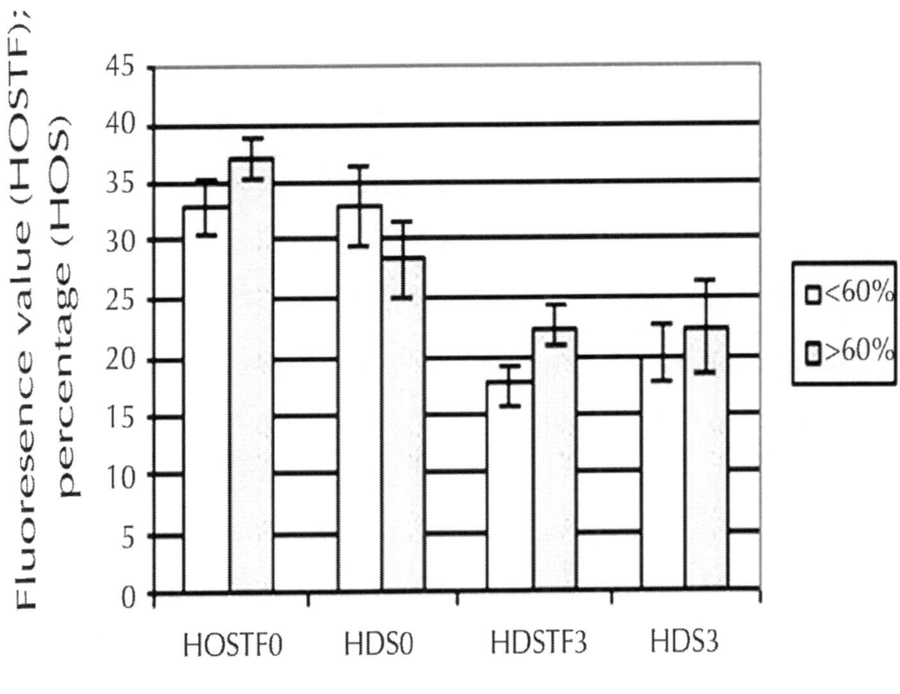

Figure 4: (Exp. 2) Mean (± s.e.m.) percentage of sperm positive for hypo-osmotic swelling test (HOST) in stallion groups with foaling rates of < 60% or > 60%. Number of mares per stallion was > 20. HOSTF0 = HOST with fluorometer after 0-h incubation; HOSTF3 = HOST with fluorometer after 3-h incubation; HOS0 = HOST with light microscopy after 0-h incubation; HOS3 = HOST with light microscopy after 3-h incubation.

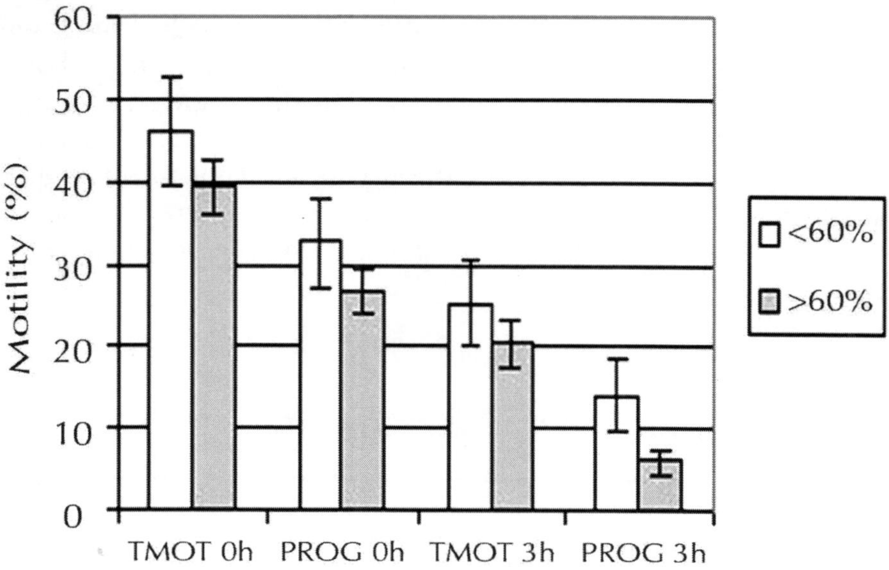

Figure 5. (Exp. 2) Mean (± s.e.m.) total (TMOT) and progressive motility (PROG) immediately after thawing and after 3-h incubation in stallion groups with foaling rates of < 60% or > 60%. Number of mares per stallion was > 7.

When the various parameters were compared, TMOT, PROG, VAP, and RAP correlated after the 0-h and 3-h incubations, correlation coefficients ranging from 0.5 to 0.8. CFDA, HOST and resazurin both by microscopy and fluorometer correlated after the 0-h and 3-h incubations with coefficients of 0.4 – 0.8, but no correlation was demonstrated between these parameters and parameters depicting motility. Before incubation, the concentration showed a significant negative correlation with CFDA/PI staining, using both light microscopy and the fluorometer, but this correlation disappeared after the 3-h incubation.

DISCUSSION

No single test was found to be a consistently reliable method for predicting the fertilizing capacity of semen. The results of Exp. 1 could not be repeated, although the stallions and methods used were partly similar. Differences in the outcome of these experiments could be explained also by different ejaculate batches.

Plasma Membrane Integrity Tests

Some tendency for the plasma membrane integrity tests to be indicators of higher foaling rates was noted in our study. Fluorometers have not been much used in the examination of stallion semen. Although no strong correlation with foaling rate was found, the various fluorometric measurements did correlate with plasma membrane integrity in light microscopy and with each other. The use of fluorometers has some advantages in comparison to the use of light microscopy: it requires less time, and more cells in the sample are assessed [14]. In boars [27] and bulls [28], fluorometric measurements significantly correlated with fertility parameters.

Neild et al. [29] found no significant connection between the HOST and fertility but a tendency for the HOST to correlate with the number or services per pregnancy. We detected both negative and positive correlations, suggesting that this test is not suitable for evaluation of frozen-thawed stallion semen.*Nie et al.* [30] reported lower pregnancy rates for HOS+ group. *Blach et al.* [12] found indirect evidence that many immotile spermatozoa possessed an intact plasma membrane, which would indicate that these two parameters do not correlate with each other. In our first experiment, plasma membrane integrity with light microscopy correlated with many other parameters, including motility. This is in disagreement with the study of *Samper* [13] who noted membrane integrity to show extremely poor correlation with motility, particularly in preserved semen. Likewise, in our second experiment correlation between motility and plasma membrane integrity was not observed.

Motility

Motility correlated with fertility in our first experiment but not in the second. One explanation can be pre-selection of semen. Most laboratories use 30% as a cut-off value when accepting semen for sale. The most important task of semen tests is to exclude semen of inferior quality, and this had already been done in the laboratories which had exported the semen. Another explanation is the use of different batches from several ejaculates from each stallion, but still the question on the accuracy of motility evaluation as a means of predicting fertility is raised. Semen from a stallion with the highest progressive motility (60%) did not produce any pregnancies in 10 inseminated mares. Motility has been claimed by other investigators to be a poor predictor of pregnancy rates [6, 31]. However, *Voss* and his coworkers [6] suggested that although the relationship between motility and fertility is poor in the stallion, spermatozoal motility and the quality of motility are still the most reliable estimates of fertility in practice. On the other hand, *Jasko et al.* [32] reported significant correlations between motility parameters and fertility.*Newcombe* [33] reported that pregnancies per insemination decreased when semen with low motility was used. VAP is not reliable or repeatable according to *Kirk et al.* [34]. The motility results immediately after thawing do not necessarily predict the results after incubation, as was seen with progressive motility in our first experiment. Longevity tests may therefore be useful in assessing viability of semen, although*Voss et al.* [6] suggested that longevity may be of limited value in predicting potential fertility. Despite these inconsistencies between studies, motility continues to have value as an easy and economical way for estimating relative cell health.

Sperm Numbers and Concentration

The total number of sperm/AI dose and concentration correlated negatively with many parameters. This can be explained by the tendency to increase AI dose and thus the concentration – the volume of one straw is limited – when low post-thaw motility is detected to increase the number of progressively motile spermatozoa and consequently the possibility of pregnancy [35]. This practice is only effective to a certain point; *Amann* [11] presented a dose-response curve showing that fertility ceases to improve as the critical number of spermatozoa needed for maximum fertility of a given male has been reached. High doses and concentration may even decrease fertility. High sperm numbers and concentration provoked more intense inflammatory responses in the uterus [36,37]. Spermatozoa at higher AI doses arrived in the oviducts later than spermatozoa contained in smaller doses [37]. Fertility dropped when the AI dose contained > 900×10^6 frozen sperm [35].

Morphology

In our study, the percentage of morphologically normal semen and foaling rates did not correlate, perhaps because semen with a high percentage of morphological abnormalities is not frozen. *Jasko et al.* [38, 32] showed the percentage of normal sperm to have a positive correlation with fertility. However, *Voss et al.* (1981) noted considerable variation in the morphologic characteristics among stallions and among ejaculates within stallions. They suggested that spermatozoal morphology may not be as valuable in evaluation of potential fertility in the stallion as it is in other large domestic animals.

Problems of Fertility Studies in Horses

Problems confronted in previous fertility studies are also obvious here. The number of mares inseminated per stallion was small, the straws were not from the same batch, foaling rates were collected during several years – fertility of stallions can vary between years and decrease with age. Insemination conditions, veterinary skills, management of stud farms, criteria for mare selection, etc. vary considerably. Many other factors in addition to semen characteristics influence fertility. Although obtaining pregnancy rates is difficult, they are more accurate and reliable than foaling rates. However, this does not eliminate other factors affecting fertility, such as management and reproductive performance of mares, their previous reproductive status, and possible genetic factors [32]. A multi-center study by *Samper et al.* [35] summarized the major factors affecting pregnancy rates of mares bred with frozen semen: the technician, mare age and status, insemination volume, timing of insemination, and number of sperm per dose. Standardizing all these variables is clearly not possible.

Development of freezing methods for stallion semen is dependant on finding dependable correlations between laboratory tests and fertility, which appears very difficult to achieve since the results of different studies in this field tend to be contradictive. The present study was unable to address the question of which laboratory tests would accurately predict fertility of commercially produced stallion semen. Objectivity, repeatability, and accuracy are basic requirements for laboratory assays, but many semen analysis tests do not meet these requirements [7]. Quality control of cryopreserved stallion semen remains to be a problem in practice where e.g. flow cytometry is not available. For practical purposes, it would be most important to identify semen samples that are likely to have poor fertilizing potential [4]. *Nie et al.* [30] concluded that evaluating fresh spermatozoa offered no advantage for pregnancy over simply inseminating with spermatozoa not selected for any particular characteristics.

The constraints in horse breeding – small numbers of mares per ejaculate and per stallion and the tremendous variations in mare management and insemination – never allow us to carry out trials similar to what the cattle industry has done in developing freezing methods and AI techniques. Fertility trials of horses are bound to be of little value because of these reasons [16].

REFERENCES

1. Colenbrander B, Gadella BM, Stout TAE: The predictive value of semen analysis in the evaluation of stallion fertility.*Reprod Dom Anim* 2003, 38:305-311.
2. Boyle MS: Artificial insemination: assessing stallion semen quality after freezing. *Equine Vet J* 1996, 28:5-6.
3. Tischner M: Evaluation of deep-frozen semen in stallions. *J Reprod Fertil* 1979, (Suppl. 27):58-59.
4. Graham JK: Assessment of sperm quality: a flow cytometric approach. *Anim Reprod Sci* 2001, 68:239-247.
5. Katila T: In vitro evaluation of frozen-thawed stallion semen: A review. *Acta vet Scand* 2001, 42:201-217.
6. Voss JL, Pickett BW, Squires EL: Stallion spermatozoal morphology and motility and their relationship to fertility. *J Am Vet Med Assoc* 1981, 178:287-289.
7. Rodriguez-Martinez H: Laboratory semen assessment and prediction of fertility: still utopia? *Reprod Dom Anim* 2003, 38:312-318.
8. Bataille B, Magistrini M, Palmer E: Analyse objective de la mobilite du sperme congele-decongele d'etalon. Essai de correlation avec la fertilite. (Objective determination of sperm motility in frozen-thawed stallion semen. Correlation with fertility). *Anim Breed Abstr* 1990, 96-106.

9. Malmgren L: Sperm morphology in stallions in relation to fertility. *Acta vet Scand* 1992, 88:39-47.
10. Watson PF: Recent developments and concepts in the cryopreservation of spermatozoa and the assessment of their post-thawing function. *Reprod Fertil Dev* 1995, 7:871-891.
11. Amann RP: Can the fertility potential of a seminal sample be predicted accurately? *J Andrology* 1989, 10:89-98.
12. Blach EL, Amann RP, Bowen RA, Frantz D: Changes in quality of stallion spermatozoa during cryopreservation: plasma membrane integrity and motion characteristics. *Theriogenology* 1989, 31:283-298.
13. Samper JC: Evaluation of cryopreserved semen: An alternative assay. *Acta vet Scand* 1992, 88:59-65.
14. Graham JK: Analysis of stallion semen and its relation to fertility. *Vet Clin North Am Equine Pract* 1996, 12:119-129.
15. Schweisguth DC, Hammerstedt RH: Evaluation of plasma membrane stability by detergent-induced rupture of osmotically swollen sperm. *J Biochem Biophys Methods* 1992, 24:81-94.
16. Amann RP: Weaknesses in reports of "fertility" for horses and other species. *Theriogenology* 2005, 63:698-715.
17. De Albuquerque Lagares M: Bestimmung der osmotischen Resistenz von Hengstsamenzellen (The determination of the osmotic resistance of stallion spermatozoa). *Thesis Hannover* 1995.
18. Vidament M, Dupere AM, Julienne P, Evain A, Noue P, Palmer E: Equine frozen semen freezability and fertility field results. *Theriogenology* 1997, 48:907-917.
19. Kenney RM, Bergman RV, Cooper WL, Morse GW: Minimal contamination techniques for breeding mares: Techniques and preliminary findings. *Proc Am Ass Equine Practnrs* 1975, 21:327-336.
20. Varner DD, Scott DV, Johnson L: Use of a computerized system for evaluation of equine spermatozoal motility. *Am J Vet Res* 1991, 52:224-230.
21. Harrison RAP, Vickers SE: Use of fluorescent probes to assess membrane integrity of mammalian spermatozoa. *J Reprod Fertil* 1990, 88:343-352.

22. Alm K, Taponen J, Dahlbom M, Tuunainen E, Koskinen E, Andersson M: A novel automatized fluorometric assay to evaluate sperm viability and fertility in dairy bulls. *Theriogenology* 2001, 56:677-684.
23. Dart MG, Mesta J, Crenshaw C, Ericsson SA: Modified resazurin reduction test for determining the fertility potential of bovine spermatozoa. *Arch Andr* 1994, 33:71 75.
24. Jeyendran RS, Van der Ven HH, Perez-Pelaez M, Crabo BG, Zaneveld LJ: Development of an assay to assess the functional integrity of the human sperm membrane and its relationship to other semen characteristics. *J Reprod Fertil* 1984, 70:219-28.
25. Watson PF: Use of Giemsa stains to detect changes in acrosomes of frozen ram spermatozoa. *Vet Rec* 1975, 97:12-13.
26. Blom E: Sygelige tilstande i konsorganen og sperma som kassationsårsag ved import og eksport af avlstyre til og fra Danmark. (Pathological conditions in genital organs and sperm as a cause for the rejection of breeding bulls for import to and export from Denmark). *Nord Vet Med* 1983, 35:105-30.
27. Juonala T, Salonen E, Nurttila T, Andersson M: Three fluorescence methods for assessing boar sperm viability. *Reprod Dom Anim* 1999, 34:83-87.
28. Januskauskas A, Johannisson A, Rodriguez-Martinez H: Assessment of sperm quality through fluorometry and sperm chromatin structure assay in relation to field fertility of frozen-thawed semen from Swedish AI bulls. *Theriogenology* 2001, 55:947-961.
29. Neild DM, Chaves MG, Flores M, Miragaya MH, Gonzalez E, Aquero A: The HOS test and its relationship to fertility in the stallion. *Andrologia* 2000, 32:351-315.
30. Nie GJ, Wenzel JGW, Johnson KE: Comparison of pregnancy outcome in mares among methods used to evaluate and select spermatozoa for insemination. *Anim Reprod Sci* 2002, 69:211-222.
31. Squires EL, Amann RP, Pickett BW: Preservation of stallion semen – Colorado experience. *Symp Equine Reprod Denmark* 1987, 49-54.

32. Jasko DJ, Little TV, Lein DH, Foote RH: Comparison of spermatozoal movement and semen characteristics with fertility in stallions: 64 cases (1987–1988). *J Am Vet Med Assoc* 1992, 200:979-985.
33. Newcombe JR: Evaluation of the fertilising capacity of frozen-thawed horse semen. *Vet Rec* 1999, 145:46-47.
34. Kirk ES, Graham JK, Bruemmer JE, Squires EL: Evaluating frozen equine semen by flow cytometry. *Anim Reprod Sci* 2001, 68:348-349.
35. Samper JC, Vidament M, Katila T, Newcombe J, Estrada A, Sargeant J: Analysis of some factors associated with pregnancy rates of frozen semen: a multi-center study. *Theriogenology* 2002, 58:647-650.
36. Kotilainen T, Huhtinen M, Katila T: Sperm-induced leukocytosis in the equine uterus. *Theriogenology* 1994, 41:629-636.
37. Fiala SM, Pimentel CA, Mattos ALG, Amaral MG, Jobim MIM, Gregory RM, Mattos RC: Sperm transport and uterine inflammatory response after insemination in the mare. *15th Int Congr Anim Reprod Porto Seguro Brazil Abstracts* 2004, 2:388.
38. Jasko DJ, Lein DH, Foote RH: Determination of the relationship between sperm morphologic classifications and fertility in stallions: 66 cases (1987–1988). *J Am Vet Med Assoc* 1990, 197:389-394.

Chapter 7

Expression and Regulation of Facilitative Glucose Transporters in Equine Insulin-Sensitive Tissue: From Physiology to Pathology

Véronique A. Lacombe

Department of Physiology Sciences, Center of Veterinary Health Sciences, Oklahoma State University, Stillwater, OK 74078, USA

ABSTRACT

Glucose uptake is the rate-limiting step in glucose utilization in mammalians and is tightly regulated by a family of specialized proteins, called the facilitated glucose transporters (GLUTs/SLC2). GLUT4, the major isoform in insulin-responsive tissue, translocates from an intracellular pool to the cell surface and as such determines insulin-stimulated glucose uptake. However, despite intensive research over 50 years, the insulin-dependent and -independent pathways that mediate GLUT4 translocation are not fully elucidated in any species. Insulin resistance (IR) is one of the hallmarks of equine metabolic syndrome and is the most common metabolic predisposition for laminitis in horses. IR is characterized by the impaired ability of insulin to stimulate glucose disposal into insulin-sensitive tissues. Similar to other species, the functional capability of the insulin-responsive GLUTs is impaired in muscle and adipose tissue during IR in horses. However, the molecular mechanisms of altered glucose transport remain elusive in all species, and there is still much to learn about the physiological and pathophysiological functions of the GLUT family members, especially in regard to class III. Since GLUTs are key regulators of whole-body glucose homeostasis, they have received considerable attention as potential therapeutic targets to treat metabolic disorders in human and equine patients.

REGULATION OF GLUCOSE TRANSPORT IN HEALTHY STATE

Glucose is of the most abundant and essential energy sources for both plants and animals, existing in various polymerized forms such as cellulose and glycogen [1]. Glucose uptake from the bloodstream into the cell is the rate-limiting step in glucose utilization primarily in insulin-sensitive tissue in all species. Striated (i.e., cardiac and skeletal) muscle is the main tissue to utilize glucose as an energy substrate, followed by adipose tissue. For instance, skeletal muscle, which makes up ~40% of the body mass in mammalian species, is the primary tissue responsible for the peripheral disposal of glucose, especially during exercise [2]. In addition, the energetic demands in the heart are extreme and as a result, the heart has the highest rate of oxygen consumption per gram of any tissue in the body [3]. In order to sustain this high energy demand, the rate of glucose utilization in the heart is greater than in skeletal muscle, adipose tissue, and lung, despite the ability of the myocardium to use other substrates (i.e., fatty acids, lactate, ketone bodies, and amino acids) [4]. Therefore, glucose transport and utilization by myocytes are critical for the maintenance of muscle function [5]. In addition, glucose absorbed from the gut stimulates the release of insulin from pancreatic β-cells, which both suppresses hepatic gluconeogenesis and promotes glucose uptake by muscle and adipose tissue [6]. Finally, glucose can regulate gene transcription, epigenetic processes, and enzyme activity, as well as glucose-sensitive neurons in the brain [1].

In all mammalian cells, blood glucose is maintained within a narrow range by homeostatic mechanisms. Since the lipid bilayers of cell membranes are impermeable to glucose, most cells take up glucose by a passive facilitative transport process, which is mediated by a family of integral membrane proteins collectively known as the glucose transporters (GLUTs) [7]. It is believed that only the epithelial cell brush border of the small intestine and the kidney proximal convoluted tubules absorb glucose by an active mechanism that uses Na^+/glucose cotransporters to transport glucose against its electrochemical gradient [8]. The equine intestinal Na^+/glucose cotransporter, SGLT1, has 85–89% homology at the nucleotide level and 84–87% at the amino acid level with SGLT1 of other species [9]. Similarly to other herbivorous and omnivorous species, there is an enhancement in the expression of the intestinal Na^+/glucose cotransporter, SGLT1, and the capacity to absorb monosaccharides in response to increased dietary carbohydrate levels in horses [10].

This paper reviews the current knowledge on the physiological and pathophysiological functions of the GLUT/SLC2 family member, as they relate to the equine species focusing on insulin-responsive tissue (e.g., striated muscle and adipose tissue).

Function and Distribution of the Facilitative Glucose Transporters

The GLUT protein family are encoded by the SLC2 genes and are a member of the major facilitator superfamily of membrane transporters, which are ubiquitous proteins with >5,000 members identified in all three kingdoms [1, 11]. Since at least one GLUT isoform is present in every cell type of the body, GLUTs are widely recognized as key regulators of whole-body glucose homeostasis. The GLUT proteins, which are comprised of ~500 amino acid residues, have 12 membrane-spanning domains, an N-linked glycosylation site, and intracellular NH_2 and COOH termini, as well as several conserved residues and motifs designated "sugar transporter signatures" [7, 12]. These facilitative GLUT proteins are expressed in a tissue-specific manner, with distinct regulatory and/or kinetic properties that reflect their specific roles in cellular and whole-body glucose homeostasis [1]. Currently, fourteen GLUT isoforms have been identified and divided into 3 different classes based on sequence similarity, as well as structural and functional characteristics: Class I (GLUTs 1–4, 14); Class II (GLUTs 5, 7, 9, and 11), and Class III (GLUTs 6, 8, 10, and 12 and HMIT). Although the major substrate(s) for several isoforms has not been identified, these facilitated transporters are capable of transporting glucose, fructose, myoinositol, and urate across the plasma membrane down-gradient. Tissue distribution and major function(s) are listed in Table 1. Since several reviews on the GLUT family have been published [1, 6–8, 13], this paper briefly summarizes key features of the major GLUTs, as they relate to the equine species. The function and distribution of two members of class I, GLUT-1 and -4, have been extensively studied [1, 14, 15]. GLUT1 is primarily located at the cell surface and thus is a basal transporter that does not require insulin stimulation for its activation. Therefore, GLUT1 is considered to be the primary transporter responsible for basal glucose uptake in many cell types. GLUT1 has a high expression in brain and erythrocytes [16], and as a consequence, ~1/3 of blood glucose is carried within the red blood cell cytoplasm [7]. Interestingly, GLUT1 is also highly abundant in the digital lamellae, indicating that this unique weight-bearing, dermoepidermal structure within the horse's hoof is a highly metabolic tissue [17, 18]. Similarly, articular chondrocytes, which express both GLUT-1 and -3, rely on glucose as the major energy substrate and as the main precursor for the synthesis of extracellular matrix glycosaminoglycans in cartilage [19, 20]. The equine small intestine is the major site of glucose absorption, with glucose transport being the highest in the duodenum, followed by the jejunum and ileum [9]. Glucose is transported across the brush-border membrane of the intestinal enterocytes by SGLT1 and then exits the cell across the basolateral membrane by the facilitated GLUT2, a low-affinity glucose and fructose transporter [10, 21]. Equine small intestine also expresses GLUT5, a fructose transporter, in the villus enterocytes with the highest levels in the duodenum and the lowest levels in the ileum [22].

Table 1: Summary of the main location and function of facilitative glucose transporter family [7, 8, 156]

Protein	Major sites of expression	Proposed function/major substrate	Major species studied
GLUT1	Many cell types (e.g., erythrocytes, brain); fetal tissues	Basal glucose uptake; transport across blood-tissue barriers	Rodents, humans, horses, cows, dogs, pigs
GLUT2	Kidney, small intestine, liver, pancreatic islets, brain	High-capacity low-affinity facilitated glucose and fructose transporter	Rodents, humans, horses, cows
GLUT3	Brain (neurons) and testis	High-affinity facilitated glucose transporter; neuronal transport	Rodents, humans, cows, dogs, pigs
GLUT4	Striated muscle, fat, heart	High-affinity facilitated glucose transporter; insulin-regulated transport; linked to IR/diabetes	Rodents, humans, horses, cows, dogs, pigs
GLUT5	Small intestine, kidney, striated muscle, fat, testis	Facilitated fructose transporter	Rodents, humans, horses, cows, dogs, pigs
GLUT6	Leukocytes, brain, spleen	Facilitated glucose transporter	
GLUT7	Small intestine, colon, testis	Transport of glucose and fructose	
GLUT8	Testis, brain, blastocyst, striated muscle, fat, liver, spleen, lung	Facilitated glucose transporter widely expressed; neuronal transport; insulin-responsive transport in blastocyst	Rodents, humans, cows, horses

GLUT9	Liver, kidney, small intestine	Facilitated urate (glucose) transporter	Rodents, humans
GLUT10	Striated muscle, lung, liver, pancreas		
GLUT11	Striated muscle	Muscle-specific; facilitated glucose/fructose transporter	Rodents, humans
GLUT12	Striated muscle, fat, prostate, mammary gland	A second insulin-responsive facilitated GLUT?	Rodents, humans, cows, horses
HMIT	Brain, fat	H+/myo-inositol cotransporter	
GLUT14	Testis	Orphan transporter	

In contrast to basal GLUTs, GLUT4 translocates from an intracellular (nonactive) pool to the cell surface (active site) to enhance glucose uptake, a process called translocation. Therefore, GLUT4 is responsible for insulin-stimulated glucose uptake [23, 24]. Since GLUT4 is predominantly expressed in insulin-sensitive tissues, it plays a crucial role in whole-body glucose homeostasis [24] and as a result is one of the most studied GLUT isoforms, including horses. The equine GLUT4 gene has been characterized in equine skeletal muscle, which shares a high degree of homology with that of other mammalians [17, 25–27]. Similar to other species, GLUT4 protein is abundantly expressed in striated muscle and adipose tissue of horses [27, 28]. In addition, GLUT4 protein is expressed in equine muscle in a fiber-type specific manner with a higher expression in type 2B fibers, compared with that in type 1 fibers [27]. In contrast, immunostaining of GLUT4 in the equine digital lamellae has produced inconclusive results [29, 30], while western blot of crude membrane and PCR showed that GLUT4 is not a predominant isoform, suggesting that this insulin-responsive GLUT is unlikely to play a substantial role in the regulation of lamellar glucose transport [17, 18]. In addition, glucose uptake was not affected by insulin, further indicating the insulin-independent nature of the equine lamellae [17].

Although it has been believed that GLUT4 translocation is the rate-limiting step for glucose uptake and utilization in insulin-sensitive tissue, GLUT4 knockout mice do not develop hyperglycemia [31], suggesting that other GLUT isoforms could be involved in the regulation of whole-body glucose homeostasis [28]. Therefore, researchers have recently focused their attention on less understood GLUTs, particularly class III transporters, such as GLUT-8 and -12 [12, 32–35]. For instance, GLUT12 has been identified as a potential novel second insulin-sensitive GLUT [36], although its function is more likely to be tissue specific as for many other isoforms. In addition, its role is not well known in any species [37]. In horses, GLUT12 is expressed in insulin-sensitive tissues, with the highest protein expression in the omental adipose tissue, similar to the distribution pattern of GLUT4 protein across tissues [28]. In addition, it has been suggested that GLUT8, a dual-specific glucose and fructose transporter, is another insulin-regulated GLUT because it is highly expressed in striated muscle and adipose tissue, in addition to other tissues such as brain, testis, spermatozoa, liver, and kidney [38]. Furthermore, GLUT8 has been identified as an insulin-responsive GLUT in blastocysts [39]. Interestingly, GLUT8 protein has been recently characterized in striated muscle and digital lamellae of horses, with similar protein expression across tissue [18]. However, further studies are required to elucidate the physiological functions of the novel GLUT-8 and -12 isoforms.

Regulation of GLUT Translocation

Despite intensive research for over 50 years (primarily in rodents), the downstream signaling pathways that mediate the translocation of GLUT4 protein from an intracellular pool to the sarcolemma (active site) are not fully elucidated in any species. GLUT4 trafficking is largely regulated by insulin-dependent processes, although other factors including calcium/contraction, catecholamines, and hypoxia can alter glucose transport in skeletal and cardiac muscles (Figure 1) [40–47]. Since there are limited reports on the equine species, most of the information presented in this section is derived from studies on humans and rodents.

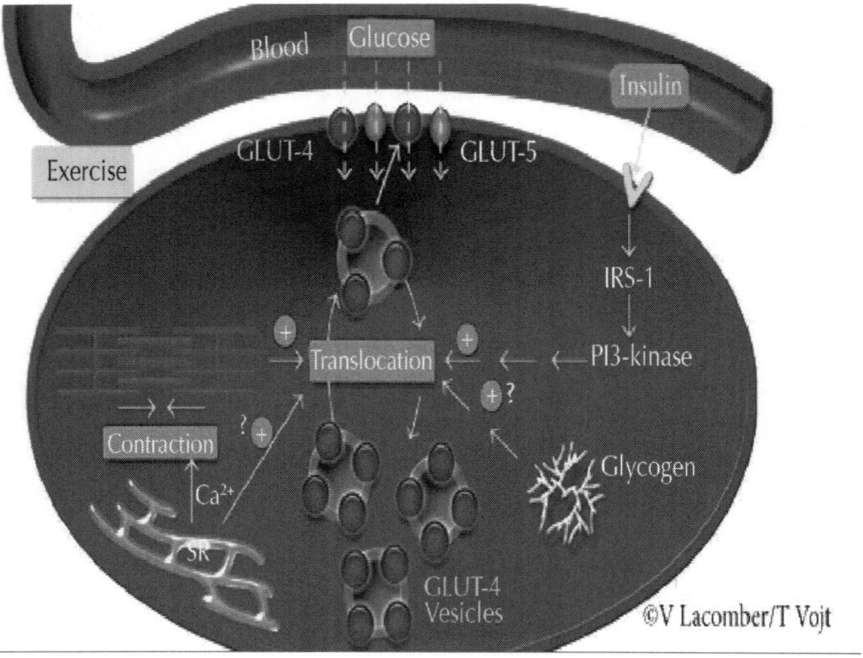

Figure 1: Regulation of glucose transport in striated muscle. GLUT4 translocation to the cell surface is mediated by both insulin-dependent and -independent pathways. GLUT: glucose transporter; PI 3-kinase: phosphatidylinositide 3-kinase; IRS: insulin receptor substrate; Ca^{2+}: calcium; SR: sarcoplasmic reticulum.

GLUT4 is a continuously recycling protein with faster endocytosis than reexocytosis, resulting in a net, but dynamic, intracellular retention [48]. The concept that insulin mobilized GLUT4 from intracellular storage vesicles to the plasma membrane was proposed by Cushman and colleagues in 1980 [49]. It has been estimated that ~5% of total GLUT4 is located at the cell surface of myocytes and adipocytes during basal conditions and that this fraction increased to ~50% after insulin stimulation (Figure 2) [6]. However, there is still some considerable debate on the regulation of GLUT trafficking by the downstream insulin signaling pathways [6]. It is known that, upon insulin release, insulin binds to the insulin receptor, thereby triggering its intrinsic protein-tyrosine kinase activity. The subsequent autophosphorylation of several insulin receptor tyrosine residues promotes tyrosine phosphorylation of insulin receptor substrates [50]. That action is followed by the activation of phosphatidylinositide 3-kinase (PI 3-kinase) and the production of phosphatidylinositol 3,4,5 triphosphate (PIP3) in the membrane (Figure 1). Increased PIP3 levels activate PDK1, a serine/threonine kinase, which in turn recruits the pivotal serine/threonine protein kinase, namely, Akt. Since it is involved in many processes, including cellular growth, survival, and fuel metabolism, Akt has 3 isoforms that directly act on several substrates [7]. Importantly, Akt2 appears to regulate AS160 (namely, Akt substrate protein of 160 kDa), which is the most distal signaling protein that has been implicated in insulin-mediated GLUT4 translocation and as such has emerged as a key regulator of GLUT trafficking. Under basal conditions, AS160 retains GLUT4 vesicles intracellularly through activity of its GTPase activating protein (GAP) domain for members of the Rab G protein family. The Rab proteins, which are guanosine triphosphate (GTP)-binding proteins, are thought to promote vesicle traffic (formation, targeting, and fusion) and may act as molecular switches, catalyzing membrane trafficking events by conversion from an inactive guanosine diphosphate-bound form to an active GTP-bound form [48]. Phosphorylation of AS160, which occurs on at least 6 different phospho-Akt-substrate (PAS) sites, suppresses or alters GAP activity, thereby elevating the GTP form of Rab, so GLUT4 exocytosis is permitted [51–53]. Although AS160 is also expressed in insulin-sensitive tissue of horses, its role in regulating GLUT trafficking has not been established [28, 54]. Finally, it has been shown that insulin-dependent GLUT4 translocation also requires dynamic remodeling of filamentous actin [48, 55]. Recently, it has also been suggested that α3(V) collagen is critical for glucose homeostasis, as mice with null alleles of the α3(V) gene Col5a3 have defective GLUT4 translocation to the plasma membrane in response to insulin [56].

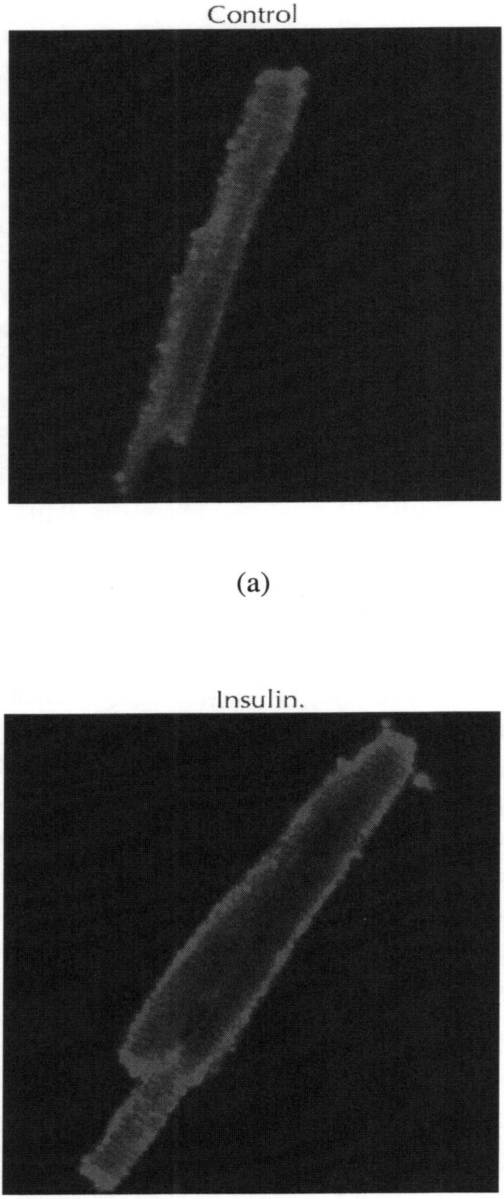

(b)

Figure 2: Insulin translocates GLUT4 from an intracellular pool (inactive site) to the cell surface (active site) in muscle, as visualized by confocal laser scanning microscopy. Adult rat cardiac myocytes were incubated without (a) or with insulin ((b), 100 μU/mL) for 30 min prior to immunofluorescent staining. Modified from [37].

Since exercise is vital for the maintenance of glucose homeostasis in diabetic patients, it has been proposed that insulin-independent pathways could be a major mechanism to regulate glucose uptake into striated muscles. Indeed, GLUT4 translocation to the cell surface can be regulated by contraction/Ca^{2+}-dependent processes in striated muscle (Figure 1). For instance, contractile activity during exercise increases glucose uptake and the number of GLUTs at the cell surface of the skeletal muscle, in the absence of insulin [40–42, 57, 58]. Holloszy and Narahara, in 1967, suggested the possibility that exercise-induced contraction and the resultant increase in cytosolic Ca^{2+} provide the signal to activate glucose transport in frog skeletal muscle [59]. In addition, exposing skeletal muscle to caffeine, which induces Ca^{2+} release from the sarcoplasmic reticulum at a concentration too low to induce contractions, results in GLUT4 translocation, suggesting that intracellular Ca^{2+} spikes are sufficient to stimulate glucose transport [60]. However, since the seminal discovery in 1967, the molecular signaling mechanisms by which contraction/Ca^{2+} regulates muscle glucose transport have remained elusive in all species. It has been hypothesized that activated PI3-kinase directly or indirectly opens Ca^{2+} channels. In striated muscle, Ca^{2+} entry subsequently initiates contraction via Ca^{2+}-induced Ca^{2+} release through the ryanodine receptors, which releases Ca^{2+} from the sarcoplasmic reticulum and subsequently activates intracellular calmodulin and calmodulin-dependent protein kinase II (CAMPKII). However, the mechanisms by which calmodulin and CAMPKII regulate glucose transport are not well known [58, 61]. Alternatively, it has been suggested that Ca^{2+} plays a direct role in the insertion of GLUT4 at the sarcolemma. Another potential candidate for contraction-stimulated glucose transport in skeletal muscle is the protein kinase C family [62]. However, the role of these potential candidates has not been well established because of the lack of specificity of most inhibitors studied [62]. Finally, during exercise, ATP is hydrolyzed to sustain the cross bridge cycle and the activity of ion channels and pumps involved in the excitation-contraction process, such as the sarcoplasmic reticulum calcium ATPase (SERCA) pump. The subsequent increase in AMP/ATP ratio has been implicated as a mediator of contraction-induced GLUT4 translocation in skeletal muscle, through activation of AMP-activated protein kinase (AMPK) [62]. There is recent evidence that activation of AMPK is involved in the regulation of AS160 through a contraction/Ca^{2+} dependent process in skeletal muscle. Indeed, AMPK phosphorylates AS160 at a site (namely, S711), which is distinct from phosphorylation sites that are modulated by insulin downstream signaling pathway [52, 63]. Although it has been shown that high-intensity exercise increases GLUT4 content in skeletal muscle of horses [64], further exploration of the molecular regulations of GLUT4 trafficking by insulin-independent pathways has not been established in this species. Only one study reported an increase in plasma AICAR (5-amino-4-imidazolecarboxamide riboside) after exercise in race horses [65]. Since AICAR activates AMPK, one could speculate that, similar to others species, AMPK-mediated metabolic regulation could be an important process for exercise-induced increased glucose transport in horses. Therefore, additional studies are needed to further understand the mechanisms of insulin-independent glucose transport.

Contribution of Glucose Transport to Muscle Glycogen Synthesis and Whole-Body Insulin Sensitivity in Healthy Horses

Similar to humans, horses rely on carbohydrate metabolism during both high- and low-to-moderate intensity exercise, where glycogen and glucose are the obligate substrates to sustain anaerobic ATP production [66]. Therefore, during exercise, the majority of circulating glucose is utilized by muscle fibers to sustain contraction. At rest, the majority of the glucose entering the cell is converted to triglycerides in adipose tissue and to glycogen in muscle fibers and liver. Therefore, the capacity to maximize muscle glycogen replenishment after exercise is an important factor for optimizing subsequent performance in horses [47]. After exercise, the feeding of a high soluble carbohydrate diet (such as grains and sweet feeds) hastens glycogen synthesis by increasing glucose availability and insulin release. Similar to other species, insulin release activates protein phosphatase, which converts glycogen synthase from its inactive form (D) to its active form (I) and inhibits glycogenolytic enzymes such as phosphorylase a (Figure 3). Since glucose is the required substrate for glycogen synthesis, insulin release also activates GLUT4 translocation to the plasma membrane to enhance glucose uptake [47, 50]. However, in contrast to other species, in which complete synthesis of the muscle glycogen pool takes 24 h, it requires 48–72 h after exhaustive exercise in horses, even after feeding a high soluble carbohydrate diet [67]. It has been proposed that the mechanisms underlying the slow rate of glycogen replenishment after exercise in horses may include limited ability for the small intestine to digest starch and slower activity of the muscle glycogen synthase enzyme compared with values reported in humans and rodents [68, 69]. In addition, there is evidence that glucose transport across the sarcolemma is the rate-limiting step for glucose uptake and subsequent glycogen synthesis in equine skeletal muscle [47, 68]. For instance, intravenous glucose infusion after exercise enhanced muscle glycogen synthesis but failed to enhance protein expression of the insulin-responsive GLUT4 in muscle 24 hours after a strenuous exercise [64]. Similarly, starch-rich meals failed to enhance GLUT4 gene expression, GLUT4 protein content, and muscle glycogen concentrations within the first 24 h after strenuous exercise [67, 70]. Finally, it was reported that in vitro insulin stimulation minimally increased GLUT4 translocation in the equine skeletal muscle, with the increase only being ~15% even after supraphysiological insulin concentrations in healthy ponies [54, 71]. These changes are much less than the ones reported in skeletal muscle of healthy human after physiological (80%) and supra-physiological (400%) insulin stimulation [71, 72]. To further evaluate in vivo glucose transport in horses, researchers used the euglycemic hyperinsulinemic clamp technique since the induced supraphysiological plasma insulin concentrations produce a maximal response of glucose uptake in insulin-sensitive tissue while inhibiting endogenous hepatic glucose production [2]. Interestingly, both short-term (i.e., 6 h) and long-term (i.e., 48 h) exogenous hyperinsulinemia in healthy horses did not affect the expression of GLUT4 gene and protein in equine skeletal muscle [18, 73]. Therefore, the observed lack of substantial increase in GLUT4 expression and/or translocation in healthy skeletal muscle in response to both in vivo and in vitro insulin stimulation may be the result of the insulin-dependent signaling pathways regulating GLUTs already being at near maximal physiologic limits for the species [54]. Alternatively, it has also been suggested that the relatively high resting muscle glycogen concentrations typical of the equine species may partially prevent further GLUT4 translocation to the plasma membrane via a negative feedback pathway [64]. Taken together, these studies demonstrated that glucose uptake across the sarcolemma is the rate-limiting step in glucose utilization and could be a major mechanism for the slow rate of muscle glycogen replenishment observed after exercise in this species [50].

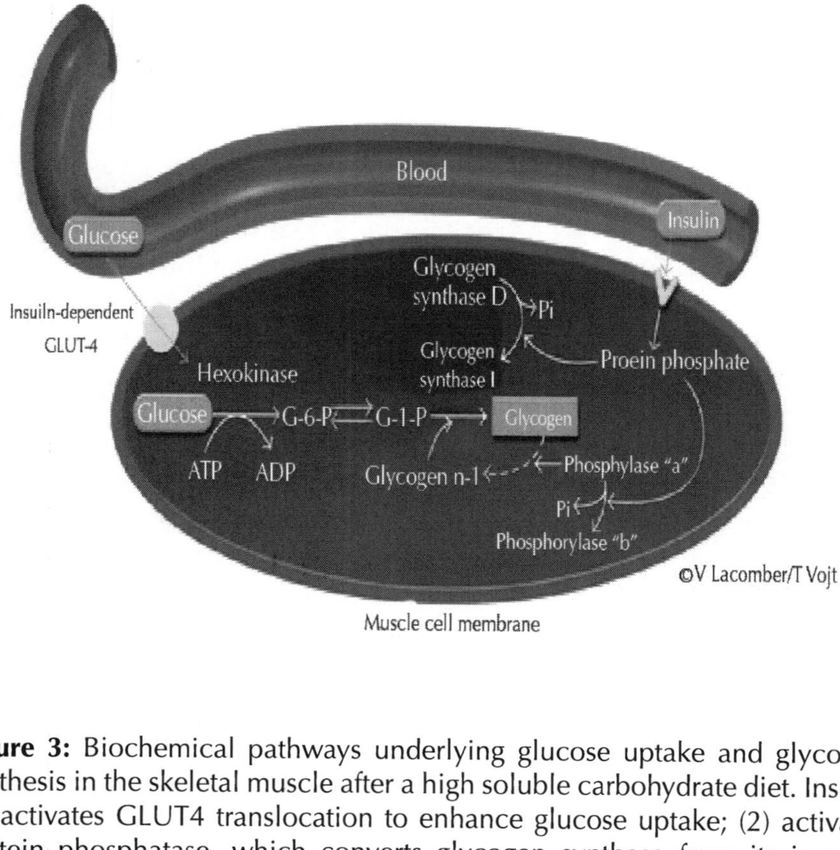

Figure 3: Biochemical pathways underlying glucose uptake and glycogen synthesis in the skeletal muscle after a high soluble carbohydrate diet. Insulin (1) activates GLUT4 translocation to enhance glucose uptake; (2) activates protein phosphatase, which converts glycogen synthase from its inactive form (D) to its active form (I); and (3) inhibits glycogenolytic enzymes such as phosphorylase a. G-6-P: glucose-6-phosphate; G-1-P: glucose-1-phosphate. Modified from [47].

The central role of adipose tissue glucose transport in regulating whole-body insulin sensitivity is becoming increasingly evident in mammalians, as adipose tissue-selective reduction of GLUT4 in mice results in impaired glucose tolerance and peripheral IR [74]. In addition, human omental adipocytes have higher GLUT4 expression and basal- and insulin-stimulated glucose uptake rate [75]. Similar to humans, GLUT4 protein expression is higher in visceral compared to subcutaneous adipose sites and skeletal muscle of insulin-sensitive horses, with the highest content present in the omental site [28]. Since GLUT4 is abundant in visceral adipose tissue, it is therefore likely to play a substantial role in the regulation of visceral glucose transport and in the maintenance of peripheral insulin sensitivity. Overall, the greater ability of insulin to promote glucose uptake in visceral compared with subcutaneous fat might be explained by higher levels of insulin receptors and downstream intermediates in the former fat depot, which could also explain the higher insulin-responsive GLUT content in this depot [76]. In support of these findings, GLUT12, a novel potential second insulin-responsive GLUT, has a higher protein content in visceral compared to subcutaneous adipose tissue and skeletal muscle in healthy horses [28]. Collectively, these findings suggest a central role for visceral GLUT-mediated glucose transport in the maintenance of peripheral insulin sensitivity in healthy horses.

GLUCOSE TRANSPORTERS: IMPLICATIONS FOR METABOLIC DYSREGULATION

Although increased insulin sensitivity has been reported with equine polysaccharide storage myopathy and equine motor neuron disease, changes in GLUT expression and/or trafficking have not been reported [21, 77]. In contrast, impaired glucose uptake appears to play a key pathogenic role during insulin resistance (IR) and other related metabolic diseases in many species, including horses, as outlined below.

Dysregulation of Glucose Transport: Parallels between Equine Metabolic Syndrome and Type 2 Diabetes in Humans

There is an emerging and growing threat as well as considerable health issues associated with insulin resistance, diabetes, and obesity, which are primary health concerns for humans and affect a wide range of economically important domesticated and/or agricultural species [78–81]. In humans, the World Health Organization has declared diabetes an epidemic disease, with worldwide prevalence expected to rise to 438 million by 2030 and projects that the number of diabetes-related deaths will increase by more than 50% worldwide in the next 10 years [82]. Prior to the development of type 2 diabetes, patients almost always suffer from "prediabetes," which is characterized by impaired glucose tolerance, increased fasting glucose (with values above the normal range but below the cutoff for the diagnosis of diabetes, 100 to 125 mg/dL), or both [83]. Development of diabetes from normal glucose tolerance is a continuous process, which may last for over a decade. Over 300 million people suffer from this preclinical stage of diabetes and this figure is expected to rise to 472 million worldwide by 2030 [83]. Insulin resistance is a core component of the preclinical stages of type 2 diabetes (i.e., "prediabetes") and is characterized by an impaired ability of insulin to stimulate glucose uptake into muscle and adipose tissue in all species. Insulin resistance first leads to compensatory oversecretion of insulin by the pancreatic β-cells and, eventually, β-cell exhaustion and development of type 2 diabetes. In addition, IR in the liver results in failure to suppress glucose production and release into the blood, further worsening the hyperglycemia. Although the development of diabetes is rarely reported in horses [84], there have been increased clinical awareness and recognition of chronic IR without marked hyperglycemia [85–88]. In addition, equine metabolic syndrome phenotype has been defined as a general clustering of obesity, IR, hyperinsulinemia, hypertriglyceridemia, and an increased risk for laminitis [85–88]. Affected patients are adult horses of both genders, from a wide range of breeds, types, and performance levels, living in distinct parts of the country [85, 88–90]. With increasing awareness, there is increasing diagnosis. Although the true prevalence of IR is not known, it has been estimated to be 10–28% (based on hyperinsulinemia) when large populations of adult horses have been studied [91]. It is anticipated that the prevalence of animals at metabolic risk of developing IR is even greater. Although there is limited work on biomarkers or panels of risk factors, environmental and physical risk factors for equine IR have been identified. Diet appears to be one important factor, as significant parallels exist between the provision of refined, nutritionally dense rations to horses and the consumption of energy dense refined foods by people in modern society [92]. In addition, increasing age, pregnancy/maternal insulin sensitivity, and obesity are also associated with equine IR [92–96]. As in other domesticated animals (e.g., dogs and cats), obesity is prevalent in horses and reported to be 19% and 32% in two independent studies of at least 300 adult horses [86]. Similar to humans, obesity promotes IR in horses, although IR occurs in nonobese equines as well [95, 96].

Although there has been increased clinical recognition of IR and diabetes, a clear understanding of the pathophysiology of these insidious diseases is still missing in horses and in other species. Cellular defects associated with IR can include reduced insulin receptor number, reduced expression and activation of insulin signaling cascade proteins (e.g., PI3K), and an impaired glucose transport process [54, 97]. Importantly, alterations in GLUT4 translocation appear to be a key pathogenic factor underlying IR in multiple species, including in horses. For example, decreased insulin-stimulated GLUT4 translocation in skeletal muscle is a hallmark of IR associated with type 2 diabetes in humans and rodents [98, 99]. Although there have been limited studies in horses, it was recently demonstrated that naturally occurring IR decreases translocation of GLUT4 to the cell surface in equine skeletal muscle, without a change in its total protein expression [54]. It is worthy to note that these horses exhibited early stage IR (with normal baseline blood glucose concentrations), suggesting that the observed alteration in muscle glucose transport is an early pathogenic event [54].

In many species, it is becoming increasingly apparent that adipose tissue plays a key pathogenic role in the overall development of IR [74]. Chronic elevation of serum free fatty acid concentrations, as observed in many humans with obesity or diabetes and horses with Cushing's or metabolic syndrome, may also contribute to the decreased uptake of glucose into peripheral tissues. It is well accepted that preferential deposition of fat into visceral deposits instead of subcutaneous deposits increases the risk of IR and diabetes in humans [100]. The "Portal Theory" suggests that IR and many of its related features could arise from visceral adipose tissue delivering free fatty acids at a high rate to the liver via the portal vein into which visceral adipose tissue directly drains. This in turn increases hepatic glucose production, reduces hepatic insulin clearance, and ultimately leads to hyperinsulinemia and IR [50]. In addition, the development of obesity-induced IR may be caused by visceral fat being more sensitive to increase in adipocyte cell size during expansion of adiposity, which may result in a relative decrease in cellular GLUT4 content as cell size increases [28, 50]. In contrast, in horses, adiposity and expansion of fat deposits in the crest and tailhead regions are associated with IR [50]. However, the importance of these regional fat sites to the pathogenesis of IR and glucose transport in horses has not been well investigated. One study reported a decrease in GLUT4 translocation in both visceral and subcutaneous adipose tissue in insulin-resistant compared to insulin-sensitive horses, suggesting an impairment of glucose transport in both of these adipose tissues [28]. Similarly, GLUT4 protein expression was lower in visceral adipose tissue of type 2 diabetic humans [101] and to a lesser extent in subcutaneous adipose tissue [102].

Since AS160 is a downstream insulin signaling protein, it could be a potential mechanism for the observed alteration in GLUT4 translocation to the cell surface during metabolic diseases. However, IR did not induce alterations in total nor phosphorylated AS160 in skeletal and adipose tissue of horses, suggesting that alterations in glucose transport occurred despite normal AS160 activation [28, 54]. Similarly, the role of AS160 in the pathogenesis of IR has not been well established in other species [6].

Overall, the early pathophysiological mechanisms underlying the long latency period preceding overt diabetes remain largely undefined in humans. Interestingly, horses are frequently affected by chronic IR and rarely decompensate to diabetes. As such, this species could provide a unique naturally occurring animal model to elucidate the chronic, pathological changes accompanying the transition from normal to impaired glucose tolerance. However, it should be pointed out that, because of its evolution as a grazing, hindgut-fermenting herbivore, the horse presents some unique features in regard to its metabolism [103]. For example, the horse derives ~30% of its energy from volatile fatty acids produced in the cecum, and acetate (the main volatile fatty acid produced in the hindgut) could account for 30% of the energy utilization by the limb of healthy horses during periods of rest [104–106]. Nonetheless, horses with chronic IR present some similarities in regard to metabolic dysregulation with human patients affected by the preclinical stages of type 2 diabetes, both at the whole tissue and molecular levels.

Dysregulated Glucose Transport and Inflammation: Potential Novel Link and Pathogenic Factor

Numerous studies in humans and animal models of metabolic diseases have demonstrated that obesity induces an inflammatory state, which plays a key pathogenic role during IR [107, 108]. With the development of obesity, adipose tissue is reported in humans and rodents to adopt a distinct inflammatory phenotype, characterized by increased gene expression and secretion of proinflammatory cytokines, such as tumor necrosis factor (TNF-α) and interleukins (IL)-1 and -6 [108]. In response to the increased proinflammatory cytokines (i.e., TNF-α), there is an increased production of suppressors of cytokine signaling (SOCS) proteins, which have been suggested to play a crucial link between inflammation and IR in the liver [109–111]. However, the feedback regulation of SOCS-3 is complex, and there are conflicting reports describing its relation with other components of the inflammatory signaling pathways, including toll-like receptors (TLR) [112], and ultimately the pathways linking inflammation to altered glucose transport remain elusive in all species [113].

It is well known that intravenous administration of endotoxin, which activates TNF- α and TLR, impairs insulin sensitivity in horses [114]. However, the role of inflammation during IR in horses has received scarce attention and findings remain controversial. It was reported that peripheral blood cells of obese hyperinsulinemic horses showed decreased endogenous proinflammatory cytokine gene expression [115]. In contrast, a correlative relationship was demonstrated between biomarkers of inflammation in the blood (i.e., TNF- α and IL-1) and obesity and IR in horses, as well as laminitis [116–118]. Dr. Burns and colleagues reported that subcutaneous depot (nuchal ligament) might be more likely to adopt an inflammatory phenotype than other adipose depots [119]. Furthermore, a significant increase in TNF- α protein expression in visceral but not subcutaneous tissue was reported in horses with compensated IR, suggesting a role for inflammation during IR [120].

Recent studies suggested that toll-like receptor (TLR) could be a key mechanism by which impaired fatty acid metabolism induces and propagates inflammation, and ultimately decreases insulin signaling and glucose transport [121]. TLRs recognize pathogen-associated molecular patterns and are of primary importance in the innate and adaptive immune system. TLR stimulation also leads to inflammation and cytokine production [121]. Although lipopolysaccharide is the key activator of TLR4 signaling, fatty acids have also been shown to be an endogenous ligand for TLR4 [122]. Activation of TLR4 signaling in adipocytes could activate JNK and NFkB signaling leading to increased production of proinflammatory cytokines, which in turn increases SOCS-3 production. Increased SOCS-3 in muscle and adipose tissue leads to decreased signal transduction through serine phosphorylation of IRS-1 and thus impairs the insulin signaling pathway, which ultimately results in dysregulation of glucose transport and homeostasis [122]. Therefore, TLR4, which is highly expressed in insulin-sensitive tissues, has been linked with the pathogenesis of IR [123, 124]. Recently, it has been shown that activation of TLR4, which is also highly expressed in striated muscle and adipose tissue of horses, was associated with an increased SOCS3 production during naturally occurring equine IR [120]. In addition, TLR4 signaling was activated in the digital lamellae of an experimental model of induced hyperinsulinemia, suggesting that inflammation contributes to the development of endocrinopathic laminitis [125]. Collectively, these findings suggest that TLR4 is a pathogenic marker during equine IR and/or metabolic dysfunction. However, further studies are required to elucidate the role of inflammation during dysregulated glucose metabolism in horses.

Complications Associated with Insulin Resistance: Potential Role of Dysregulated Glucose Transport

In humans, it is well accepted that IR even without overt diabetes can lead to multiorgan dysfunction and increased mortality [126, 127]. Evidence suggests that a similar state of inflammatory and multiple tissue complications occur in insulin-resistant horses [85, 87]. For instance, IR is thought to be involved not only in the pathogenesis of equine metabolic syndrome and diabetes mellitus, but also in the pathogenesis of pars intermedia dysfunction, hyperlipemia, endotoxemia, osteoarthritis and osteochondrosis dissecans [19, 128]. Importantly, IR is well known to be a direct and independent risk factor for a painful, debilitating peripheral vascular limb disease in horses, namely, laminitis, with some similarities to peripheral vascular disease and ischemic necrosis of the foot in human diabetic patients [85, 87, 88]. The prognosis and outcomes for horses with laminitis are poor, varying from 8 to 20% dying or being euthanized after 1 year, and it has been suggested that hyperinsulinemic laminitis is ultimately not reversible [129]. Therefore, a better understanding of the early pathophysiological effects could improve our capacity to predict and prevent this debilitating disease. Although the proposed mechanisms involved in the pathogenesis of laminitis are numerous and interrelated, IR is at the forefront of current investigations [130–133]. To this end, the development of experimental models of hyperinsulinemia-induced laminitis in the horse has provided further insights into the pathogenesis of endocrinopathic laminitis, especially as it relates to the altered glucose metabolism [27, 131,134]. This is particularly germane as the regulation of glucose transport in the lamellae in the healthy and laminitic horse remains scarce and controversial. Although GLUT1 has been consistently reported within lamellar keratinocytes, its expression during laminitis is variable [17, 18, 30]. An immunohistochemical study demonstrated loss of lamellar GLUT1 during chronic laminitis [29]. In contrast, lamellar GLUT1 gene and protein expression was unaffected in horses and ponies treated with a prolonged supraphysiologic infusion of insulin (which induces laminitis) suggesting that endocrinopathic laminitis is unlikely due to impaired glucose uptake and subsequent glucose deprivation in lamellae [17, 18]. Interestingly, it has been recently reported that both novel GLUT-8 and -12 (members of class III) proteins were upregulated in the equine lamellae following prolonged insulin infusion [18]. Interestingly, it has been recently suggested that GLUT8 mediates the deleterious metabolic effects associated with insulin resistance in mice fed a high-fructose diet [135]. However, it remains to be determined whether glucotoxicity contributes to the development of hyperinsulinemic laminitis in horses. In addition, it is not well established whether insulin resistance is required for the induction of endocrinopathic laminitis. Therefore, further studies are required to elucidate the pathogenesis of endocrinopathic laminitis, including additional potential mechanisms such as oxidative stress and vascular perturbations to the digit.

To further understand the impact of impaired glucose transport during diabetes, researchers have focused their attention on mechanisms by which chronic hyperglycemia induced micro- and macrovascular damages. Four main hypotheses have been proposed: (1) increased polyol pathway flux, (2) activation of protein kinase C isoforms, (3) increased hexosamine pathway flux, and (4) increased advanced glycation end products (AGEs) [136]. Importantly, chronic hyperglycemia accelerates the reaction between glucose and proteins and leads to the formation of advanced glycation end products, which form irreversible cross-links throughout the lifetime of many large proteins (such as collagen and hemoglobin), covalently modifying their structure and function [137–139]. In diabetes, and to a lesser extent during aging, AGEs accumulate at an accelerated rate in various cell types (in days to weeks) and cause multiple organ dysfunction [137, 139]. Once AGEs are formed, they are irreversible. At the organ level, AGEs stimulate collagen deposition, which ultimately leads to increased tissue fibrosis [137–141]. AGEs can also initiate alterations in cellular function by binding to a specific receptor known as the receptor for advanced glycation end products (RAGE), which is found on the surface of many cells, including macrophages, epithelial and endothelial cells, and smooth muscle cells. Although there is evidence that RAGE activation could occur early during the pathophysiological process, the role of RAGE and AGEs during metabolic dysfunction in horses has received scarce attention, in contrast to the extensive studies performed in human and rodents. Recently, one study reported a modest accumulation of AGE in the lamellar tissue of horses after 48 h of hyperinsulinemia-induced laminitis, suggesting a potential pathogenic role [142].

GLUCOSE TRANSPORTERS: POTENTIAL THERAPEUTIC TARGETS

Since GLUTs are key regulators of whole-body glucose homeostasis during physiologic and pathophysiologic states, they have received considerable attention as potential therapeutic targets to treat metabolic disorders in humans, such as during diabetes and IR. However, despite the increasing clinical awareness, research on new pharmacologic approaches for equine IR is limited and effective insulin-sensitizing strategies are lacking.

As in humans, careful dietary management and increasing physical activity are suggested in horses to promote insulin sensitivity [86]. However, the difficulty of encouraging exercise and weight loss in a recurrently laminitic horse can make the management very challenging or even be contraindicated. Therefore, there is a need for pharmacological intervention in horses, and levothyroxine sodium (i.e., T4) has been prescribed to induce weight loss and to improve insulin sensitivity [143]. In other species, it has been shown that thyroid hormone increases glucose uptake in insulin-sensitive tissue, in part by the activation of GLUTs [144]. In addition, veterinarians have increasingly prescribed the off-label use of human medications, such as metformin, a biguanide [145]. Although the main mechanism of action of metformin is through the suppression of hepatic gluconeogenesis, its spectrum of action is wide and remains not completely understood [146]. Importantly, metformin activates AMPK, which induces GLUT4 translocation to the cell surface, and thereby increases insulin sensitivity by enhancing peripheral glucose uptake. However, no clinical effect was observed with oral doses of 11–16 mg/kg/day [147], and either no effect or only modest increases in insulin sensitivity were observed in insulin-resistant horses following 30 mg/kg/day oral metformin [145, 148]. In addition, long-term results appear to be variable, and possible adverse drug effects have been reported [147,148]. This lack of prolonged therapeutic effect could be in part explained by the poor bioavailability of metformin in horses (36–52% lower than in humans) and thus, chronic dosing may not achieve therapeutic blood concentrations [146, 149]. Recently, pioglitazone, an FDA-approved thiazolidinedione to treat type 2 diabetes, has been evaluated in healthy horses. It is absorbed after oral administration without any clinically detectable adverse effects or any abnormalities in hematological and biochemical analyses [150]. Its mechanism of action relies on the activation of peroxisome proliferators-activated receptor gamma (i.e., PPAR-γ agonist). PPAR-γ, which is expressed in adipose tissue and muscle, is an intracellular transcription factor that controls the transcription of genes regulating glucose homeostasis [151, 152]. In particular, pioglitazone increases the efficiency of insulin-stimulated glucose uptake from blood into insulin-sensitive tissue by targeting GLUT proteins [153]. This increase in glucose uptake following pioglitazone treatment would in turn increase whole-body insulin sensitivity. In addition, pioglitazone possesses some anti-inflammatory properties including reduction of inflammatory markers (i.e., IL6, TNF-α), as well as prevention of SOCS-3 upregulation in the liver of insulin-resistant rodents fed a high fat/fructose diet [109], although similar effects have not been demonstrated in horses yet [154]. Pioglitazone could become an affordable therapeutic option for IR in horses since a generic preparation is going to be available soon [150]. However, only a few studies have investigated its therapeutic efficacy in horses. Although twelve days of pioglitazone treatment (1 mg/kg bodyweight PO) did not improve basal insulin-sensitivity, an increased skeletal muscle tissue transcript abundance of GLUT1 and insulin receptor was reported [155]. Therefore, further investigation of different dosing regimens of pioglitazone and metformin might be warranted in horses [146], as well as the investigation of alternative insulin-sensitizing strategies.

CONCLUSIONS

Glucose uptake is the rate-limiting step in whole-body glucose utilization and is tightly regulated by a family of specialized proteins, the glucose transporters. Insulin resistance is characterized by an impaired ability of insulin to stimulate glucose uptake into insulin sensitive tissues (i.e., muscle and adipose tissue) in all species. As for other species, the functional capability of the insulin-responsive glucose transporter GLUT4 is impaired in skeletal muscle and adipose tissue during naturally occurring IR in horses. Therefore, these insulin-responsive GLUTs provide molecular tool to further understand the pathophysiology of metabolic diseases across species and constitute potential therapeutic targets for equine patients affected by IR. However, despite intensive research for over 50 years, the molecular mechanisms of altered glucose transport remain elusive, and further research is required to characterize impairments of the downstream signaling pathways regulating GLUT4 translocation. Importantly, there is still much to learn about the physiological and pathophysiological functions of the GLUT family member, especially in regard to class III, and such knowledge will be essential in understanding the pathogenesis of IR and metabolic syndrome. Finally, future studies could also investigate novel physical, nutritional, and/or therapeutic strategies to activate GLUTs, which may be beneficial for both healthy equine athletes and horses with IR.

ACKNOWLEDGMENTS

The author is grateful to Tim Vojt for his excellent assistance with the medical illustrations, as well as to members of her laboratory, in particular Dr. Amanda Waller and Dr. Melody de Laat, for valuable discussions. This work was supported by grants from the United States Equestrian Federation Equine Health Research Fund, the Animal Health Foundation, and the National Institutes of Health (K01RR023083).

REFERENCES

1. B. Thorens and M. Mueckler, "Glucose transporters in the 21st Century," The American Journal of Physiology—Endocrinology and Metabolism, vol. 298, no. 2, pp. E141–E145, 2010.
2. J. H. van der Kolk, K. E. P. M. Rijnen, F. Rey, E. de Graaf-Roelfsema, G. C. M. Grinwis, and I. D. Wijnberg, "Evaluation of glucose metabolism in three horses with lower motor neuron degeneration,"American Journal of Veterinary Research, vol. 66, no. 2, pp. 271–276, 2005.
3. C. E. Grueter, E. Van Rooij, B. A. Johnson et al., "A cardiac MicroRNA governs systemic energy homeostasis by regulation of MED13," Cell, vol. 149, no. 3, pp. 671–683, 2012.
4. W. C. Stanley, F. A. Recchia, and G. D. Lopaschuk, "Myocardial substrate metabolism in the normal and failing heart," Physiological Reviews, vol. 85, no. 3, pp. 1093–1129, 2005.
5. R. W. Schwenk, J. J. F. P. Luiken, A. Bonen, and J. F. C. Glatz, "Regulation of sarcolemmal glucose and fatty acid transporters in cardiac disease," Cardiovascular Research, vol. 79, no. 2, pp. 249–258, 2008.
6. J. S. Bogan, "Regulation of glucose transporter translocation in health and diabetes," Annual Review of Biochemistry, vol. 81, pp. 507–532, 2012.
7. M. Mueckler and B. Thorens, "The SLC2 (GLUT) family of membrane transporters," Molecular Aspects of Medicine, vol. 34, no. 2-3, pp. 121–138, 2013.

8. F.-Q. Zhao and A. F. Keating, "Expression and regulation of glucose transporters in the bovine mammary gland," Journal of Dairy Science, vol. 90, pp. E76–E86, 2007.
9. J. Dyer, E. Fernandez-Castaño Merediz, K. S. H. Salmon, C. J. Proudman, G. B. Edwards, and S. P. Shirazi-Beechey, "Molecular characterisation of carbohydrate digestion and absorption in equine small intestine," Equine Veterinary Journal, vol. 34, no. 4, pp. 349–358, 2002.
10. J. Dyer, M. Al-Rammahi, L. Waterfall et al., "Adaptive response of equine intestinal Na^+/glucose co-transporter (SGLT1) to an increase in dietary soluble carbohydrate," Pflugers Archiv European Journal of Physiology, vol. 458, no. 2, pp. 419–430, 2009.
11. S. S. Pao, I. T. Paulsen, and M. H. Saier Jr., "Major facilitator superfamily," Microbiology and Molecular Biology Reviews, vol. 62, no. 1, pp. 1–34, 1998.
12. S. Schmidt, H.-G. Joost, and A. Schürmann, "GLUT8, the enigmatic intracellular hexose transporter,"The American Journal of Physiology—Endocrinology and Metabolism, vol. 296, no. 4, pp. E614–E618, 2009.
13. V. Douard and R. P. Ferraris, "Regulation of the fructose transporter GLUT5 in health and disease," The American Journal of Physiology—Endocrinology and Metabolism, vol. 295, no. 2, pp. E227–E237, 2008.
14. H.-G. Joost and B. Thorens, "The extended GLUT-family of sugar/polyol transport facilitators: nomenclature, sequence characteristics, and potential function of its novel members," Molecular Membrane Biology, vol. 18, no. 4, pp. 247–256, 2001.
15. E. Karnieli and M. Armoni, "Transcriptional regulation of the insulin-responsive glucose transporter GLUT4 gene: from physiology to pathology," The American Journal of Physiology—Endocrinology and Metabolism, vol. 295, no. 1, pp. E38–E45, 2008.
16. T. Arai, T. Washizu, M. Sagara et al., "D-glucose transport and glycolytic enzyme activities in erythrocytes of dogs, pigs, cats, horses, cattle and sheep," Research in Veterinary Science, vol. 58, no. 2, pp. 195–196, 1995.

17. K. E. Asplin, J. D. Curlewis, C. M. Mcgowan, C. C. Pollitt, and M. N. Sillence, "Glucose transport in the equine hoof," Equine Veterinary Journal, vol. 43, no. 2, pp. 196–201, 2011.
18. M. A. de Laat CKC, C. C. Pollitt, C. M. McGowan, M. N. Sillence, and V. A. Lacombe, "Regulation of glucose transport during equine hyperinsulinaemia," in Proceeding of the American College of Veterinary Internal Medecine Forum, 2013.
19. A. Mobasheri, S. J. Vannucci, C. A. Bondy et al., "Glucose transport and metabolism in chondrocytes: a key to understanding chondrogenesis, skeletal development and cartilage degradation in osteoarthritis,"Histology and Histopathology, vol. 17, no. 4, pp. 1239–1267, 2002.
20. T. Phillips, I. Ferraz, S. Bell, P. D. Clegg, S. D. Carter, and A. Mobasheri, "Differential regulation of the GLUT1 and GLUT3 glucose transporters by growth factors and pro-inflammatory cytokines in equine articular chondrocytes," Veterinary Journal, vol. 169, no. 2, pp. 216–222, 2005.
21. N. A. Benders, J. Dyer, I. D. Wijnberg, S. P. Shirazi-Beechey, and J. H. van der Kolk, "Evaluation of glucose tolerance and intestinal luminal membrane glucose transporter function in horses with equine motor neuron disease," American Journal of Veterinary Research, vol. 66, no. 1, pp. 93–99, 2005.
22. E. Fernandez-Castaño Merediz, J. Dyer, K. S. H. Salmon, and S. P. Shirazi-Beechey, "Molecular characterisation of fructose transport in equine small intestine," Equine Veterinary Journal, vol. 36, no. 6, pp. 532–538, 2004.
23. N. J. Bryant, R. Govers, and D. E. James, "Regulated transport of the glucose transporter GLUT4,"Nature Reviews Molecular Cell Biology, vol. 3, no. 4, pp. 267–277, 2002.
24. A. Zisman, O. D. Peroni, E. D. Abel et al., "Targeted disruption of the glucose transporter 4 selectively in muscle causes insulin resistance and glucose intolerance," Nature Medicine, vol. 6, no. 8, pp. 924–928, 2000.
25. Y. S. Nout, K. W. Hinchcliff, E. Jose-Cunilleras, L. R. Dearth, G. S. Sivko, and J. W. DeWille, "Effect of moderate exercise immediately followed by induced hyperglycemia on gene expression and content of the glucose transporter-4 protein in skeletal muscles

of horses," American Journal of Veterinary Research, vol. 64, no. 11, pp. 1401–1408, 2003.

26. E. Jose-Cunilleras, K. A. Hayes, R. E. Toribio, L. E. Mathes, and K. W. Hinchcliff, "Expression of equine glucose transporter type 4 in skeletal muscle after glycogen-depleting exercise," American Journal of Veterinary Research, vol. 66, no. 3, pp. 379–385, 2005.
27. K. G. van Dam, E. van Breda, G. Schaart et al., "Investigation of the expression and localization of glucose transporter 4 and fatty acid translocase/CD36 in equine skeletel muscle," American Journal of Veterinary Research, vol. 65, no. 7, pp. 951–956, 2004.
28. A. P. Waller, K. Kohler, T. A. Burns, M. C. Mudge, J. K. Belknap, and V. A. Lacombe, "Naturally occurring compensated insulin resistance selectively alters glucose transporters in visceral and subcutaneous adipose tissues without change in AS160 activation," Biochimica et Biophysica Acta, vol. 1812, no. 9, pp. 1098–1103, 2011.
29. A. Mobasheri, K. Critchlow, P. D. Clegg, S. D. Carter, and C. M. Canessa, "Chronic equine laminitis is characterised by loss of GLUT1, GLUT4 and ENaC positive laminar keratinocytes," Equine Veterinary Journal, vol. 36, no. 3, pp. 248–254, 2004.
30. O. Wattle and C. C. Pollitt, "Lamellar metabolism," Clinical Techniques in Equine Practice, vol. 3, no. 1, pp. 22–33, 2004.
31. E. B. Katz, A. E. Stenbit, K. Hatton, R. DePinho, and M. J. Charron, "Cardiac and adipose tissue abnormalities but not diabetes in mice deficient in GLUT4," Nature, vol. 377, no. 6545, pp. 151–155, 1995.
32. S. C. D'Cruz, R. Jubendradass, and P. P. Mathur, "Bisphenol a induces oxidative stress and decreases levels of insulin receptor substrate 2 and glucose transporter 8 in rat testis," Reproductive Sciences, vol. 19, no. 2, pp. 163–172, 2012.
33. P. A. Dawson, J. C. Mychaleckyj, S. C. Fossey, S. J. Mihic, A. L. Craddock, and D. W. Bowden, "Sequence and functional analysis of GLUT10: a glucose transporter in the type 2 diabetes-linked region of chromosome 20q12–13.1," Molecular Genetics and Metabolism, vol. 74, no. 1-2, pp. 186–199, 2001.
34. O. Gómez, B. Ballester-Lurbe, J. E. Mesonero, and J. Terrado, "Glucose transporters GLUT4 and GLUT8 are upregulated after

facial nerve axotomy in adult mice," Journal of Anatomy, vol. 219, no. 4, pp. 525–530, 2011.

35. A. Scheepers, H.-G. Joost, and A. Schürmann, "The glucose transporter families SGLT and GLUT: molecular basis of normal and aberrant function," Journal of Parenteral and Enteral Nutrition, vol. 28, no. 5, pp. 364–371, 2004.
36. S. H. Purcell, L. B. Aerni-Flessner, A. R. Willcockson, K. A. Diggs-Andrews, S. J. Fisher, and K. H. Moley, "Improved insulin sensitivity by GLUT12 overexpression in mice," Diabetes, vol. 60, no. 5, pp. 1478–1482, 2011.
37. A. P. Waller, M. George, A. Kalyanasundaram et al., "GLUT12 functions as a basal and insulin-independent glucose transporter in the heart," Biochimica et Biophysica Acta-Molecular Basis of Disease, vol. 1832, no. 1, pp. 121–127, 2013.
38. L. Aerni-Flessner, M. Abi-Jaoude, A. Koenig, M. Payne, and P. W. Hruz, "GLUT4, GLUT1, and GLUT8 are the dominant GLUT transcripts expressed in the murine left ventricle," Cardiovascular Diabetology, vol. 11, article 63, 2012.
39. M. O. Carayannopoulos, M. M.-Y. Chi, Y. Cui et al., "GLUT8 is a glucose transporter responsible for insulin-stimulated glucose uptake in the blastocyst," Proceedings of the National Academy of Sciences of the United States of America, vol. 97, no. 13, pp. 7313–7318, 2000.
40. J. T. Brozinick Jr., G. J. Etgen Jr., B. B. Yaspelkis III, and J. L. Ivy, "The effects of muscle contraction and insulin on glucose-transporter translocation in rat skeletal muscle," Biochemical Journal, vol. 297, no. 3, pp. 539–545, 1994.
41. L. J. Goodyear, M. F. Hirshman, and E. S. Horton, "Exercise-induced translocation of skeletal muscle glucose transporters," The American Journal of Physiology—Endocrinology and Metabolism, vol. 261, no. 6, pp. E795–E799, 1991.
42. T. Hayashi, J. F. P. Wojtaszewski, and L. J. Goodyear, "Exercise regulation of glucose transport in skeletal muscle," The American Journal of Physiology—Endocrinology and Metabolism, vol. 273, no. 6, pp. E1039–E1051, 1997.
43. T. Kolter, I. Uphues, A. Wichelhaus, H. Reinauer, and J. Eckel, "Contraction-induced translocation of the glucose transporter Glut4 in isolated ventricular cardiomyocytes," Biochemical and

Biophysical Research Communications, vol. 189, no. 2, pp. 1207–1214, 1992.

44. M. Till, T. Kolter, and J. Eckel, "Molecular mechanisms of contraction-induced translocation of GLUT4 in isolated cardiomyocytes," American Journal of Cardiology, vol. 80, no. 3, pp. 85A–89A, 1997.
45. M. Till, D. M. Ouwens, A. Kessler, and J. Eckel, "Molecular mechanisms of contraction-regulated cardiac glucose transport," Biochemical Journal, vol. 346, no. 3, pp. 841–847, 2000.
46. A. Zorzano, L. Sevilla, M. Camps et al., "Regulation of glucose transport, and glucose transporters expression and trafficking in the heart: studies in cardiac myocytes," American Journal of Cardiology, vol. 80, no. 3, Supplement 1, pp. 65A–76A, 1997.
47. V. A. Lacombe, K. W. Hinchcliff, and L. E. Taylor, "Interactions of substrate availability, exercise performance, and nutrition with muscle glycogen metabolism in horses," Journal of the American Veterinary Medical Association, vol. 223, no. 11, pp. 1576–1585, 2003.
48. A. Klip, "The many ways to regulate glucose transporter 4," Applied Physiology, Nutrition and Metabolism, vol. 34, no. 3, pp. 481–487, 2009.
49. S. W. Cushman and L. J. Wardzala, "Potential mechanism of insulin action on glucose transport in the isolated rat adipose cell. Apparent translocation of intracellular transport systems to the plasma membrane," Journal of Biological Chemistry, vol. 255, no. 10, pp. 4758–4762, 1980.
50. V. A. Lacombe, "Glucose metabolism in insulin-sensitive tissue: from health to disease (vol 31, pg 578, 2011)," Journal of Equine Veterinary Science, vol. 32, no. 2, pp. 116–116, 2012.
51. M. Larance, G. Ramm, J. Stöckli et al., "Characterization of the role of the Rab GTPase-activating protein AS160 in insulin-regulated GLUT4 trafficking," Journal of Biological Chemistry, vol. 280, no. 45, pp. 37803–37813, 2005.
52. H. F. Kramer, C. A. Witczak, N. Fujii et al., "Distinct signals regulate AS160 phosphorylation in response to insulin, AICAR, and contraction in mouse skeletal muscle," Diabetes, vol. 55, no. 7, pp. 2067–2076, 2006.

53. H. F. Kramer, E. B. Taylor, C. A. Witczak, N. Fujii, M. F. Hirshman, and L. J. Goodyear, "Calmodulin-binding domain of AS160 regulates contraction- but not insulin-stimulated glucose uptake in skeletal muscle," Diabetes, vol. 56, no. 12, pp. 2854–2862, 2007.
54. A. P. Waller, T. A. Burns, M. C. Mudge, J. K. Belknap, and V. A. Lacombe, "Insulin resistance selectively alters cell-surface glucose transporters but not their total protein expression in equine skeletal muscle,"Journal of Veterinary Internal Medicine, vol. 25, no. 2, pp. 315–321, 2011.
55. I. Talior-Volodarsky, V. K. Randhawa, H. Zaid, and A. Klip, "α-actinin-4 is selectively required for insulin-induced GLUT4 translocation," Journal of Biological Chemistry, vol. 283, no. 37, pp. 25115–25123, 2008.
56. G. Huang, G. Ge, D. Wang et al., "α3(V) Collagen is critical for glucose homeostasis in mice due to effects in pancreatic islets and peripheral tissues," Journal of Clinical Investigation, vol. 121, no. 2, pp. 769–783, 2011.
57. A. G. Douen, T. Ramlal, G. D. Cartee, and A. Klip, "Exercise modulates the insulin-induced translocation of glucose transporters in rat skeletal muscle," The FEBS Letters, vol. 261, no. 2, pp. 256–260, 1990.
58. D. C. Wright, P. C. Geiger, J. O. Holloszy, and D.-H. Han, "Contraction- and hypoxia-stimulated glucose transport is mediated by a Ca^{2+}-dependent mechanism in slow-twitch rat soleus muscle," The American Journal of Physiology—Endocrinology and Metabolism, vol. 288, no. 6, pp. E1062–E1066, 2005.
59. J. O. Holloszy and H. T. Narahara, "Enhanced permeability to sugar associated with muscle contraction. Studies of the role of Ca^{++}," Journal of General Physiology, vol. 50, no. 3, pp. 551–562, 1967.
60. J. H. Youn, E. A. Gulve, and J. O. Holloszy, "Calcium stimulates glucose transport in skeletal muscle by a pathway independent of contraction," The American Journal of Physiology—Cell Physiology, vol. 260, no. 3, pp. C555–C561, 1991.
61. D. C. Wright, C. A. Fick, J. B. Olesen, K. Lim, B. R. Barnes, and B. W. Craig, "A role for calcium/calmodulin kinase in insulin

stimulated glucose transport," Life Sciences, vol. 74, no. 7, pp. 815–825, 2004.

62. N. Jessen and L. J. Goodyear, "Invited review: contraction signaling to glucose transport in skeletal muscle," Journal of Applied Physiology, vol. 99, no. 1, pp. 330–337, 2005.
63. J. T. Treebak, E. B. Taylor, C. A. Witczak et al., "Identification of a novel phosphorylation site on TBC1D4 regulated by AMP-activated protein kinase in skeletal muscle," The American Journal of Physiology—Cell Physiology, vol. 298, no. 2, pp. C377–C385, 2010.
64. V. A. Lacombe, K. W. Hinchcliff, and S. T. Devor, "Effects of exercise and glucose administration on content of insulin-sensitive glucose transporter in equine skeletal muscle," American Journal of Veterinary Research, vol. 64, no. 12, pp. 1500–1506, 2003.
65. M. A. Robinson, Y. Liu, C. E. Uboh, and L. R. Soma, "Exercise increases plasma AICAR (5-amino-4-imidazolecarboxamide riboside) in the horse," The FASEB Journal, vol. 26, 2012.
66. V. A. Lacombe, K. W. Hinchcliff, R. J. Geor, and C. R. Baskin, "Muscle glycogen depletion and subsequent replenishment affect anaerobic capacity of horses," Journal of Applied Physiology, vol. 91, no. 4, pp. 1782–1790, 2001.
67. V. A. Lacombe, K. W. Hinchcliff, C. W. Kohn, S. T. Devor, and L. E. Taylor, "Effects of feeding meals with various soluble-carbohydrate content on muscle glycogen synthesis after exercise in horses,"American Journal of Veterinary Research, vol. 65, no. 7, pp. 916–923, 2004.
68. D. M. Votion, R. Navet, V. A. Lacombe et al., "Muscle energetics in exercising horses," Equine and Comparative Exercise Physiology, vol. 4, no. 3/4, pp. 105–118, 2007.
69. J. L. Ivy and C.-H. Kuo, "Regulation of GLUT4 protein and glycogen synthase during muscle glycogen synthesis after exercise," Acta Physiologica Scandinavica, vol. 162, no. 3, pp. 295–304, 1998.
70. E. Jose-Cunilleras, K. W. Hinchcliff, V. A. Lacombe et al., "Ingestion of starch-rich meals after exercise increases glucose kinetics but fails to enhance muscle glycogen replenishment in horses," Veterinary Journal, vol. 171, no. 3, pp. 468–477, 2006.

71. R. Duehlmeier, A. Hacker, A. Widdel-Bigdely, W. V. Engelhardt, and H.-P. Sallmann, "Insulin stimulates GLUT4 translocation in the semitendinosus muscle of Shetland ponies," Veterinary Journal, vol. 184, no. 2, pp. 176–181, 2010.
72. J. W. Ryder, J. Yang, D. Galuska et al., "Use of a novel impermeable biotinylated photolabeling reagent to assess insulin- and hypoxia-stimulated cell surface GLUT4 content in skeletal muscle from type 2 diabetic patients," Diabetes, vol. 49, no. 4, pp. 647–654, 2000.
73. J. K. Suagee, B. A. Corl, M. W. Hulver, L. J. McCutcheon, and R. J. Geor, "Effects of hyperinsulinemia on glucose and lipid transporter expression in insulin-sensitive horses," Domestic Animal Endocrinology, vol. 40, no. 3, pp. 173–181, 2011.
74. E. D. Abel, O. Peroni, J. K. Kim et al., "Adipose-selective targeting of the GLUT4 gene impairs insulin action in muscle and liver," Nature, vol. 409, no. 6821, pp. 729–733, 2001.
75. K. A. Virtanen, P. Lönnroth, R. Parkkola et al., "Glucose uptake and perfusion in subcutaneous and visceral adipose tissue during insulin stimulation in nonobese and obese humans," Journal of Clinical Endocrinology and Metabolism, vol. 87, no. 8, pp. 3902–3910, 2002.
76. R. MacLaren, W. Cui, S. Simard, and K. Cianflone, "Influence of obesity and insulin sensitivity on insulin signaling genes in human omental and subcutaneous adipose tissue," Journal of Lipid Research, vol. 49, no. 2, pp. 308–323, 2008.
77. E. J. Annandale, S. J. Valberg, J. R. Mickelson, and E. R. Seaquist, "Insulin sensitivity and skeletal muscle glucose transport in horses with equine polysaccharide storage myopathy," Neuromuscular Disorders, vol. 14, no. 10, pp. 666–674, 2004.
78. L. M. Chagas, M. C. Lucy, P. J. Back et al., "Insulin resistance in divergent strains of Holstein-Friesian dairy cows offered fresh pasture and increasing amounts of concentrate in early lactation," Journal of Dairy Science, vol. 92, no. 1, pp. 216–222, 2009.
79. H. Ohtsuka, M. Koiwa, A. Hatsugaya et al., "Relationship between serum TNF activity and insulin resistance in dairy cows affected with naturally occurring fatty liver," Journal of Veterinary Medical Science, vol. 63, no. 9, pp. 1021–1025, 2001.

80. J. R. Feldhahn, J. S. Rand, and G. Martin, "Insulin sensitivity in normal and diabetic cats," Journal of Feline Medicine and Surgery, vol. 1, no. 2, pp. 107–115, 1999.
81. A. J. German, M. Hervera, L. Hunter et al., "Improvement in insulin resistance and reduction in plasma inflammatory adipokines after weight loss in obese dogs," Domestic Animal Endocrinology, vol. 37, no. 4, pp. 214–226, 2009.
82. L. Chen, D. J. Magliano, and P. Z. Zimmet, "The worldwide epidemiology of type 2 diabetes mellitus—present and future perspectives," Nature Reviews Endocrinology, vol. 8, no. 4, pp. 228–236, 2012.
83. A. G. Tabak, C. Herder, W. Rathmann, E. J. Brunner, and M. Kivimaki, "Prediabetes: a high-risk state for diabetes development," The Lancet, vol. 379, no. 9833, pp. 2279–2290, 2012.
84. A. E. Durham, K. J. Hughes, H. J. Cottle, D. I. Rendle, and R. C. Boston, "Type 2 diabetes mellitus with pancreatic beta cell dysfunction in 3 horses confirmed with minimal model analysis," Equine Veterinary Journal, vol. 41, no. 9, pp. 924–929, 2009.
85. N. Frank, R. J. Geor, S. R. Bailey, A. E. Durham, and P. J. Johnson, "Equine metabolic syndrome,"Journal of Veterinary Internal Medicine, vol. 24, no. 3, pp. 467–475, 2010.
86. R. J. Geor and P. Harris, "Dietary management of obesity and insulin resistance: countering risk for laminitis," Veterinary Clinics of North America, vol. 25, no. 1, pp. 51–65, 2009.
87. R. Geor and N. Frank, "Metabolic syndrome-From human organ disease to laminar failure in equids,"Veterinary Immunology and Immunopathology, vol. 129, no. 3-4, pp. 151–154, 2009.
88. P. J. Johnson, C. E. Wiedmeyer, A. LaCarrubba, V. K. Seshu Ganjam, and N. T. Messer, "Laminitis and the equine metabolic syndrome," Veterinary Clinics of North America, vol. 26, no. 2, pp. 239–255, 2010.
89. N. Frank, S. B. Elliott, L. E. Brandt, and D. H. Keisler, "Physical characteristics, blood hormone concentrations, and plasma lipid concentrations in obese horses with insulin resistance," Journal of the American Veterinary Medical Association, vol. 228, no. 9, pp. 1383–1390, 2006.

90. K. H. Treiber, D. S. Kronfeld, T. M. Hess, B. M. Byrd, R. K. Splan, and W. B. Staniar, "Evaluation of genetic and metabolic predispositions and nutritional risk factors for pasture-associated laminitis in ponies," Journal of the American Veterinary Medical Association, vol. 228, no. 10, pp. 1538–1545, 2006.
91. R. J. Geor, C. D. Thatcher, R. S. Pleasant, F. Elvinger, L. Gay, and S. R. Werre, "Prevalence of hyperinsulinemia in mature horses: relationship to adiposity," Journal of Veterinary Internal Medicine, vol. 21, no. 3, p. 601, 2007.
92. R. M. Hoffman, R. C. Boston, D. Stefanovski, D. S. Kronfeld, and P. A. Harris, "Obesity and diet affect glucose dynamics and insulin sensitivity in Thoroughbred geldings," Journal of Animal Science, vol. 81, no. 9, pp. 2333–2342, 2003.
93. L. A. George, W. B. Staniar, K. H. Treiber, P. A. Harris, and R. J. Geor, "Insulin sensitivity and glucose dynamics during pre-weaning foal development and in response to maternal diet composition,"Domestic Animal Endocrinology, vol. 37, no. 1, pp. 23–29, 2009.
94. S. L. Ralston, C. F. Nockels, and E. L. Squires, "Differences in diagnostic test results and hematologic data between aged and young horses," American Journal of Veterinary Research, vol. 49, no. 8, pp. 1387–1392, 1988.
95. S. R. Bailey, J. L. Habershon-Butcher, K. J. Ransom, J. Elliott, and N. J. Menzies-Gow, "Hypertension and insulin resistance in a mixed-breed population of ponies predisposed to laminitis," American Journal of Veterinary Research, vol. 69, no. 1, pp. 122–129, 2008.
96. S. R. Bailey, N. J. Menzies-Gow, P. A. Harris et al., "Effect of dietary fructans and dexamethasone administration on the insulin response of ponies predisposed to laminitis," Journal of the American Veterinary Medical Association, vol. 231, no. 9, pp. 1365–1373, 2007.
97. Y. Kitamura and D. Accili, "New insights into the integrated physiology of insulin action," Reviews in Endocrine and Metabolic Disorders, vol. 5, no. 2, pp. 143–149, 2004.
98. A. Handberg, A. Vaag, P. Damsbo, H. Beck-Nielsen, and J. Vinten, "Expression of insulin regulatable glucose transporters

in skeletal muscle from Type 2 (non-insulin-dependent) diabetic patients,"Diabetologia, vol. 33, no. 10, pp. 625–627, 1990.

99. J. R. Zierath, K. L. Houseknecht, L. Gnudi, and B. B. Kahn, "High-fat feeding impairs insulin-stimulated GLUT4 recruitment via an early insulin-signaling defect," Diabetes, vol. 46, no. 2, pp. 215–223, 1997.

100. M. J. Cartwright, T. Tchkonia, and J. L. Kirkland, "Aging in adipocytes: potential impact of inherent, depot-specific mechanisms," Experimental Gerontology, vol. 42, no. 6, pp. 463–471, 2007.

101. W. T. Garvey, L. Maianu, J.-H. Zhu, J. A. Hancock, and A. M. Golichowski, "Multiple defects in the adipocyte glucose transport system cause cellular insulin resistance in gestational diabetes: heterogeneity in the number and a novel abnormality in subcellular localization of GLUT4 glucose transporters,"Diabetes, vol. 42, no. 12, pp. 1773–1785, 1993.

102. L. Maianu, S. R. Keller, and W. T. Garvey, "Adipocytes exhibit abnormal subcellular distribution and translocation of vesicles containing glucose transporter 4 and insulin-regulated aminopeptidase in type 2 diabetes mellitus: implications regarding defects in vesicle trafficking," Journal of Clinical Endocrinology and Metabolism, vol. 86, no. 11, pp. 5450–5456, 2001.

103. M. J. Glinsky, R. M. Smith, H. R. Spires, and C. L. Davis, "Measurement of volatile fatty acid production rates in the cecum of the pony," Journal of Animal Science, vol. 42, no. 6, pp. 1465–1470, 1976.

104. D. W. Pethick, R. J. Rose, W. L. Bryden, and J. M. Gooden, "Nutrient utilisation by the hindlimb of thoroughbred horses at rest," Equine Veterinary Journal, vol. 25, no. 1, pp. 41–44, 1993.

105. M. J. S. Moore-Colyer, J. J. Hyslop, A. C. Longland, and D. Cuddeford, "Intra-caecal fermentation parameters in ponies fed botanically diverse fibre-based diets," Animal Feed Science and Technology, vol. 84, no. 3-4, pp. 183–197, 2000.

106. H. F. Hintz, R. A. Argenzio, and H. F. Schryver, "Digestion coefficients, blood glucose levels and molar percentage of volatile acids in intestinal fluid of ponies fed varying forage-grain ratios," Journal of Animal Science, vol. 33, no. 5, pp. 992–995, 1971.

107. K. Clément, N. Viguerie, C. Poitou et al., "Weight loss regulates inflammation-related genes in white adipose tissue of obese subjects," The FASEB Journal, vol. 18, no. 14, pp. 1657–1669, 2004.

108. N. Rasouli and P. A. Kern, "Adipocytokines and the metabolic complications of obesity," Journal of Clinical Endocrinology and Metabolism, vol. 93, no. 11, supplement 1, pp. S64–S73, 2008. View at Publisher · View at Google Scholar · View at Scopus

109. M. Collino, M. Aragno, S. Castiglia et al., "Pioglitazone improves lipid and insulin levels in overweight rats on a high cholesterol and fructose diet by decreasing hepatic inflammation," British Journal of Pharmacology, vol. 160, no. 8, pp. 1892–1902, 2010.

110. G. C. Farrell, "Signalling links in the liver: knitting SOCS with fat and inflammation," Journal of Hepatology, vol. 43, no. 1, pp. 193–196, 2005.

111. K. Ueki, T. Kondo, Y.-H. Tseng, and C. R. Kahn, "Central role of suppressors of cytokine signaling proteins in hepatic steatosis, insulin resistance, and the metabolic syndrome in the mouse," Proceedings of the National Academy of Sciences of the United States of America, vol. 101, no. 28, pp. 10422–10427, 2004.

112. L. Liu, H. Gu, Y. Zhao, and F. Yu, "Study on SOCS-3, PPARgamma and ACO mRNA expression of adipose tissues in obese rats with leptin resistance," Wei Sheng Yan Jiu, vol. 37, no. 1, pp. 40–42, 2008.

113. A. Yoshimura, T. Naka, and M. Kubo, "SOCS proteins, cytokine signalling and immune regulation,"Nature Reviews Immunology, vol. 7, no. 6, pp. 454–465, 2007.

114. F. Tóth, N. Frank, S. B. Elliott, R. J. Geor, and R. C. Boston, "Effects of an intravenous endotoxin challenge on glucose and insulin dynamics in horses," American Journal of Veterinary Research, vol. 69, no. 1, pp. 82–88, 2008.

115. T. C. Holbrook, T. Tipton, and D. McFarlane, "Neutrophil and cytokine dysregulation in hyperinsulinemic obese horses," Veterinary Immunology and Immunopathology, vol. 145, no. 1-2, pp. 283–289, 2012.

116. M. M. Vick, A. A. Adams, B. A. Murphy et al., "Relationships among inflammatory cytokines, obesity, and insulin sensitivity in

the horse," Journal of Animal Science, vol. 85, no. 5, pp. 1144–1155, 2007.

117. R. A. Carter, K. H. Treiber, R. J. Geor, L. Douglass, and P. A. Harris, "Prediction of incipient pasture-associated laminitis from hyperinsulinaemia, hyperleptinaemia and generalised and localised obesity in a cohort of ponies," Equine Veterinary Journal, vol. 41, no. 2, pp. 171–178, 2009.

118. K. Treiber, R. Carter, L. Gay, C. Williams, and R. Geor, "Inflammatory and redox status of ponies with a history of pasture-associated laminitis," Veterinary Immunology and Immunopathology, vol. 129, no. 3-4, pp. 216–220, 2009.

119. T. A. Burns, R. J. Geor, M. C. Mudge, L. J. McCutcheon, K. W. Hinchcliff, and J. K. Belknap, "Proinflammatory cytokine and chemokine gene expression profiles in subcutaneous and visceral adipose tissue depots of insulin-resistant and insulin-sensitive light breed horses," Journal of Veterinary Internal Medicine, vol. 24, no. 4, pp. 932–939, 2010.

120. A. P. Waller, L. Huettner, K. Kohler, and V. A. Lacombe, "Novel link between inflammation and impaired glucose transport during equine insulin resistance," Veterinary Immunology and Immunopathology, vol. 149, no. 3-4, pp. 208–215, 2012.

121. A. C. Könner and J. C. Brüning, "Toll-like receptors: linking inflammation to metabolism," Trends in Endocrinology and Metabolism, vol. 22, no. 1, pp. 16–23, 2011.

122. J. K. Kim, "Fat uses a TOLL-road to connect inflammation and diabetes," Cell Metabolism, vol. 4, no. 6, pp. 417–419, 2006.

123. T. Suganami, T. Mieda, M. Itoh, Y. Shimoda, Y. Kamei, and Y. Ogawa, "Attenuation of obesity-induced adipose tissue inflammation in C3H/HeJ mice carrying a Toll-like receptor 4 mutation," Biochemical and Biophysical Research Communications, vol. 354, no. 1, pp. 45–49, 2007.

124. D. M. L. Tsukumo, M. A. Carvalho-Filho, J. B. C. Carvalheira et al., "Loss-of-function mutation in toll-like receptor 4 prevents diet-induced obesity and insulin resistance," Diabetes, vol. 56, no. 8, pp. 1986–1998, 2007.

125. M. A. de Laat, C. K. Clement, C. M. McGowan, M. N. Sillence, C. C. Pollitt, and V. A. Lacombe, "Toll-like receptor and pro-inflammatory cytokine expression during prolonged

hyperinsulinaemia in horses: implications for laminitis," Veterinary Immunology and Immunopathology, vol. 157, no. 1-2, pp. 78–86, 2014.

126. J. B. Meigs, D. M. Nathan, R. B. D›Agostino Sr., and P. W. F. Wilson, "Fasting and postchallenge glycemia and cardiovascular disease risk: the framingham offspring study," Diabetes Care, vol. 25, no. 10, pp. 1845–1850, 2002.

127. J. D. Sorkin, D. C. Muller, J. L. Fleg, and R. Andres, "The relation of fasting and 2-h postchallenge plasma glucose concentrations to mortality: data from the Baltimore Longitudinal Study of Aging with a critical review of the literature," Diabetes Care, vol. 28, no. 11, pp. 2626–2632, 2005.

128. A. M. Firshman and S. J. Valberg, "Factors affecting clinical assessment of insulin sensitivity in horses,"Equine Veterinary Journal, vol. 39, no. 6, pp. 567–575, 2007.

129. P. J. Cripps and R. A. Eustace, "Factors involved in the prognosis of equine laminitis in the UK," Equine Veterinary Journal, vol. 31, no. 5, pp. 433–442, 1999.

130. C. S. Venugopal, S. Eades, E. P. Holmes, and R. E. Beadle, "Insulin resistance in equine digital vessel rings: an in vitro model to study vascular dysfunction in equine laminitis," Equine Veterinary Journal, vol. 43, no. 6, pp. 744–749, 2011.

131. M. A. de Laat, C. M. McGowan, M. N. Sillence, and C. C. Pollitt, "Equine laminitis: induced by 48 h hyperinsulinaemia in Standardbred horses," Equine Veterinary Journal, vol. 42, no. 2, pp. 129–135, 2010.

132. D. M. Walsh, "Field treatment and management of endocrinopathic laminitis in horses and ponies,"Veterinary Clinics of North America, vol. 26, no. 2, pp. 379–390, 2010. View at Publisher · View at Google Scholar · View at Scopus

133. K. E. Asplin, M. N. Sillence, C. C. Pollitt, and C. M. McGowan, "Induction of laminitis by prolonged hyperinsulinaemia in clinically normal ponies," Veterinary Journal, vol. 174, no. 3, pp. 530–535, 2007.

134. M. A. de Laat, M. T. Kyaw-Tanner, A. R. Nourian, C. M. McGowan, M. N. Sillence, and C. C. Pollitt, "The developmental and acute phases of insulin-induced laminitis involve minimal

metalloproteinase activity," Veterinary Immunology and Immunopathology, vol. 140, no. 3-4, pp. 275–281, 2011.

135. B. J. Debosch, Z. Chen, B. N. Finck, M. Chi, and K. H. Moley, "Glucose transporter-8 (GLUT8) mediates glucose intolerance and dyslipidemia in high-fructose diet-fed male mice," Molecular Endocrinology, vol. 27, no. 11, 2013.

136. S. Boudina and E. D. Abel, "Diabetic cardiomyopathy revisited," Circulation, vol. 115, no. 25, pp. 3213–3223, 2007.

137. M. E. Cooper, "Importance of advanced glycation end products in diabetes-associated cardiovascular and renal disease," American Journal of Hypertension, vol. 17, no. 12, pp. 31S–38S, 2004.

138. J. Liu, M. R. Masurekar, D. E. Vatner et al., "Glycation end-product cross-link breaker reduces collagen and improves cardiac function in aging diabetic heart," The American Journal of Physiology—Heart and Circulatory Physiology, vol. 285, no. 6, pp. H2587–H2591, 2003.

139. A. L. Kranstuber, C. Del Rio, B. J. Biesiadecki et al., "Advanced glycation end product cross-link breaker attenuates diabetes-induced cardiac dysfunction by improving sarcoplasmic reticulum calcium handling," Frontiers in Physiology, vol. 3, article 292, 2012.

140. M. Asif, J. Egan, S. Vasan et al., "An advanced glycation endproduct cross-link breaker can reverse age-related increases in myocardial stiffness," Proceedings of the National Academy of Sciences of the United States of America, vol. 97, no. 6, pp. 2809–2813, 2000.

141. P. V. Vaitkevicius, M. Lane, H. Spurgeon et al., "A cross-link breaker has sustained effects on arterial and ventricular properties in older rhesus monkeys," Proceedings of the National Academy of Sciences of the United States of America, vol. 98, no. 3, pp. 1171–1175, 2001.

142. M. A. de Laat, M. T. Kyaw-Tanner, M. N. Sillence, C. M. McGowan, and C. C. Pollitt, "Advanced glycation endproducts in horses with insulin-induced laminitis," Veterinary Immunology and Immunopathology, vol. 145, no. 1-2, pp. 395–401, 2012.

143. N. Frank, C. S. Sommardahl, H. Eiler, L. L. Webb, J. W. Denhart, and R. C. Boston, "Effects of oral administration of levothyroxine

sodium on concentrations of plasma lipids, concentration and composition of very-low-density lipoproteins, and glucose dynamics in healthy adult mares," American Journal of Veterinary Research, vol. 66, no. 6, pp. 1032–1038, 2005.

144. S. S. Teixeira, A. K. Tamrakar, F. Goulart-Silva, C. Serrano-Nascimento, A. Klip, and M. T. Nunes, "Triiodothyronine acutely stimulates glucose transport into l6 muscle cells without increasing surface GLUT4, GLUT1, or GLUT3," Thyroid, vol. 22, no. 7, pp. 747–754, 2012.

145. K. D. Tinworth, S. Edwards, P. A. Harris, M. N. Sillence, L. P. Hackett, and G. K. Noble, "Pharmacokinetics of metformin after enteral administration in insulin-resistant ponies," American Journal of Veterinary Research, vol. 71, no. 10, pp. 1201–1206, 2010.

146. A. E. Durham, "Metformin in equine metabolic syndrome: an enigma or a dead duck?" Veterinary Journal, vol. 191, no. 1, pp. 17–18, 2012.

147. M. M. Vick, D. R. Sessions, B. A. Murphy, E. L. Kennedy, S. E. Reedy, and B. P. Fitzgerald, "Obesity is associated with altered metabolic and reproductive activity in the mare: effects of metformin on insulin sensitivity and reproductive cyclicity," Reproduction, Fertility and Development, vol. 18, no. 6, pp. 609–617, 2006.

148. A. E. Durham, D. I. Rendle, and J. R. Newton, "The effect of metformin on measurements of insulin sensitivity and β cell response in 18 horses and ponies with insulin resistance," Equine Veterinary Journal, vol. 40, no. 5, pp. 493–500, 2008.

149. J. L. Hustace, A. M. Firshman, and J. E. Mata, "Pharmacokinetics and bioavailability of metformin in horses," American Journal of Veterinary Research, vol. 70, no. 5, pp. 665–668, 2009.

150. J. M. G. Wearn, M. V. Crisman, J. L. Davis et al., "Pharmacokinetics of pioglitazone after multiple oral dose administration in horses," Journal of Veterinary Pharmacology and Therapeutics, vol. 34, no. 3, pp. 252–258, 2011.

151. S.-Y. Ding, Z.-F. Shen, Y.-T. Chen, S.-J. Sun, Q. Liu, and M.-Z. Xie, "Pioglitazone can ameliorate insulin resistance in low-dose streptozotocin and high sucrose-fat diet induced obese rats," Acta Pharmacologica Sinica, vol. 26, no. 5, pp. 575–580, 2005.

152. A. Hammarstedt, V. Rotter Sopasakis, S. Gogg, P.-A. Jansson, and U. Smith, "Improved insulin sensitivity and adipose tissue dysregulation after short-term treatment with pioglitazone in non-diabetic, insulin-resistant subjects," Diabetologia, vol. 48, no. 1, pp. 96–104, 2005.
153. I. M. El-Kebbi, S. Roser, and R. J. Pollet, "Regulation of glucose transport by pioglitazone in cultured muscle cells," Metabolism, vol. 43, no. 8, pp. 953–958, 1994.
154. J. G. Wearn, J. K. Suagee, M. V. Crisman et al., "Effects of the insulin sensitizing drug, pioglitazone, and lipopolysaccharide administration on markers of systemic inflammation and clinical parameters in horses," Veterinary Immunology and Immunopathology, vol. 145, no. 1-2, pp. 42–49, 2012.
155. J. K. Suagee, B. A. Corl, J. G. Wearn et al., "Effects of the insulin-sensitizing drug pioglitazone and lipopolysaccharide administration on insulin sensitivity in horses," Journal of Veterinary Internal Medicine, vol. 25, no. 2, pp. 356–364, 2011.
156. D. Bucci, G. Isani, M. Spinaci et al., "Comparative immunolocalization of GLUTs 1, 2, 3 and 5 in boar, stallion and dog spermatozoa," Reproduction in Domestic Animals, vol. 45, no. 2, pp. 315–322, 2010.

Chapter 8

Recent Advances in Reproductive Biotechnologies in Sheep and Goat

Basil Alexander[1,2], Gabriela Mastromonaco[1,3], and W. Allan King[1]

[1]Department of Biomedical Sciences, Ontario Veterinary College (OVC), University of Guelph, Ontario, Canada

[2]Department of Farm Animal Production and Health, Faculty of Veterinary Medicine and Animal Science, University of Peradeniya, Sri Lanka

[3]Reproductive Physiology, Toronto Zoo, 361A Old Finch Avenue, Scarborough, ON, M1B 5K7

CONTENTS

This review focuses on the platform of recent advances in reproductive biotechnologies in sheep and goat. Here, we discuss some aspects of veterinary and biomedical importance in artificial insemination using sexed semen, in vitro/in vivo fertilization, interspecies in vitro fertilization, multiple ovulation and embryo transfer (MOET), somatic cell nuclear transfer and transgenic animal production in sheep and goat. Some of these technologies are already widely used in the cattle industry, and some are new to the goat and sheep industry.

INTRODUCTION

The world sheep and goat populations in 2006 were recorded as 416 and 489 million, respectively [1]. Reproductive biotechnologies are playing an increasingly important role in the production and management of these species. Animal biotechnology encompasses the application of science and engineering principles to the processing or production of materials to provide services or goods for human use [2]. Examples of current animal biotechnologies include artificial insemination using fresh, frozen or sexed semen, embryo transfer using fresh or frozen in vivo or in vitro produced embryos, cloning using somatic cell nuclear transfer procedures and production of transgenic animals. Recent advances in reproductive biotechnologies have shown important developments in the technologies and their delivery that promise to yield significant benefits for their application within the livestock industry as well as in biomedical sciences. This review focuses on the recent advances of biotechnologies in sheep and goats.

METHODS

Artificial Insemination (AI)

Artificial insemination is the procedure involving the mechanical deposition of pre-collected semen into the uterus of an estrous female by a technician. The widespread commercial application of AI, a robust tool in livestock breeding, began in earnest in the 1950's after researchers developed methods to successfully freeze cattle semen [3]. This technology, which is the most extensively applied reproductive biotechnology in the world, has many valuable advantages such as reducing venereal diseases, rapidly increasing genetic merits of the production animals through selective breeding and eliminating lethal alleles. The potential to pass high genetic merits of a selected male to thousands of females makes this a far more efficient technology for producing large numbers (1.5 x 10^8) of offspring per year compared to female based technologies, such as embryo transfer (ET), which can only produce a few progeny from a selected female. More recently, the advent of separation of sperm into X- and Y-chromosome fractions using flow cytometry has added a new dimension to livestock production [4].

Since the first report of live rabbit pups of predetermined sex using X and Y-enriched sorted semen over 20 years ago [5], there have been more than 40,000 births of live animals resulting from the so- called Beltsville sperm sexing technology [4]. This sperm sexing technology has proven to be a reliable and more efficient method of obtaining predetermined sex in animals compared to other relatively wasteful methods of embryo sexing and pre-implantation genetic diagnosis [6 - 8]. Live offspring born from fresh sex- sorted semen have been reported in many species including cattle [9], pigs [10,11], horses [12,13] and sheep [14,15]. As the sorting procedure can separate sperm only at a speed of approximately 10 million per hour, inseminations have to be carried out using limited numbers of sperm in each insemination dose compared to the conventional standards for AI. To obtain high success rates with sorted semen AI, most trials have been carried out using fresh sorted semen, nevertheless, use of frozen sorted semen is ultimately more beneficial to the livestock industry as it can be stored for long duration and easy to transport anywhere in the world.

Semen Sexing Technology

Semen sexing is the process of separating spermatozoa into two subpopulations containing X-chromosome and Y-chromosome bearing spermatozoa. In theory, use of the X-bearing spermatozoa fraction for insemination will result in female progeny, while the Y-bearing spermatozoa fraction will give male progeny. Considerable efforts have been made in this area over the past 30-40 years, but only recently has there been considerable progress, particularly in cattle [16]. The most commonly applied technique for the separation of a fresh semen sample into X and Y-chromosome bearing fractions is fluorescence activated cell sorting (FACS). The concept behind this technique is described below:

Fluorescence Activated Cell Sorting (FACS)

This technique involves the separation of X- and Y- bearing spermatozoa in small quantities based on the DNA content of the spermatozoa so that they can then be used in in vitro fertilization and AI programs [17]. The procedure is relatively slow and requires expensive infrastructure at least for mass scale commercial application. The technique is based on the biological principle that the DNA content of the X and Y chromosomes as X-chromosome has 3.8% more DNA than Y-chromosome [9]. This difference can, nonetheless, be detected with FACS technique. Before the spermatozoa are passed through the cell sorter, the sample is exposed to a nontoxic DNA dye that specifically binds to DNA to allow measurement of the DNA content of each spermatozoa. The cell suspension is then passed through an extremely fine nozzle that vibrates at high frequency causing the fluid stream to disperse into micro-drops which, optimally holds only one spermatozoa after the conditions are calibrated. When the stream of micro-droplets is passing through a UV laser beam, the already stained DNA will start to glow or emit fluorescence. The strength (intensity) of the florescence is measured by a detector, and if the florescence is in the range designated for the Y-bearing spermatozoa, that micro-drop is given an electric charge. Furthermore, if the intensity is within the range for X-bearing spermatozoa, the micro-drop is given an opposite electric charge. The charged micro-drops fall between two charged plates, resulting in two groups of droplets to be separated into different pools (Figure 1). Droplets that fall outside of the fluorescence range for X or Y are collected into a third group where the sex cannot be determined. The disadvantages of the technique are its relatively slow process and increased wastage of unsorted spermatozoa. The advantage is it can give up to 95% purity sexed semen samples.

Application of Sexed Semen in Goat and Sheep Production

Although the sexed semen technology is gaining in popularity in commercial cattle industries, its use has yet to be developed in the sheep and goat industries. Nevertheless recent attempts to separate the X- and Y-chromosomal fractions using flow cytometry on ram semen has been attempted and yielded fraction purity greater than 90% [18]. In flow cytometry, the sperm extending medium plays a critical role in the efficiency of separation and the viability of the sperm after sorting [17,19,20]. Ram sperm have to be diluted 20- fold before sorting and a further 200-fold dilution takes place when it passes through the cell sorter resulting in capacitation-like changes that lead to reduced fertility of sexed sheep semen [17,20]. It has also been shown that suspension of ram semen in Tris-based medium without egg- yolk, improves the staining of the DNA and efficiency of separation of sperm without reducing its viability [8,18,21].

When working with frozen sex- sorted semen in sheep, it is believed that the semen should be deposited in the oviduct or deep within the uterus to obtain high success rates, although it appears to be not as critical in cattle [16]. In sheep, frozen semen is usually deposited laparoscopically into the uterus and these same methods have been used effectively to produce offspring from frozen sexsorted semen [15]. Oviductal deposition of frozen semen in sheep is not practical if large numbers of sheep are to be inseminated. To our knowledge, there have been no reports of attempts to inseminate sheep or goat using sex- sorted semen in the cervix or transcervically.

The minimum number of sperm in an intrauterine AI dose in sheep varies between 5 x 10^6 and 25 x 10^6, but in Australia it has been suggested as 25 x 10^6 motile spermatozoa. Although it is not known exactly the minimum number of frozen sex-sorted sperm for intrauterine insemination of sheep, it is expected that it should be in the range of standard commercial intrauterine AI semen dose [20]. However, it is acceptable that the number of sperm in frozen sex sorted semen should be increased in line with the negative effects of the sorting process to obtain high efficiency.

The timing of AI also plays a significant role in AI success in sheep but recent findings have suggested that the best results can be achieved with sex–sorted frozen sperm when inseminated just before the expected ovulation time in ovulation- synchronized progesterone treated ewes. Using sex sorted frozen semen (40 million sperm per AI dose), optimal results can be expected when ewes are inseminated at 58 h after sponge removal or 36 h after GnRH injection [20].

Embryo Production and Transfer

Multiple ovulation and embryo transfer (MOET): This breeding model has been extensively used to multiply genetically superior goats and sheep and many protocols have been developed to optimize its application in research as well as in commercial practice [22-25]. In most domestic farm animals, especially in cattle, the genetic gain is limited on the female side due to low reproductive rate with only one calf being produced per year and also relatively long intervals between generations. To overcome these limitations MOET has been developed. Using this method, a female is hormonally stimulated to have multiple ovulations (superovulation). Most MOET programs in sheep and goat consist of a 14 to 17 day progesterone exposure, with FSH injections beginning 2 days before the removal of the progesterone releasing device. Following six or eight FSH injections given twice daily, the animals are allowed to breed naturally or by artificial insemination. The ovulated ova are allowed to fertilize in vivo following artificial insemination or natural mating. After fertilization and initiation of embryo development, 6-7 day old embryos (morula/ blastocyst stage) are recovered from within the uterus using embryo flushing techniques. In sheep, this is done surgically [26]. These embryos are then transferred to non-pregnant estrus-synchronized recipients 6-7 days post estrus or frozen in liquid nitrogen (-196i° C) for future use.

It is well-known that the superovulation protocols in small ruminants do not guarantee the recovery of quality transferable embryos due to various factors that affect the success of the program [25]. These factors can be listed as extrinsic and intrinsic factors. The extrinsic factors include: a) source and purity of the gonadotrophins, b) protocol of gonadotrophin injection, and c) the type of progesterone treatment protocol [25]. Intrinsic factors include: age, breed, nutrition and reproductive status of the animals [25]. However, despite all the achievements in the MOET programs in small ruminants so far, the success of obtaining high quality transferable embryos still remains

Figure 1: Schematic representation of the concept behind the Florescent Activated Cell Sorting technique used in separation of X- and Y-bearing chromosomes in a fresh semen sample. low and more studies are needed to investigate the optimization of these programs.

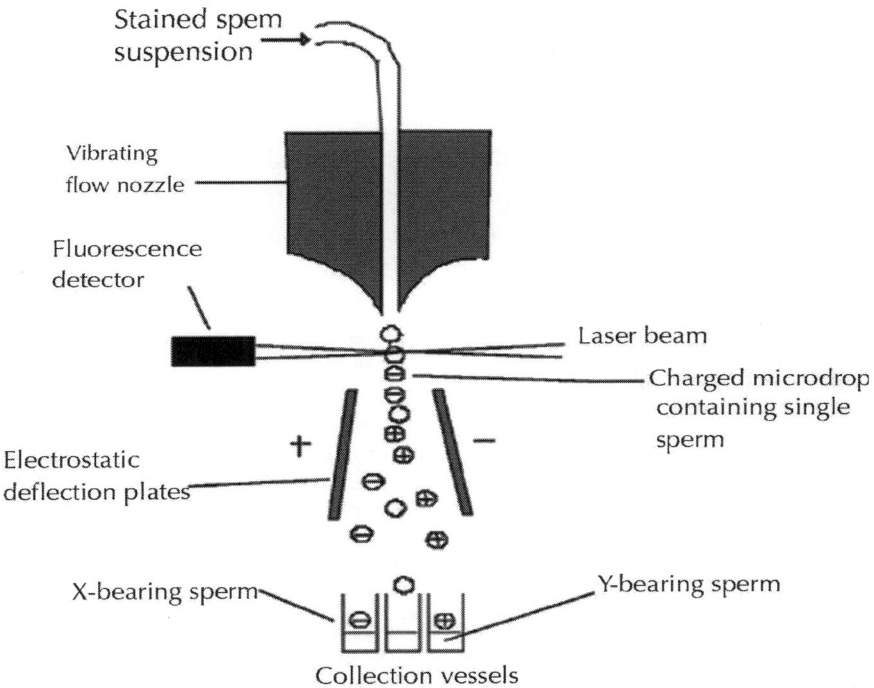

Figure 1: Schematic representation of the concept behind the Florescent Activated Cell Sorting technique used in separation of X- and Y-bearing chromosomes in a fresh semen sample.

Embryo Transfer (ET)

According to the available data from the International Embryo Transfer Society (IETS), the number of embryo transfers carried out in small ruminants is shown in Table 1. In sheep and goat, ET is usually carried out by laparoscopic surgery 6-7 days post estrus [27], (Figure 2). Estrus is generally synchronized in sheep as follows. On day-1 of the program, progesterone releasing intravaginal sponges (Veramix®, 60mg medroxyprogesterone acetate, Pharmacia & Upjohn,

Orangeville, Canada) are inserted in to the vagina. On day- 14, the sponges are removed and 300 IU PMSG (Folligon®, Intervet) are injected intramuscularly to each ewe at the time of sponge withdrawal. Vasectomised rams are introduced on day-15 and ewes in estrus are identified between 12-36 h post PMSG injections. Surgical embryo transfer is then performed on day-22 of the program [27].

The embryos are usually evaluated for morphology according to the IETS criteria [28] and only the excellent quality blastocysts/morulae are transferred into recipient ewes. Ewes are anesthetized using xylazine (0.2mg/kg) injection intravenously, and are secured on a laparoscopic cradle. An incision of approximately 1 cm is made in the skin approximately 3 cm to the left of the mid line and approximately 5cm from the udder, using a scalpel blade (Figure 2B-D). A trochar and cannula are inserted into the abdominal cavity through the incision made in the skin (Figure 2E-F). The uterine horns and the ovaries with corpora lutea are visualized using a laparoscope (Figure 2G). The uterine horn is punctured close to the utero-tubular junction using a blunt 18-gauge needle and the embryos are loaded into an embryo transfer catheter and transferred into the lumen of the uterine horn (Figure 2H). The ewes are then monitored postoperatively for a few hours and released to the paddocks.

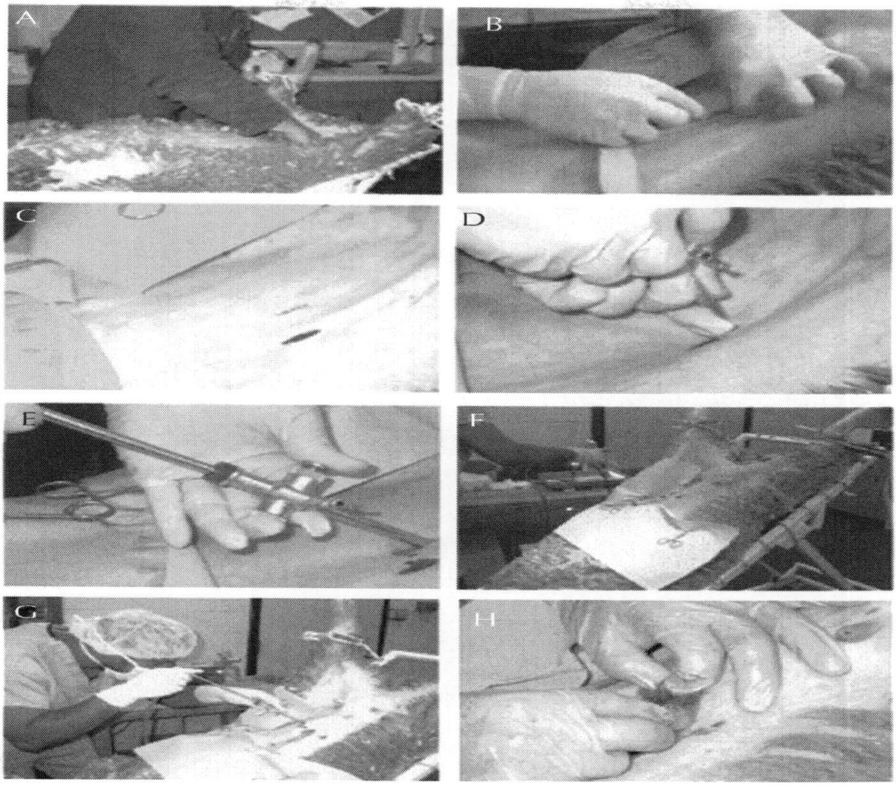

Figure 2: Embryo Transfer in sheep and goat. Embryo Transfer in sheep and goats (A–H): (A), preparation of anesthetized ewe on a cradle; (B) and (C), two skin incisions (each 1cm) are made on either side of the mid ventral line, 5 cm away from the udder; (D, E and F), insertion of trocar and cannula, cannula is left on the abdomen through which endoscope is inserted into the abdomen; (G), insertion of the endoscope through the cannula to visualize the ovaries, corpora lutea and reproductive tract; (H), a uterine horn is punctured close to the utero-tubular junction using a blunt-end 18 Gauge needle, embryos are loaded into an ET catheter and transferred into the lumen.

Table 1: World embryo transfer activity in small ruminants in 2008

Species	Transferable embryos	Transferred embryos		
		Fresh	Frozen	Total

Sheep	18828	4793	433	5226
Goat	3141	824	278	1102
Cervids	980	840	0	840

Source: Embryo transfer Newsletter, IETS, September 2009

Recently, a goat ET group in Sri Lanka reported that they have produced ET born goat kids (Figure 2B) from fresh embryos in a field embryo transfer program without using sophisticated equipment [22], thus validating the field application of the technique in veterinary practice to multiply genetically valuable goats to establish an elite goat herd under local production conditions. Moreover, ET in small ruminants is still carried out using the conventional ET techniques employing laparoscopic techniques with an average pregnancy rate of 60% with fresh embryo transfers. The pregnancy rates can vary due to many factors such as donor, recipient, embryo and operator. The transcervical ET procedure seems to be not practical in these species due to the problems associated with handling of the cervix and its anatomy. Recently, a research group [29] reported that anestrus sheep cervix can be dilated using prostaglandin 12 h prior to the insertion of AI gun into the uterus suggesting possibility of transcervical ET in sheep. However, more studies are needed to optimize this technique in small ruminants to obtain high success rates.

In Vitro Embryo Production in Sheep and Goat

In vitro embryo production in sheep and goat provides an alternate source of low cost embryos for transfer in breeding programs such as MOET. The process consists of 3 main steps: 1) oocyte collection and In vitro maturation (IVM) of cumulus-oocyte complexes (COCs), 2) In vitro fertilization (IVF) and 3) in vitro culture of embryos. These steps have been reviewed in detail by others [30 -33]. Here we will highlight the important differences between species.

Oocyte Collection and in Vitro Maturation

Prior to in vitro fertilization, COCs are collected either by minimally invasive laparoscopic ovum pick up (LOPC) or postmortem from slaughtered females [32,34]. Cumulus-oocyte complexes are collected from live sheep by a laparotomy followed by aspiration of oocytes from ovaries using an aspiration pump. This method is often called as laparoscopic ovum pick-up (LOPU) and seems to be very efficient for the recovery and quality of the COCs obtained in sheep and goats. Usually, in sheep, a short repeated gonadotrophin treatment is followed by LOPU [35-38]. In contrast, goats can be stimulated with a 'one shot' regime of gonadotrophins (one shot of follicular stimulating hormone (FSH) plus equine chorionic gonadotrophin (eCG), compared to the traditional multi-dose gonadotrophin regimes. The results revealed no differences in the efficiency of COCs recovered and their quality [36,39]. It has also been shown that 'one shot' regime can be performed as a 4-day treatment regime followed by LOPU in sheep and goats without reducing the efficiency in oocyte recovery and quality [40]. The most common method of oocyte collection is from abattoir derived ovaries from sheep or goat. Ovaries are transported to the laboratory at 37°C in phosphate buffered saline (PBS) after which they are finely sliced with a scalpel blade and rinsed in oocyte collection medium consisting of 2% steer serum in Ham's F10 medium [34].

In vitro maturation of abattoir derived oocytes from sheep and goats (for comprehensive reviews see 32, 31) rely on methods based on bi-carbonate buffered TCM 199 medium supplemented with L-glutamine, ovine FSH (10 µg/ml), ovine LH (10 µg/ml, estrogen (1 µg/ml) and 10% fetal bovine serum [34]. Some researchers have used mature follicular fluid supplementation in the IVM medium to enhance the maturation of sheep oocytes [31]. Under these conditions, goat and sheep oocytes tend to extrude first polar body between 16-24 h of in vitro maturation [41]. In contrast, it is accepted that supplementation of the glutathione precursor cysteamine (100 µM) in IVM medium enhances the in vitro maturation process of goat oocytes [41]. In addition, a recent study [42] showed that cysteamine and BSA added to IVM medium for sheep, resulted in high blastocyst rates (42% blastocyst rate from total cultured oocytes) and high survival rate of blastocysts after embryo transfer. It is obvious that artificial oocyte maturation and culture systems have detrimental effects on embryo development compared to their in vivo counterparts. Recent fluorescent in situ hybridization cytogenetic studies from our laboratory using whole chromosome painting probes have revealed that high incidence of chromosomal abnormalities in sheep blastocysts derived from IVP systems, compared to in vivo derived blastoctsts [43] emphasizing the inherent differences in the two production methods.

In Vitro Fertilization

In vitro fertilization of the oocytes is usually carried out following 24 h maturation in the IVM medium. Surrounding cumulus cells are removed by gentle pippetting and washing in fertilization medium and groups of 40-50 oocytes are placed in 4-well dishes in 500 µl of synthetic oviductal fluid (SOF) covered by 200 µl of mineral oil [31,43]. Motile sperm are obtained by centrifugation of frozen-thawed semen in Percoll gradient (45%/90%) at 500 g for 10 min in room temperature. Percoll gradient separation of spermatozoa seems to be an effective means of yielding motile sperm from frozen-thawed semen [44]. Motile sperm are collected from the bottom of the 90% fraction and diluted to a concentration of 107 spermatozoa/ml in media. Recent studies have shown that incubation of spermatozoa for a further 1 h period in media supplemented with heat-inactivated estrus serum enhances the capacitation process of spermatozoa (sheep and goat : [41]; deer : [45,46]). In our laboratory we routinely add heat – inactivated sheep serum (2%) to the IVF medium and incubate oocytes with motile spermatozoa for 17 hours resulting acceptable levels of blastocyst development [43]. Although 17 h co-incubation is practiced in IVF, it has been shown that even 4 h co-incubation was enough to obtain acceptable cleavage and blastocyst rates in sheep [41]. Further application of in vitro fertilization in obtaining sex pre-determined offspring will be an advantage for the livestock industry [20,47]. In vitro fertilization of prepubertal oocytes and oocytes recovered from LOPU [37] are also important areas to be developed further.

In Vitro Culture

Following in vitro fertilization, embryos are washed several times and then placed in in vitro culture (IVC) media for further development.

There are 3 methods available for embryo culture after fertilization, such as co-culture with somatic cells, culture in semi-defined media and culture of embryos in in vivo systems (oviducts) of the same or different species [41]. Co-culture systems in sheep and goat are usually based on including oviductal cells in TCM-199 medium. Semi-defined medium is also used often in small ruminant IVC based on the components of the sheep oviductal fluid (SOF), a medium containing essential and non-essential amino acids supplemented with BSA [43,48]. In our laboratory, sheep embryos cultured in SOF medium supplemented with amino acids and BSA at 38°C in 5% O2, 5% CO2, 90% N2 humidified atmosphere resulted in 19.2% blastocyst rates from total oocytes cultured [43]. This rate is confirmed by [38], who showed that SOF culture systems supplemented with BSA and amino acids produce high quality blastocysts in sheep. Addition of fetal bovine serum (FBS) on day 2 or 3 of culture does result in high embryo survival post-embryo transfer and normal viable offspring [41]. However, some studies have reported that sheep embryos reduce their viability by 15%–25% when produced in SOF systems supplemented with serum compared to co-culture [48] or in in vivo systems of culturing the embryos in oviducts [49]. It has been noted that adding steer serum or human serum to sheep and goat IVC media may attribute to many abnormalities in the offspring [50,51].

Interspecies in Vitro Fertilization

Investigating interspecies fertilization provides valuable insights into the role of cytoplasmic and nuclear events that regulate full term development. Due to species specific molecular, morphological and chronological markers these embryo models are unique for examining the paternal and maternal interactions and their vital role in development. Interesting findings from our laboratory revealed that ram spermatozoa is not able to fertilize bovine oocytes in vivo, however, in vitro fertilization occurs and the resulting hybrid embryos, confirmed by cytogenetic analysis (Figure 3), arrested at 4-8 cell stage [52] even when zygotes were transferred to sheep oviducts for early development. Similar developmental arrest occurs with the reverse cross. Hybridization between sheep and goats through cross or chance breeding like many species, appears to be polar with the success or efficiency dependent of the parent of origin [53]. Goats bred to rams conceive and pregnancies will progress to second trimester while in the case of the reverse cross, sheep oocytes exposed to buck sperm in vivo do not fertilize [52]. However, a few cases of sheep X goat hybrids born to goats have been documented [54]. In vitro sheep and goat oocytes, could be fertilized by buck or ram sperm and embryos developed to the blastocyst stage, hatched and, following transfer into the uteri of sheep or goats, they established pregnancies. However, retarded fetal growth, defects in placentome formation and pregnancy failure during the second month of gestation were observed [52]. The in vitro production of hybrid embryos is particularly amenable to facilitate further study of the reproductive barriers and species differences in imprinted and epigenetic, regulation of early embryo development that are key to embryo survival and development.

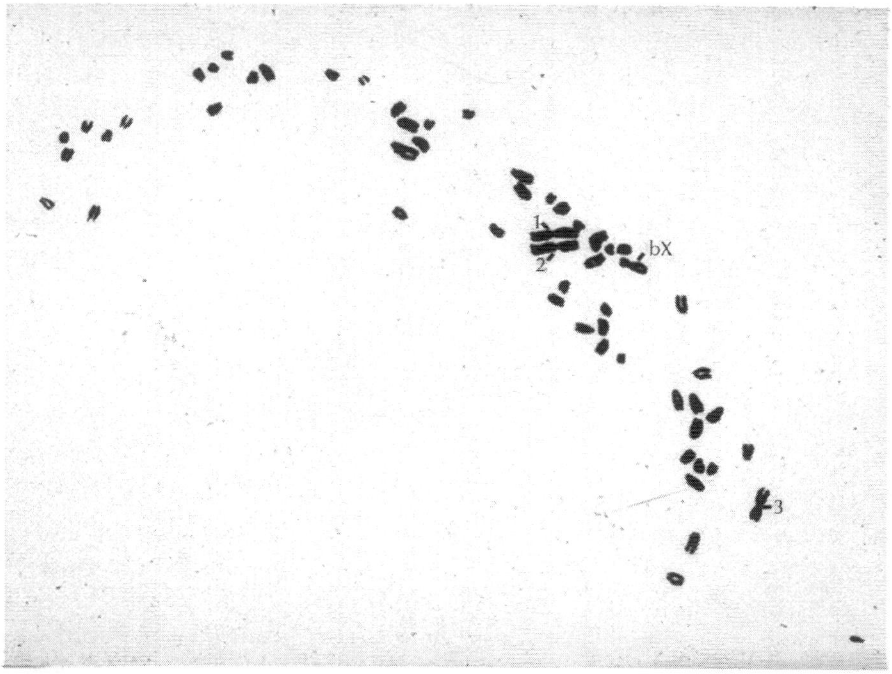

Figure 3: Metaphase spread from a 4-cell sheep-cattle hybrid embryo showing 57 chromosomes (30 cattle and 27 sheep). Note the 3 metacentric sheep chromosomes labeled 1,2 and 3 and the cattle X chromosome labeled bX. (King and Kelk, unpublished data).

Somatic Cell Nuclear Transfer (Cloning)

A new era in reproductive biotechnology began when Wilmut and colleagues produced the first somatic cell nuclear transfer (SCNT) derived viable sheep, "Dolly", from transplanting an adult somatic cell into an enucleated sheep oocyte [55]. Following this breakthrough, theoretically, it seems to be a promising technology to produce unlimited numbers of genetic copies from an adult animal or a fetus; and so far many species including farm, pet and endangered animals have been cloned using this technology [56]. Obtaining a viable offspring through this technology still imposes a great challenge for researchers due to its relatively low success rate and in some instances compromised health status of offspring [57,58]. At present, cloning is carried out for biomedical and research purposes, and agriculture production. Although extensive reviews are available on animal cloning, here we emphasize some recent findings that are important in small ruminant cloning.

The standard SCNT technique in sheep/goat in most of the laboratories follows some common steps such as oocyte maturation, removal of cumulus cells from oocytes, enucleation, transplantation of the somatic cell into the perivitelline space of the oocyte, electrofusion of the cell couplet, activation of the embryo and in vitro embryo culture. When the embryos develop to blastocyst, they are transplanted into the uteri of estrus-synchronized surrogate animals 6-7 day post estrus [27]. In most cases, the oocytes are collected from abattoir ovaries using the slicing method and undergo IVM for 17h (goat: [59-61], Sheep: [27,34]). Some laboratories that conduct goat SCNT programs preferred in vivo derived oocytes either following ovulation [62,63] or LOPU [64,65]. This may be due to the decreased availability of goat abattoirs in different countries or the higher success rates from in vivo matured oocytes. Following maturation, the cumulus cells are removed by vortexing in 3% Sodium citrate medium [27] for 1-2 minute or in 0.01% hyaluronidase. Cumulus –free oocytes with first polar body extrusion are selected and after a short exposure to cytochalasin B and Hoechst stain, enucleation is carried out in a micromanipulator equipped with UV light [27,61,64,65]. Following oocyte enucleation, cell cycle-synchronized donor cells are transplanted into the perivitelline space of the oocytes in a manner that both cell membranes attach firmly to each other. The cellcouplets are then electrofused in a 0.3

M mannitol fusion medium. One hour following fusion, cell-couplets are activated by culturing for 5 min in ionomycin containing medium followed by culturing them in 6-DMAP or cycloheximide containing medium [27,34,61]. Recent studies in our laboratory revealed that a greater incidence of chromosomal abnormalities occur when SCNT-sheep embryos are cultured in 6-DMAP containing medium compared to cycloheximide [27,34]. After activation, embryos are cultured in IVC medium and are surgically transferred into uteri of estrus –synchronized ewes [27] or into the oviducts of the does [61]. Pregnancy confirmation is done by ultrasound scanning beginning on day 35 of pregnancy. Pregnancy loss in sheep following SCNT-derived embryo transfer can be monitored by ultrasound imaging combined with serum progesterone levels [27].

Recently, there has been some controversy on the biological age of the SCNT-derived offspring, and whether they may susceptible for pre-mature death compared to their age-matched control counterparts [56]. A good example of this was the premature death of "Dolly". The hypothesis behind this is that donor somatic cells from adults may correlate with offspring carrying shortened telomere lengths compared to normal controls. Telomeres are located at the end of the chromosomes and become shorter in each cell cycle when somatic cells replicate. When the telomere length reaches a critical length the cell either enters senescence or enters a 'crisis' state associated with the development of cancer cells. This phenomenon does not happen in the germ line and in embryonic cells as these cells posses telomerase, an enzyme that adds telomere sequences to chromosomes during cell replication thus preventing telomere shortening from occurring. In most somatic cells, the telomerase enzyme is not present, leading to continuous telomere shortening when cells replicate [66].

Recent findings in telomere lengths in animal clones revealed cases of shorter [67, 68] not different [69-71] and surprisingly even longer lengths compared to those measured in their age matched control counterparts [72]. These findings have triggered much speculation on the fate of clones. However, this makes animal clones derived from adult somatic cells appropriate models for studying cellular rejuvenation and aging in vivo since they are generated from aged and culture propagated somatic cells known to contain shorten telomeres. Following SCNT, the differentiated donor nucleus undergoes extensive remodeling and reprogramming by the recipient oocyte cytoplasm

[73], which has been shown to cause altered gene expression profiles [74] and chromatin modifications [75] that likely contribute to the high incidence of abnormalities, prenatal and post natal losses found in clones [73]. Altered expression of telomerase activity [71] and donor cell type-dependent telomere length differences [76] further support inappropriate genome reprogramming, however, the precise etiology of altered telomere lengths in vivo are not clear for clones. Recent studies from our laboratory on SCNT-derived small ruminants showed that shortened telomere lengths in sheep cloned using adult donor cells compared to controls [67] and a similar phenomenon was observed in SCNTderived goats [77]. Interestingly, the offspring derived from natural breeding between cloned parents, did not show any discrepancies in telomere length [67] suggesting that telomere length was reset in the germ line of the cloned offspring. To date we do not possess enough data on telomere length of clones and "Dolly" cannot be considered the only incidence in this nature, thus more research is needed to investigate the lifespan of cloned offspring; at this stage the data available is inconclusive.

Production of Transgenic Sheep and Goats

Transgenic animals are produced either to carry an exogenous gene or to have a "knock out" gene from their own genome. Many transgenic animals have been produced for biomedical research interests as well as to test their application in livestock production [78]. There are many techniques available for the production of transgenic animals, such as pronuclear microinjection [37,79,80], sperm-mediated transgenesis [81] and somatic cell nuclear transfer[65,82,83]. During the last decade, research has focused on producing transgenic animals which secrete recombinant proteins in their milk. These animals produce relatively high quantities of recombinant proteins compared to other conventional methods due to the physiological nature of the mammary gland for its unique ability to synthesize proteins [78,84,85,86,87,88]. A few examples of transgenic small ruminants producing recombinant proteins in milk for pharmaceutical and biomedical interest are sheep producing human clotting factor VIII [89] and factor IX [82] and goats synthesizing human antithrombin III [90], human alpha-fetoprotein [91], human monoclonal antibodies [92, 93], malaria antigens [94] spider silks [95], human granulocyte colony stimulating factor (96) and human butyryl-cholinesterase [97,98]. Although these animals have shown high expression of the transgene product in the milk, a recent report suggests that the transgene may have some negative effects on the physiology of mammary gland function, leading to a compromised situation [87]. However, the first protein produced by transgenic animals, ATryn, a recombinant human anti-thrombinproduced in transgenic goats' milk, received approval for use in humans in 2009.

CONCLUSIONS

In this review, we have focused on some aspects of reproductive biotechnology that are of veterinary and biomedical importance in sheep and goat that have been reported in the recent past. It is well known that most biotechnologies take many years to come into full practice after enormous amounts of laboratory and field research. Therefore, more focus should be carried out in emerging areas like artificial insemination of sheep and goat using sexed semen, in vitro and in vivo embryo production systems, transgenic animal production and cloning using stem cells.

ACKNOWLEDGEMENTS

The authors gratefully acknowledge the assistance provided by Ed R Reyes, Elizabeth St. John, Pamela Hasson in the University of Guelph, the MITACS Accelerate internship program, Canada, the Canadian Commonwealth Scholarship Plan and the University of Peradeniya in preparation of this manuscript.

REFERENCES

1. Zygoyiannis D (2006) Sheep production in the world and in Greece. Small Rumin Res 62: 143-147.
2. Ghadar F, Spindler H (2005) The growth of biotechnology. Industrial Management 47: 19-26.
3. Polge C (1968) Frozen semen and the A.I. Programme in Proc. 2nd Tech. Conf. Artif. Insem. Reprod. NAAB, Columbia, MO: 46-51.

4. Johnson LA, Rath D, Vazquez JM, Maxwell WMC, Dobrinsky JR (2005) Preselection of sex of offspring in swine for production: current status of the process and its application.Theriogenology 63: 615-624.
5. Johnson LA, Flook JP, Hawk HW (1989) Sex preselection in rabbits: live births from X and Y sperm separated by DNA and cell sorting. Biol Reprod 41: 199-203.
6. Garner DL (2001) Sex-sorting mammalian sperm: concept to application in mammals. J Androl 22: 519-526.
7. Seidel GE Jr, Garner DL (2002) Current status of sexing mammalian spermatozoa. Reproduction 124: 733-743.
8. Evans G, Hollinshead FK, Maxwell WMC (2004) Preservation and artificial insemination of sexed semen in sheep. Reprod Fertil Dev 16: 455-464.
9. Seidel GE, Schenk JL, Herickhoff LA, Doyle SP, Brink Z, et al. (1999) Insemination of heifers with sexed sperm. Theriogenology 52: 1407-1420.
10. Vazquez JM, Martinez EA, Parrilla I, Roca J, Gill MA, et al. (2003) Birth of piglets after deep intrauterine insemination with flow cytometrically sorted boar spermatozoa. Theriogenology 59: 1605-1614.
11. Rath D, Ruiz S, Sieg B (2003) Birth of female piglets following intrauterine insemination of a sow using flow cytometrically sexed boar semen. Vet Rec 152: 400-401.
12. Buchanan BR, Seidel GE, McCue PM, Schenk JL, Heickhoff LA, et al. (2000) Insemination of mares with low numbers of either unsexed or sexed spermatozoa. Theriogenology 53: 1333-1344.
13. Lindsey AC, Schenk JL, Graham JK, Bruemmer JE, Squires EL (2002) Hysteroscopic insemination of low numbers of flow sorted fresh and frozen thawed stallion spermatozoa. Equine Vet J 34: 121-127.
14. Catt SL, Catt JW, Gomez MC, Maxwell WMC, Evans G (1996) The birth of a male lamb derived from an in vitro matured oocyte fertilized by intra-cytoplasmic injection of a single presumptive male sperm. Vet Rec 139: 494-495.
15. Hollinshead FK, O'Brien JK, Maxwell WMC, Evans G (2002) Production of lambs of pre-determined sex after the insemination

of ewes with low numbers of X- or Y-chromosome bearing spermatozoa. Reprod Fertil Dev 14: 503-508.

16. Garner DL, Seidel GE Jr (2003) Past, present and future perspectives on sexing sperm. Can J Anim Sci 83: 375-384.
17. Maxwell WMC, Johnson LA (1997) Chlortetracycline analysis of boar spermatozoa after incubation, flow cytometric sorting, cooling or cryopreservation. Mol Reprod Dev 46: 408-418.
18. Hollinshead FK, O' Brien JK, Gillan L, Mayers M, Maxwell WMC, et al. (2004) Liquid storage of
19. flow cytometrically sorted ram spermatozoa. Theriogenology 62: 587-605.
20. Catt SL, O'Brian JK, Maxwell WMC, Evans G (1997) Assessment of ram and boar spermatozoa during cell-sorting by flow cytometry. Reprod Domestic Anim 32: 251- 258.
21. Hollinshead FK, Gillan L, O'Brian JK, Evans G, Maxwell WMC (2003) In vitro and in vivo assessment of functional capacity of flow cytometrically sorted ram spermatozoa after freezing and thawing. Reprod Fertil Dev 15: 351-359.
22. De Graaf SP, Gillan L, Evans G, Maxwell WMC, O'Brian JK (2004). The effect of the sheath fluid on the quality of sex-sorted ram spermatozoa. Reprod Fertil Dev 16: 284-285.
23. Perera GDRK, Pushpakumara PGA, De Silva LNA, Alexander B (2008) Production of genetically superior goats through embryo transfer technology in Sri Lanka. Tropi Agri Res 20: 177-184.
24. Bartlewski PM, Alexander BD, Rawlings NC, Barrett DMW, King WA (2008) Ovarian responses, hormonal profiles and embryo yields in anoestrus ewes superovulated with Folltropin-V after pretreatment with medroxyprogesterone acetate (MAP)- releasing vaginal sponges and a single dose of estradiol-17ß (E2-17ß). Reprod Domest Anim 43: 299 – 307.
25. Bartlewski PM, Alexander BD, King WA (2008a) Ovarian and endocrine determinants of superovulatory responses in anestrous ewes. Small Rumin Res 75: 210-216.
26. Gonzalez-Bulnes A, Baird DT, Campbell BK, Cocero MJ, Garcia-Garcia RM, et al. (2004) Multiple factors affecting the efficiency of multiple ovulation and embryo transfer in sheep and goats. Reprod Fertil Dev 16: 421-435.

27. Menchaca A, Vilarino M, Pinczak A, Kmaid S, Saldana JM (2009) Progesterone treatment, FSH plus eCG, GnRH administration, and Day 0 Protocol for MOET programs in sheep. Theriogenology 72: 477-483.
28. Alexander B, Coppola G, Mastromonaco GF, John ES, Reyes ER, et al. (2008) Early Pregnancy Diagnosis by Serum Progesterone and Ultrasound in Sheep Carrying Somatic Cell Nuclear Transfer - Derived Pregnancies. Repro Domest Anim 43: 207-211.
29. String fellow and Seidel (1998) Manual of the International Embryo Transfer Society.
30. Candappa IBR, Bainbridge HC, Price NT, Hourigan KR, Bartlewski PM (2009) A preliminary study on the suitability of Cervidil to induce cervical dilation for artifi cial insemination in ewes. Res Vet Sci 87: 204-206.
31. Garcia-Garcia R, Ward F, Fair S, O'Meara C, Wade M, et al. (2007) Development and quality of sheep embryos cultured in commercial G1.3/G2. 3 sequential media. Anim Reprod Sci 98: 233-240.
32. Cognie Y, Poulin N, Locatelli Y, Mermillod P (2004) State-of-the-art production, conservation and transfer of in-vitro-produced embryos in small ruminants. Reprod Fertil Dev 16: 437-445.
33. Wani NA (2002) In vitro maturation and in vitro fertilization of sheep oocytes. Small Rumin Res 44: 89-95.
34. Wang S, Liu Y, Holyoak GR, Evans RC, Bunch TD (1998) A protocol for in vitro maturation and fertilization of sheep oocytes. Small Rum Res 29: 83-88.
35. Alexander B, Coppola G, Di Berardino D, Rho GJ, St John E, et al. (2006) The effect of 6-dimethylaminopurine (6-DMAP) and cycloheximide (CHX) on the development and chromosomal complement of sheep parthenogenetic and nuclear transfer embryos. Mol Reprod Dev 73: 20-30.
36. Alberio R, Olivera J, Roche A, Alabart J, Folch J (2002) Performance of a modified ovum pick-up system using three different FSH stimulation protocols in ewes. Small Rumin Res 46: 81-87.
37. Baldassarre H, Wang B, Kafi di N, Keefer C, Lazaris A, et al. (2002) Advances in the production and propagation of transgenic goats using laparoscopic ovum pickup and in vitro embryo production technologies. Theriogenology 57: 275-284.

38. Baldassarre H, Wang B, Kafi di N, Gauthier M, Neveu N, et al. (2003) Production of transgenic goats by pronuclear microinjection of in vitro produced zygotes derived from oocytes recovered by laparoscopy. Theriogenology 56: 83-839.
39. Wan PC, Haoa ZD, Zhoub P, Wua Y, Yanga L (2009) Effects of SOF and CR1 media on developmental competence and cell apoptosis of ovine in vitro fertilization embryos. Anim Reprod Sci 114: 279-288.
40. Baldassarre H, Furnus CC, De Matos DG, Pessi H (1996) In vitro production of sheep embryos using laparoscopic folliculocentesis: Alternative gonadotrophin treatments for stimulation of oocyte donors. Theriogenology 45: 707-717.
41. Gibbons A, Bonnet FP, Cueto MI, Catala M, Salamone DF, et al. (2007) Procedure for maximizing oocyte harvest for in vitro embryo production in small ruminants. Reprod Dom Anim 42: 423-440.
42. Cognie Y, Baril G, Poulin N, Mermillod P (2003) Current status of embryo technologies in sheep and goat. Theriogenology 59: 171-188.
43. Accardo C, Dattena M, Pilichi S, Mara L, Chessa B, et al. (2004) Effects of recombinant human FSH and LH on in vitro maturation of sheep oocytes: embryo development and viability. Anim Reprod Sci 81: 77-86.
44. Coppola G, Alexander B, Di Berardino D, St John E, Basrur PK, et al. (2007) Use of cross-species in-situ hybridization (ZOO-FISH) to assess chromosome abnormalities in day-6 in vivo- or in vitro-produced sheep embryos. Chromosome Res 15: 399-408.
45. Rho GJ, Hahnel AC, Betteridge KJ (2001) Comparison of oocyte maturation times and of three methods of sperm preparation for their effects on the production of goat embryos in vitro. Theriogenology 56: 503-516.
46. Comizzoli P, Mermillod P, Cognie Y, Chal N, Legendre X, et al. (2001) Successful in vitro production of embryos in red deer (Cervus elaphus) and the sika deer (Cervus nippon). Theriogenology 55: 649-659.
47. Berg DK, Thompson JG, Asher GW (2002) Development of In Vitro Embryo Production Systems for Red Deer (Cervus Elaphus).

Part 3. In Vitro Fertilisation Using Sheep Serum as a Capacitating Agent and the Subsequent Birth of Calves. Anim Reprod Sci 70: 85-98.

48. O' Brien JK, Hollinshead FK, Maxwell WMC (2004) In vivo development capacity of in vitro produced embryos derived from sex-sorted and re-cryopreserved frozen-thawed ram-sperm. Reprod Fertil Dev 16: 286.
49. Hoshi H (2003) In vitro production of bovine embryos and their application for embryo transfer.Theriogenology 59: 675-685.
50. Holm P, Walker SK, Seamark RF (1996) Embryo viability, duration of gestation and birth weight in sheep after transfer of in vitro matured and in vitro fertilized zygotes cultured in vitro or in vivo. J Reprod Fertil 107: 175-181.
51. Sinclair KD, McEvoy TG, Maxfi eld EK, Maltin CA, Young LE, et al. (1999) Aberrant fetal growth and development after in vitro culture of sheep zygotes. J Reprod Fertil 116: 177-186.
52. Walker S, Hill J, Kleeman D, Nancarrow C (1996) Development of ovine embryos in synthetic oviductal fluid containing amino acids at oviductal fluid concentrations. Biol Reprod 55: 703-708.
53. Kelk DA (1997) Development characteristics of interspecific hybrid embryos. PhD Thesis. University of Guelph, Ontario, Canada.
54. Anderson GB (1988) Interspecific pregnancy: barriers and prospects. Biol Reprod 38: 1-15.
55. Pinheiro LEL, Guimaraes SEF, Almeida IL, Mikich AB (1989) The natural occurrence of sheep X goat hybrids. Theriogenology 32: 987 – 994.
56. Wilmut I, Schnieke AE, McWhir J, Kind AJ, Campbell KH (1997) Viable offspring derived from fetal and adult mammalian cells. Nature 385: 810-813.
57. Vajta G, Gjerris M (2006) Science and technology of farm animal cloning: state of the art. Anim Reprod Sci 92: 211-230.
58. Hill JR, Roussel AJ, Cibelli JB, Edwards JF, Hooper NL, et al. (1999) Clinical and pathological features of cloned transgenic calves and fetuses (13 case studies). Theriogenology 51: 1451-1465.

59. Rho GJ, Coppola G, Sosnowski J, Kasimanickam R, Johnson WH, et al. (2007) Use of somatic cell nuclear transfer to study meiosis in female cattle carrying a sex-dependent fertility-impairing X-chromosome abnormality. Cloning Stem Cells 9: 118-29.
60. Ma S, Lan G, Miao Y, Wang Z, Chang Z, et al. (2003) Hypoxanthine (HX) inhibition of in vitro meiotic resumption in goat oocytes. Mol Reprod Dev 66: 306-313.
61. Lan GC, Han D, Wu YG, Han ZB, Ma SF, et al. (2005) Effects of duration, concentration and timing of ionomycin and 6-dimethylaminopurine (6-DMAP) treatment on activation of goat oocytes. Mol Reprod Dev 71: 380-388.
62. Lan GC, Chang ZL, Luo MJ, Jiang YL, Han D, et al. (2006) Production of Cloned Goats by Nuclear Transfer of Cumulus Cells and Long-Term Cultured Fetal Fibroblast Cells Into Abattoir-Derived Oocytes. Mol Reprod Dev 73: 834-840.
63. Zou X, Wang Y, Cheng Y, Yang Y, Ju H, et al. (2002) Generation of cloned goats (Capra hircus) from transfected foetal fibroblast cells, the effect of donor cell cycle. Mol Reprod Dev 61: 164-172.
64. Behboodi E, Memili E, Melican DT, Destrempes MM, Overton SA, et al. (2004) Viable transgenic goats derived from skin cells. Transgenic Res 13: 215-224.
65. Keefer CL, Stone RK, Bhatia B, Lazaris A, Begin I, et al.(2000) Efficient production of viable goat offspring following nuclear transfer using adult somatic cells. Biol Reprod 62: 192.
66. Keefer CL, Baldassarre H, Keyston R, Wang B, Bhatia B, et al. (2001) Generation of dwarf goat (Capra hircus) clones following nuclear transfer with transfected and nontransfected fetal fi broblasts and in vitro-matured oocytes. Biol Reprod 64: 849-856.
67. Xu J, Yang X (2003) Will cloned animals suffer premature aging - the story at the end of clone's chromosomes. Reprod Biol Endocrinol 1: 105-110.
68. Alexander B, Coppola G, Perrault SD, Peura TT, Betts DH, et al. (2007) Telomere length of sheep clones and their offspring. Mol Reprod Dev 74: 1525-1537.
69. Shiels PG, Jardine AG (2003) Dolly, no longer the exception: Telomeres and implications for transplantation. Cloning stem cells 5: 157-160.

70. Jiang L, Carter DB, Xu J, Yang X, Prather RS, et al. (2004) Telomere lengths in cloned transgenic pigs. Biol Reprod 70: 1589-1593. Betts DH, Bordingnon V, Hill JR, Winger Q, Westhusing ME, et al. (2001) Reprogramming of telomerase activity and rebuilding of telomere length in cloned cattle. Proc Natl Acad Sci USA 98: 1077-1082.
71. Betts DH, Bordingnon V, Hill JR, Winger Q, Westhusing ME, et al. (2001) Reprogramming of telomerase activity and rebuilding of telomere length in cloned cattle. Proc Natl Acad Sci USA 98: 1077-1082.
72. Tian XC, Xu J, Yang X (2000) Normal telomere lengths found in cloned cattle. Nat Genet 26: 272-273.
73. Lanza R, Cibelli JB, Blackwell C, Cristofalo VJ, Francis MK, et al. (2000) Extension of cell life- span and telomere length in animals cloned from senescent somatic cells. Science 288: 665-669.
74. Reik W, Dean W (2002) Epigenetic reprogramming: back to the beginning. Nature 420: 127.
75. Humpherys D, Eggan K, Akatsu H, Friedman A, Hoechedlinger K, et al. (2002) Abnormal gene expression in cloned mice derived from embryonic stem cell and cumulus cell nuclei. Proc Natl Acad Sci USA 99: 12889-12894.
76. Dean W, Santos F, Stojkovic M, Zakhartchenko V, Walter J, et al. (2001) Conservation of methylation reprogramming in mammalian development: aberrant reprogramming in cloned embryos. Proc Natl Acad Sci USA 98: 13734- 13738.
77. Miyashita N, Shiga K, Yonai M, Keneyama K, Kobayashi S, et al. (2002) Remarkable differences in telomere lengths among cloned calves derived from different cell types. Biol Repro 66: 1649-1655.
78. Betts DH, Perrault SD, Petrik J, Lin L, Favetta LA, et al. (2005) Telomere length analysis in goat clones and their offspring. Mol Reprod Dev 72: 461-470.
79. Wheeler MB, Walters EM, Clark SG (2003) Transgenic animals in biomedicine and agriculture: outlook for the future. Anim Reprod Sci 79: 265-289.
80. Ebert KM, Selgrath JP, DiTullio P, Denman J, Smith TE, et al. (1991) Transgenic production of a variant of human tissue-type

plasminogen activator in goat milk: generation of transgenic goats and analysis of expression. Biotechnology 9: 835- 838.

81. Baldassarre H, Wang B, Gauthier M (1999) Embryo transfer in a commercial transgenic production program using BELE® goat embryos. Theriogenology 51: 415.

82. Celebi C, Guillaudeux T, Auvray P, Vallet-Erdtmann V, Jegou B (2003) The making of "transgenic spermatozoa". Biol Reprod 68: 1477-1483.

83. Schnieke AE, Kind AJ, Ritchie WA, Mycock K, Scott AR, et al. (1997) Human Factor IX transgenic sheep produced by nuclear transfer of nuclei form transfected fetal fibroblasts. Science 278: 2130-2133.

84. Keefer CL, Lazaris A, Keyston R (2002) Cloning using somatic cells for the production and propagation of transgenic Nigerian dwarf and dwarf-crossed goats. Theriogenology 57: 422.

85. Houdebine LM (2000) Transgenic animal bioreactors Transgenic Res 9: 305-320.

86. Keefer CL (2004) Production of bioproducts through the use of transgenic animal models. Anim Reprod Sci 82: 5-12.

87. H, Wang B, Pierson J, Neveu N, Sneek L, et al. (2004) Prepubertal Propagation of Transgenic Cloned Goats by Laparoscopic Ovum Pick-Up and in Vitro Embryo Production. Cloning Stem Cells 6: 25-29.

88. H, Hockley DK, Dore M, Brochu E, Hakier B, et al. (2008a) Lactation performance of transgenic goats expressing recombinant human butyrylcholinesterase in the milk. Transgenic Res 17: 73-84.

89. Baldassarre H, Hockley DK, Olaniyan B, Brochu E, Zhao X, et al. (2008b) Milk composition studies in transgenic goats expressing recombinant human butyrylcholinesterase in the mammary gland. Transgenic Res 17: 863-872.

90. Niemann H, Halter R, Carnwath JW, Herrmann D, Lemme E, et al. (1999) Expression of blood clotting factor VIII in the mammary gland of transgenic sheep. Transgenic Res 8: 237-247.

91. Zhou Q, Kyazike J, Echelard Y, Meade HM, Higgins E, et al. (2005) Effect of

92. genetic background on glycosylation heterogeneity in human antithrombin
93. produced in the mammary gland of transgenic goats. J Biotechnol 117: 57-72.
94. Parker MH, Birck-Wilson E, Allard G, Masiello N, Day M, et al. (2004) Purification and characterization of a recombinant version of human alpha-fetoprotein expressed in the milk of transgenic goats. Protein Expr Purif 38: 177-183.
95. Young MW, Meade H, Curling JM, Ziomek CA, Harvey M (1998) Production of recombinant antibodies in the milk of transgenic animals. Res Immunol 149: 609- 610.
96. Pollock DP, Kutzko JP, Birck-Wilson E, Williams JL, Echerlard Y, et al. (1999) Transgenic milk as a method for the production of recombinant antibodies. J Immunol Methods 231: 147-157.
97. Behboodi E, Ayres SL, Memili E, O'Coin M, Chen LH, et al. (2005) Health and reproductive profi les of malaria antigen-producing transgenic goats derived by somatic cell nuclear transfer.Cloning Stem Cells 7: 107-118.
98. Karatzas CN, Zhou FJ, Huang Y, Duguay F, Chretien N, et al. (1999) Production of recombinant spider silk (BioSteel®) in the milk of transgenic animals. Transgenic Res 8: 476-477.
99. Ko JH, Lee CS, Kim KH, Pang MG, Koo JS, et al. (2000) Production of biologically active human granulocyte colony stimulating factor in the milk of transgenic goat. Transgenic Res 9: 215-222.
100. Cerasoli DM, Griffi ths EM, Doctor BP, Saxena A, Fedorko JM, et al. (2005) In vitro and in vivo characterization of recombinant human butyrylcholinesterase (Protexia) as a potential nerve agent bioscavenger. Chem Biol Interact 158: 363- 365.
101. Huang YJ, Huang Y, Baldassarre H, Wang B, Lazaris A, et al. (2007) Recombinant human butyrylcholinesterase from milk of transgenic animals to protect against organophosphate poisoning. Proc Natl Acad Sci USA 104: 13603-13608.

Chapter 9

Changes in Adenylate Nucleotides Concentration and Na+, K+-ATPase Activities in Erythrocytes of Horses in Function of Breed and Sex

Maria Suska and Ewa Skotnicka

Department of Physiology, Faculty of Life Sciences, University of Szczecin, Piastów 40 B, av, bl. 6, 71-065 Szczecin, Poland

ABSTRACT

The aim of this study was to examine the relationships between the concentrations of ATP, ADP, AMP (HPLC methods), total nucleotide pool (TAN), adenylate energy charge (AEC) and Na^+, K^+-ATPase erythrocytic activities (by Choi's method) of horses as a function of breed and sex.

The studies were conducted on 54 horses (stallions and mares) of different constitution types: breathing constitution (Wielkopolska and Hanoverian breed) and digestive constitution (Ardenian breed). Horse erythrocytes, independently of examined breed, present low ATP concentration in comparison to other mammal species while retaining relatively high AEC. Erythrocytes of breathing constitution type horses appear to have a more intensive glucose metabolism and a more efficient energetic metabolism when compared to digestive constitution type horses. The conclusions may be proven by significantly higher ATP concentration, higher TAN and significantly higher AEC in breathing constitution type horses compared to the digestive constitution type. Sex does not significantly influence adenine nucleotides concentration in the erythrocytes of the examined horses, however, stallions have slightly higher values in comparison to mares. A positive correlation was found between Na^+, K^+, -ATPase activity, ATP, ADP and AMP concentration and TAN in Wielkopolska and Ardenian breeds, which was not confirmed for the Hanoverian breed.

INTRODUCTION

The horse (Equus caballus L.) is the only mammal that went through evolution in the steppes. Lacking an active protection mechanism against predators, escape is the only way to protect its life and thus to guarantee the survival of the species. To allow for an intensive run, during which oxygen consumption can be up to 35 times higher than in resting tomes, both the anatomical structure and the overall metabolism of horses have been optimized during evolution to favour energy supply to the muscles. Contemporary horses, selected by man according to his needs or likes, did not lose their elementary cell characteristic of quick energy delivery and high energy consumption. This also holds true for erythrocytes, which play a key physiological function in oxygen binding and transport to the tissues.

The study of purine nucleotide metabolism is very important for the understanding of disruptions in energy metabolism as the purine nucleotides participate in most energy-requiring metabolic reactions and act as coenzymes [1, 2]. Characteristic compounds in the erythrocyte energy metabolism are the adenylate nucleotides (ATP, ADP, AMP) which undergo reversible changes in glycolysis and in pentose phosphate pathway [3, 4]. They are involved in the control of the correct shape of red blood cells, active transport through the membrane, phosphorylation of proteins and phospholipids, and the synthesis of glutathione and pyridine coenzymes Moreover, ATP plays a significant role in transferring energy within the cell, diffusing from where it is produced to where it is utilized. ATP in erythrocytes is utilized in ion transport processes that account for almost 30% of the total ATP consumption. Na^+ and K^+ transport utilizes a lot of ATP, while Ca^{2+} transport requires markedly less energy. There is no consensus in literature on the dependence of Na^+,K^+-ATPase (EC 3.6.1.37) and Ca^+-ATPase (EC 3.6.1.3) on ATP. For this reason we also attempted to find out the relations between the ATP concentration and the activity of Na^+,K^+-ATPase (EC 3.6.1.37) [5–9]. Mathematic modelling suggests that during changes in ATP-consuming processes, adenylate metabolism may regulate the adenylate energy charge (AEC) of the cell [10].

The rate of glucose metabolism and the concentration of metabolites of the glycolytic pathway in the erythrocytes of various species of mammals, as well as the concentration of the adenylate nucleotides, are genetically determined [11] and also depend on species and age [12–14]. Different exogenous (heavy metal ion influence; such as fluorine, lead) and endogenous (physical effort, pregnancy, morbidity such as diabetes) factors may also influence these values [15–18].

The aim of this study was to compare the erythrocyte energy metabolism in stallions and mares of three horse breeds of different constitution and different functional characteristics (Wielkopolska breed, Hanoverian breed, Ardenian breed). The study was to determine the relationships between the ATP, ADP, AMP and Na^+,K^+-ATPase activities on one hand, and the level of TAN and AEC values on the other, in the erythrocytes as a function of breed and sex.

MATERIALS AND METHODS

Animals and Management Practices

The studies were conducted for 54 clinically healthy horses aged 3-4 years of different constitution type: Wielkopolska breed (W: n = 8 stallions and w: n=8 mares), Hanoverian breed (H: n = 8 stallions and h: n = 10 mares), Ardenian breed (A: n = 10 stallions and a: i= 10 mares). The horses came from environmentally clean areas, were not in training and were fed and treated equally. The animals had a standard diet with respect to their age. The horses did not show any sign of particular stress during blood sampling. All studies were approved by the Local Ethics Committee.

Blood Sampling

In order to eliminate the influence of physical strain and circadian changes on some biochemical indices, 2mL of blood per heparinized test tube (250 IU heparine from Polfa Poland) was taken from the external jugular vein early in the morning before feeding. The blood was delivered to the laboratory in ice flasks and immediately analyzed.

HPLC Separation of Purine

Chemicals: Purines used as chromatographic standards were obtained from Sigma-Aldrich. HPLC grade acetonitrile was obtained from Merck. HPLC grade potassium dihydrogen orthophosphate, potassium chloride and tripotassium orthophosphate were obtained from Fluka Chemie GmbH. HPLC grade water was prepared using a Milli-Q (Millipore purification system). All HPLC solvents were filtered through 0.22 μm nylon filters (Supelco) before use.

Instrumentation: For the HPLC analysis, a Hewlett Packard chromatographic system was used. The HP series 1100 chromatographic system consisted of a quaternary pump system with a degasser and a continuous seal wash option (G1311A), a variable-wavelength detector (G1314) and a thermostatted column compartment (G1316A). The analytical column (100 × 4.6mm LC) was packed with 18.3μm Hypersil BDS-C (Hewlett Packard). Samples were introduced using a Rheodyne 7725 injection valve equipped with a 20μm loop. Sample peaks were integrated and quantified using an HPLC chromatography data system operating on Chemstation Software for Windows 98 (Hewlett Packard).

HPLC separation of adenine nucleotides: The samples (500μL) were deproteinized with 500μL of 1.3M perchloric acid in 1.5mL Eppendorf tubes. Extract mixtures were centrifuged (16000g for 10 minutes, at 4°C). The supernatant (600 Jll) was neutralized with approximately

60–90μL of 3M potassium orthophosphate solution (pH range of the sample at 6.3). The neutralized extract was centrifuged again and filtered through a nylon filter of 0.22 μm. The obtained clear filtrate was used directly for the HPLC assay or stored at –80°C.

Purine nucleotide: determination: Concentrations of purine nucleotides: ATP, ADP, and AMP were measured by the HPLC method of Smolenski et al. [19]. Sample aliquots (100μL) were injected into the chromatograph column and the nucleotides were separated using a linear phosphate buffer gradient system at the flow rate of 0.666mL/min (buffer A: 150 mM KH_2PO_4, 150mM KCl adjusted to pH 6.0 with K_2HPO_4; buffer B: 15% v/v solution of acetonitrile in buffer A). Peaks were detected by absorption measurements at 254nm. The composition of the mobile phase was controlled by a low-pressure gradient mixing device. The cycle time was 12.8 minutes between injections. The analytical column was maintained at constant temperature of 20.5°C. The adenine nucleotide concentrations (μM in the whole blood) were calculated according to factors given in the method of Smolenski et al. [19]. Then the adenine nucleotide concentrations in the erythrocytes were calculated using the value of the packed cell volume (PCV).

The total adenylate nucleotides (TAN) and the adenylate energy charge (AEC) were calculated according to the formulas:

$$\begin{aligned} TAN &= [ATP] + [ADP] + [AMP] \\ AEC &= \frac{1}{2} * \frac{[ADP] + 2[ATP]}{[ATP] + [ADP] + [AMP]}. \end{aligned} \tag{1}$$

MEASUREMENTS OF ATPASE ACTIVITIES

The Na^+,K^+-ATPase activities were determined on erythrocyte plasma membranes by Choi's method [20]. For the determination of membrane ATPase, aliquots of a 25μL membrane suspension, containing 25–50μg of protein, were preincubated at 37°C for 5 minutes in the following media: 20mM KCl; 100mM NaCl; 0.5mM EGTA; 30mM histidine-imidasole buffer (pH 7.0); 0.5mM $MgCl_2$. The enzymatic reaction was started by adding 2mM ATP. After 30 minutes of incubation at 37°C, the reaction was stopped by adding 1mL of ice cold 20% trichloric acid. Then the mixture was centrifuged at 20000G for 2 minutes and the inorganic phosphate released into the supernatant was measured, according to the Goldenberg and Fernandez method [21]. Enzyme activity is expressed as of nmol of P_i per mg membrane proteins per 60 minutes determined according to Lowry et al. [22].

Statistical Evaluation

The results are given as mean values $(\overline{x})$ and standard deviations (SD). The statistical significance of differences among the groups was determined with the monofactor analysis of variance (ANOVA) using the evaluation of statistical significance of differences for many means and NIR Tukey's test (paired design). The Pearson's correlation coefficient was determined in all the groups (according to the Statistica PL software) for all adenylate nucleotide, TAN and ATPase activity, as well as the value of the AEC. The regression lines with marked values of correlation coefficients [r] were drawn for the significant relationships within the groups.

RESULTS

Mean values and standard deviations determined for the adenine nucleotides concentrations, nucleotides pool and adenylate energy charge in the erythrocytes and in chosen haematological indicators (RBC, Hb) of stallions: Wielkopolska breed (W), Hanoverian breed (H), Ardenian breed (A) were gathered in Table 1, and for mares (w, h, a) in Table 2.

Table 1: Concentration of adenine nucleotides: ATP, ADP, AMP (μM), total adenylate nucleotide pool (TAN) and values of the adenylate energy charge (AEC) in erythrocytes of stallions Wielkopolska breed (W), Hanoverian breed (H), Ardenian breed (A) Legend: $(\overline{x})$-mean; ±SD—standard deviation; **-significant difference ($P<.01$); *-significant difference ($P<.05$), n-group size

Group	n		ATP	ADP	AMP	TAN	AEC	RBC [1012/L]	Hb [g/L]
			μM RBC						
W	8	x	178.3	28.3	5.5	212.1	0.91	8.31	98
		±SD	12.5	3.8	1.6	14.7	0.013	0.39	9.1
H	8	x	155.0	24.9	4.3	184.2	0.91	8.01	91
		±SD	11.3	4.2	0.8	13.0	0.012	0.76	3.8
A	10	x	148.7	29.5	5.5	183.8	0.89	7.71	77
		±SD	12.9	2.8	0.5	15.3	0.006	0.97	2.8
Statistical significance of the group differences			W, A** W, H*	A, H*	A, H*	W, H* W, A*	H, A** W, A*	W, A*	W, A* A, H*

Table 2: Concentration of adenine nucleotides: ATP, ADP, AMP (μM), total adenylate nucleotide pool (TAN) and values of the adenylate energy charge (AEC) in erythrocytes of mares Wielkopolska breed (w), Hanoverian breed (h), Ardenian breed (a) Legend: $\overline{(x)}$-mean; ±SD—standard deviation; **- significant difference (P < .01); *- significant difference (P < .05), n-group size

Group	n		ATP	ADP	AMP	TAN	AEC	RBC [1012/L]	Hb [g/L]
			μM RBC						
w	8	x	175.4	27.8	6.1	209.3	0.90	8.27	92
		±SD	9.6	3.2	1.1	10.7	0.004	0.61	7.5
h	10	x	150.4	24.0	4.0	178.5	0.91	8.05	88
		±SD	21.5	1.8	0.5	21.0	0.013	0.77	2.2
a	10	x	147.3	28.0	5.4	180.7	0.89	7.53	73
		±SD	21.2	2.9	0.6	23.0	0.010	0.81	7.1
Statistical significance of the group differences			w, a* w, h*	h, a** w, h*	h, a** w, h**	w, h* w, a*	h, a**	w, a*	w, a* h, a*

We determined statistically significant differences in ATP concentrations in stallions and mares of all the breeds, respectively, at *P*<.05 and *P*<.01 (Tables 1 and 2). The highest ATP concentration was determined in Wielkopolska stallions (178.3 ± 12.5$\mu M_{0x0039cRBC}$) and mares (175.4 ± 9.6$\mu M_{0x0039cRBC}$). The lowest ATP values were found in the Ardenian horses, both stallions (148.7 ± 12.5 $\mu M0x0039c$RBC), and mares (147.3 ± 21.2$\mu M_{0x0039cRBC}$), while average values were found in the Hanoverian breed (stallions-155.1 ± 11.3$\mu M_{0x0039cRBC}$, mares-150.4 ± 21.5$\mu M_{0x0039cRBC}$). Wielkopolska stallions have significantly higher ATP concentrations in comparison to Hanoverian ($P<.05$) and Ardenian breed ($P<.01$). The difference of ATP concentration between Hanoverian and Ardenian breeds was not statistically significant. Slightly higher ATP erythrocyte concentrations were found in stallions in comparison to mares regardless of breed (Tables 1 and 2).

ADP and AMP concentrations in the erythrocytes of Hanoverian stallions were the lowest among the examined breeds. However, significant differences for the determined parameters were found between Hanoverian and Ardenian stallions $P<.01$ (Table 1).

Nucleotides pool values (TAN) in the erythrocytes of stallions and mares of Wielkopolska breed have a higher value in comparison to Hanoverian and Ardenian breeds (stallions-212.1 ± 14.7$\mu M_{0x0039cRBC}$, mares-209.3 ±10.7$\mu M_{0x0039cRBC}$). The differences were statistically significant at $P<.05$ (Table 1). Stallions of all the examined breeds have higher adenine nucleotides pool (TAN) in comparison to mares. However, in none of the examined groups statistically significant differences were found. No significant differences in adenylate energy charge (AEC) were found between stallions and mares (Tables 1 and 2).

A significant intra-group positive correlation between the ATP erythrocyte concentration and the nucleotides pool TAN was found in stallions and mares of all three breeds. Statistically significant correlation was found between ATP and adenylate energy charge (AEC) values in the Hanoverian and Ardenian, whereas in the Wielkopolska mares the correlation coefficient value although significant, was the lowest (Table 3).

Table 3: Correlation coefficient (r) between ATP concentration and total adenylate nucleotide pool (TAN) and values of the adenylate energy charge (AEC) in erythrocytes of stallions and mares Wielkopolska breed (W,w), Hanoverian breed (H,h), Ardenian breed (A, a); *-significant difference (P < .05)

ATP						
	W	H	A	w	h	a
TAN (μM RBC)	0.93	0.94	0.99	0.96	1.00	0.99
AEC	0.65	0.97	0.76	0.67	0.97	0.77

The lowest Na^+,K^+-ATPase activity of erythrocytes was found in the Ardenian horses, both stallions (0.22 ±0.05μMP^i/mg protein/h) and mares (0.19±0.02μMP^i/mg protein/h). Both Wielkopolska and Hanoverian stallions presented similar activity of the examined enzyme, respectively, 0.34 ± 0.06μMP^i/mg protein/h and 0.34 ± 0.01μMP^i/mg protein/h; the enzyme activity in Wielkopolska mares was (0.28 ± 0.02μMP^i/mg protein/h) and in Hanoverian mares, 0.33 ± 0.04 (μMP^i/mg protein/h) (Table 4). One-way analysis of variance and Tukey's test allowed us to find significantly higher Na^+,K^+-ATPase activity in Hanoverian stallions in comparison to Ardenian stallions at $P<.001$. While the difference between Wielkopolska and Ardenian stallions was significant at $P<.01$. A significantly higher erythrocyte Na^+,K^+-ATPase activity was found in Hanoverian mares in comparison to Wielkopolska mares at $P<.05$, while the difference between Wielkopolska and Ardenian mares was significant at $P<.001$.

Table 4: The Na^+, K^+-ATPase activities of the erythrocytes and $Na^+ : K^+$ ions ratio in blood serum of stallions and mares Wielkopolska breed (W, w), Hanoverian breed (H, h), Ardenian breed (A, a)

Group	n		Na+,K+-ATPase	Na+ : K+
			µmolPi/mg protein/h	
W	8	x	0.34	32.30
		±SD	0.06	
H	8	x	0.34	34.80
		±SD	0.01	
A	10	x	0.22	37.70
		±SD	0.05	
w	8	x	0.28	34.20
		±SD	0.02	
h	10	x	0.33	34.70
		±SD	0.04	
a	10	x	0.19	39.20
		±SD	0.02	

Correlation coefficients (r) concerning intra-group relationships analysis between Na^+,K^+-ATPase activity and ATP, ADP, AMP, TAN concentrations and AEC values in the erythrocytes of the examined horse breeds are presented in Table 5. Positive significant relationship was found between ATP erythrocyte concentration and Na^+,K^+-ATPase activity of erythrocytes in the groups of Wilekopolska (r=0.65) and Ardenian stallions (r=0.85). Moreover, significant correlation between AMP concentration and ATPase activity was found in the stallions of all the examined breeds: respectively, Wielkopolska breed r=0.66, Ardenian breed r=0.66,Hanoverian breed r=0.53. In Hanoverian horses no significant correlations between ADP concentration and Na^+,K^+-ATPase activity was found. Such correlation was found in the Ardenian horses (r=0.65). In Wielkopolska and Ardenian stallions a significant correlation was found between adenine nucleotides pool (TAN) and ATPase activity. Coefficient *r* was respectively 0.76 for Wielkopolska breed and 0.85 for Ardenian breed. We found significant correlation between ADP concentration and ATPase activity in the group of Wielkopolska (r=0.77) and Ardenian (r=0.62) mares. Significant correlations between adenylate energy charge (AEC) and Na^+,K^+-ATPase activity values were not found for the examine breeds (Table 5).

Table 5: Correlation coefficient (r) between adenine nucleotides concentration (μM), total adenylate nucleotide pool (TAN), values of the adenylate energy charge (AEC) in erythrocytes and the Na^+, K^+-ATPase activities of stallions and mares Wielkopolska breed (W, w), Hanoverian breed (H, h), Ardenian breed (A, a); *-significant difference ($P<.05$)

Dependent variable		Independent variable									
		ATP		ADP		AMP		TAN		AEC	
		µM RBC									
Na+, K+-ATPase µmolPi/ mgprotein/h		stallions	mares	stallions	Mares	stallions	mares	stallions	mares	stallions	mares
	W, w	0.65*	0.35	0.49	0.76*	0.66*	0.56*	0.76*	0.48	-0.37	-0.09
	H, h	0.10	0.40	0.43	0.20	0.53*	0.01	0.26	0.43	-0.46	0.32
	A, a	0.85*	0.47	0.65*	0.66*	0.66*	0.36	0.85*	0.52*	0.23	0.52*

DISCUSSION

The history of horses' evolution goes back 40-million years. The representatives of horses appeared on Earth millions of years before Homo erectus. Horse's ancestor was Hyracotherium (Eohippus), which lived at the area of present Northern America. Its rear limbs had 3 digits, while the anterior limbs had 4 digits. During the evolution process many indirect forms arose (such as Mesohippus, Merychippus i Philohippus).

The modern horse is the result of a long-lasting evolution process which resulted from the natural adaptation of the animals to the environment. The appearance of the horse on steppes and the necessity of grass feeding determined the adaptation direction for millions of years. Extensive empty spaces did not provide the horse with an appropriate shelter that was why it had to learn to escape its enemy quickly and efficiently. The effects of which may be seen in the adaptation of the motor system to the fast run and unusual resistance of the organism to hypoxia and high acidity resulting from the intensive run. The above is possible due to an immense concentration of the erythrocytes in the spleen which are ready for use the moment there is a necessity to provide muscles with the oxygen.

Moreover multigenerational selection of horses by man for different usage purposes has brought into existence many horse breeds different not only in structure, size and beautiful appearance, but also in the rate of cell metabolism.

The initial material for modern horse breeding of Wielkopolska horses were local, primitive forest horses, which were at first crossbred with heavy horses and then improved by oriental (Persian and Arabic) blood horses as well as by the Thoroughbred horses. Since the XVIII century the breed was created mostly by Trakehner and other horses from eastern Europe, and only partially by Hanoverian and other German half-breed horses. The selection of Wielkopolska breed was leading to forming a horse of a high weight, appropriate and efficient movement and gentle nature—suitable for drawing. Modern Wielkopolska horses are mainly functional animals, with the majority of riding characteristics.

Hanoverian horses are recognized as the best sport horses bred in Germany. They appeared at the beginning of the XVIII century. Their appearance was greatly influenced by a state owned stud in Celle, where, at the beginning, Holsteiner stallions were used as sires. After the Second World War the Hanoverian horse breeding led to the creation of sport horse and for that reason it was crossbred with Trakehners (resistance improvement) and with Thoroughbred horses (the improvement of courage and movement). Modern Hanoverian horses are characterized by high strength, appropriate movement, gentle nature and good boniness. The Hanoverian horse is good for competitive sport, especially for dressage and horse jumping. Although the Hanoverian is not a sprinter due to being a functional animal; thanks to its strength and efficient movement it is as effective as other breeds when in a run.

The Ardenian breed derived from the ancient horses coming from Solutré. In France the following types are recognized: French Arden (called Eastern); trait du nord (Northen Arden) i auxois. The functional characteristics of the Ardenian horses were influenced by Belgian horses, small Brabansons, Percherons, Boulonnais and Norman horses. This obedient, calm, massive, strong and muscular horses are perfect for physical works. All the Ardenian horses are mainly used for meat. Belgian, Luxemburg and Swedish Ardens also belong of the group of the Ardenian horses.

Comparing individual average adenine nucleotides concentration values in red blood cells of the examined horses it may be assumed that the ATP concentration is several dozen times higher than the AMP concentration, and ADP is of average value. Relationships among ATP, ADP and AMP concentrations determine the adenylate energy charge (AEC) value, which under physiological conditions, is always 0.8-0.9, regardless of cell type and generic features [23].

Based on the literature high interspecies changeability of the erythrocytic ATP concentration may be assumed. Approximate ATP, ADP, and AMP contents in chosen mammals are presented in Table 6.

Table 6: Concentration of adenine nucleotides: ATP, ADP, AMP (μM) in erythrocytes of chosen animal species (the own study based on the references [11] [B], [12][C], [14][D], [25][A])

Species of mammals	human	Pig	horse	goat	dog
ATP [μM RBC]	1650A	2220A	120A	710A	590A
	1438B		184.9D		639B
	1519C				
ADP [μM RBC]	216B		28.8D		138B
	171C				
AMP [μM RBC]	21B		5.7D		40B
	12C				

The obtained research results explicitly suggest that among the examined mammals, horses, regardless of breed, have relatively low physiological ATP concentration in the erythrocytes, which was also confirmed by other authors [24, 25]. Despite low ATP erythrocytic concentration, energy charge (AEC) value was relatively constant and comprised within the 0.89–0.92 range. Adenine nucleotides pools (TAN) of the examined horses, on the other hand, varied depending on breed and sex.

The relatively low ATP concentration of erythrocytes found in horses compared to other animal species may be the result of the erythrocytes size, the diameter of which is about 5μm [26]. Therefore, the hypothesis that a connection may exist between small erythrocyte size, low ATP concentration and lively breathing of the organism may find confirmation in our data.

The highest adenine nucleotides pool (TAN) was found in stallions and mares of breathing constitution type horses of Wielkopolska breed, and the lowest in digestive constitution type horses of Ardenian breed. The ATP concentration which decides about adenylate pool in erythrocytes was significantly higher in Wielkopolska horses in comparison to Hanoverian and Ardenian breeds. Leyko et al. [27] found that in the erythrocytes adenine nucleotides concentration, TAN values and AEC are determined genetically, which was also proven by our study. The changes of the ATP concentration in the erythrocytes of the examined horses may possibly be connected with the changes of the hematological indicators' values of the examined animals since the highest amount of red blood cells and hemoglobin were found in Wielkopolska horses (stallions: RBC—8.31×10^{12}/L ±0.39, Hb—98 g/L ± 9.1; mares: RBC—8.27×10^{12}/L ± 0.61, Hb—92 g/L ± 7.5), najnisz u rasy ardeskiej (stallions: RBC—7.71×10^{12}/L ± 0.97, Hb—77 g/L ± 2.8 mares: RBC—7.53×10^{12}/L ± 0.81, Hb—73 g/L ± 7.1). Genetically determined higher amount of red blood cells is favorable for a better adaptation of the horse to a physical effort of a high-speed type and for more effective gas exchange connected with an adaptation to a long run [11, 27, 28]. The observed differences were formed during a long, multigenerational selection of horses. They prove better predispositions and adaptation to a high-speed effort in breathing constitution type horses (Wielkopolska and Hanoverian breeds) compared to digestive constitution type (Ardenian breed) which is rather predisposed to endurance exertion

Harvey and Kaneko [28] indicate that in physiological conditions there are certain generic differences in the utilization of glucose in the process of glycolysis. Horse erythrocytes have a higher hexokinase activity (HK, EC 2.7.1.1) in comparison to other animals which may influence the rate of metabolic utilization of glucose. However, the glucose utilization rate in horse erythrocytes is half the rate of humans and dogs, and 2/3 in comparison to cat's erythrocytes [28]. Still as much as 13% of glucose used by horses is metabolized in the pentose phosphate pathway, while humans, cats and dogs only use half (about 6%). Glucose-6-phosphate (G-6-P), created in the reaction catalyzed by HK, acting as an allosteric inhibitor of the enzyme, may reduce glucose utilization in the process of glycolysis [29]. It was proven that G-6-P regulation depends on intracellular pH. Optimal pH value for the glycolysis process is 8.2, and for pentose phosphate pathway: 7.6 [28].

A relatively high glucose utilization in the pentose phosphate pathway [28] and a low glucose utilization in the process of glycolysis in horses may result in a relatively low ATP concentration in horses in comparison to other species [5]. Breathing constitution type horses' erythrocytes (Wielkopolska and Hanoverian breeds) may be subjected to more intensive glucose changes and more effective energetic metabolism of the erythrocytes in comparison to digestive constitution type horses (Ardenian breed). This is suggested by our data, which have proven the existence of higher ATP concentration, higher adenine nucleotides pools (TAN) and a significantly higher adenylate energy charge (AEC), which may make breathing constitution type horses more suitable for long distance runs [30]. Moreover, higher erythrocytic ATP concentration and higher TAN values of breathing constitution type horses may be the result of a higher adenylate kinase activity (AK, EC 2.7.4.3) catalyzing the reaction 2 ADP = ATP + AMP. In the short term this mechanism protects cells against an excessive drop of ATP concentration and nucleotides pool [31].

Some mammals (a rat, a mouse, a rabbit, a human, a dog, a pig) have significant amounts of 2,3-BPG in the erythrocytes compared to a sheep and a cow [11]. This metabolite is responsible for intraerythrocytic regulatory mechanism of oxygen releasing from the blood to the cells. It also participates in the regulation of RBC metabolism [4, 32, 33]. The increase of 2,3-BPG amount in blood indicates the decrease of hemoglobin's affinity for oxygen and the increase of P_{50} value (partial oxygen pressure at which 50%of the hemoglobin is saturated with oxygen). This leads to the increased ability for oxygen delivery to the tissues and more intensive metabolism. The amount of glucose metabolized to create 2,3-BPG in human erythrocytes under physiological conditions was estimated for 19% and it depends on ADP concentration in RBC [34]. With the decrease of ADP concentration in the erythrocytes 2,3-BPG concentration increases, if, however, the ADP concentration compared to ATP is high, 2,3-BPG decrease may be observed. The regulatory mechanism of 2,3-BPG concentration by ADP results from the fact that ADP and 2,3-BPG are the reagents in the reaction of phosphoglicerine kinase (PGK, EC 2.7.2.3) and the changes of their concentrations may influence the content of 1,3-BPG [33].

Keeping higher 2,3-BPG concentration in the erythrocytes is energetically expensive but it allows for a proper regulation of hemoglobin's affinity for oxygen to the speed of the metabolism. It is physiologically favorable as lower oxygen affinity (higher P_{50} values) allows for easier oxygen delivery to the tissues in animals characterized by more intensive metabolism.

Sex does not have a significant influence on adenine nucleotides concentration (ATP, ADP, AMP) in red blood cells of the examined horses, however, stallions have slightly higher values in comparison to mares.

A positive correlation between ATP, ADP, AMP, and TAN concentrations and Na^{+},K^{+}-ATPase activity of the erythrocytes was found in Wielkopolska and Ardenian horses, which was not confirmed in Hanoverian breed. Na^+,K^+-ATPase activity depends on the breed. The highest enzyme activity was found in Wielkopolska breed, and the lowest in Ardenian horses. The interbreed differences in the enzyme activity were also observed in humans [35].

Na^+,K^+-ATPase activity regulation is influenced by many endogenous factors [36]. The enzyme activity depends on the saturation degree of the substrates binding sites and on the cytoplasmatic products of the enzymatic reaction—ADP and P_i concentration [37].

The inhibit influence of ADP on the enzyme activity based on competition between ADP and ATP for enzyme protein binding sites. The effect of ADP and Na^+,K^+-ATPase binding is lowered when the ATP concentration is higher [37]. Both in vitro and in vivo researches have shown that the K^+ concentration increase in the erythrocytes results in a higher Na^+,K^+-ATPase activity. However, lowering of the K^+ concentration in the solution of the cell, or partial saturation of Na^+,K^+-ATPase binding sites, results in the restrain of the enzyme activity [37, 38]. Na^+,K^+-ATPase activity of the membrane cell is significantly influenced by pH (the highest activity at pH = 9.5, the lowest activity at pH = 6.0). Enzyme activity also depends on Ca^{2+} concentration. Ca^{2+}may compete with K^+ or Mg^+ (reaction cofactors) for enzyme receptor site [39]. We found lower Na^+,K^+-ATPase activity in the examined mares in comparison to stallions, with a simultaneous increase of K^+concentration and decrease of Na^+ concentration in serum. It may be related to the hormonal state of the mares' organisms [40].

ACKNOWLEDGMENTS

The author's wishes to thank Mr. Anna Piorkowska for her help in translation.

REFERENCES

1. W. Dudziska and A. J. Hłyczak, "Purine nucleotides of human erythrocytes—metabolism and regulation," Postepy Biochemii, vol. 50, no. 4, pp. 353–362, 2004.

2. W. Dudziska, A. J. Hłyczak, E. Skotnicka, and M. Suska, "The purine metabolism of human erythrocytes," Biochemistry, vol. 71, no. 5, pp. 467–475, 2006.
3. F. I. Ataullakhanov, V. M. Vitvitskii, S. V. Komarova, and E. V. Mosharov, "Energy-dependent processes and adenylate metabolism in human erythrocytes," Biochemistry, vol. 61, no. 2, pp. 197–203, 1996.
4. K. V. Fokina, M. Y. Yazykova, P. V. Danshina, E. V. Schmalhausen, and V. I. Muronetz, "Participation of glyceraldehyde-3-phosphate dehydrogenase in the regulation of 2,3-diphosphoglycerate level in erythrocytes," Biochemistry, vol. 65, no. 4, pp. 463–468, 2000.
5. T. Arai, T. Washizu, M. Sagara, et al., "D-glucose transport and glycolytic enzyme activities in erythrocytes of dogs, pigs, cats, horses, cattle and sheep," Research in Veterinary Science, vol. 58, no. 2, pp. 195–196, 1995.
6. C. Brugnara, "Erythrocyte membrane transport physiology," Current Opinion in Hematology, vol. 4, no. 2, pp. 122–127, 1997.
7. J. F. Hoffman, "ATP compartmentation in human erythrocytes," Current Opinion in Hematology, vol. 4, no. 2, pp. 112–115, 1997.
8. W. G. Siems, O. Sommerburg, and T. Grune, "Erythrocyte free radical and energy metabolism," Clinical Nephrology, vol. 53, supplement 1, pp. S9–S17, 2000.
9. V. Bennett and A. J. Baines, "Spectrin and ankyrin-based pathways: metazoan inventions for integrating cells into tissues," Physiological Reviews, vol. 81, no. 3, pp. 1353–1392, 2001.
10. A. Joshi and B. O. Palsson, "Metabolic dynamics in the human red cell—part IV: data prediction and some model computations," Journal of Theoretical Biology, vol. 142, no. 1, pp. 69–85, 1990.
11. J. W. Harvey, "The erythrocyte: physiology, metabolism, and biochemical disordes," in Clinical Biochemistry of Domestic Animals, J. J. Kalenko, J. W. Harvey, and M. L. Bruss, Eds., pp. 125–142, Academic Press, New York, NY, USA, 1997.
12. T. W. Traut, "Physiological concentrations of purines and pyrimidines," Molecular and Cellular Biochemistry, vol. 140, no. 1, pp. 1–22, 1994.

13. H. Brommer, M. M. SloetVan Oldruitenborgh-Oosterbaan, and B. Kessels, "Haematological and blood biochemical characteristics of dutch warmblood foals managed under three different rearing conditions from birth to 5 months of age," Veterinary Quarterly, vol. 23, no. 2, pp. 92–95, 2001.
14. M. Suska, E. Skotnicka, W. Dudziska, W. Orowicz, and M. Brzeziska, "Adenylate nucleotides and 2,3-biphosphoglycerate concentration in erythrocytes of growing Wielkopolska stallions," Acta Veterinaria Brno, vol. 75, no. 1, pp. 13–20, 2006.
15. M. Suska, "The effect of sodium fluoride on the adenine nucleotide pool in erythrocytes of wistar rats,"International Journal of Occupational Medicine and Environmental Health, vol. 14, no. 4, pp. 369–373, 2001.
16. M. Suska, "Energy metabolism of erythrocytes in lambs chronically exposed to fluorine compounds,"Acta Veterinaria Brno, vol. 71, no. 3, pp. 313–317, 2002.
17. W. Dudzi ska and A. J. Hłyczak, "Purine nucleotides and their metabolites in erythrocytes of streptozotocin diabetic rats," Diabetes and Metabolism, vol. 30, no. 6, pp. 557–567, 2004.
18. E. Skotnicka, I. Baranowska-Bosiacka, W. Dudziska, et al., "The effect of exhaustive exercise on the concentration of purine nucleotides and their metabolites in erythrocytes," Biology of Sport, vol. 25, no. 1, pp. 35–55, 2008.
19. R. T. Smolenski, D. R. Lachno, S. J. M. Ledingham, and M. H. Yacoub, "Determination of sixteen nucleotides, nucleosides and bases using high-performance liquid chromatography and its application to the study of purine metabolism in hearts for transplantation," Journal of Chromatography, vol. 527, no. 2, pp. 414–420, 1990.
20. S. J. Choi, M. A. Taylor, and R. Abrams, "Depression, ECT, and erythrocyte adenosinetriphosphatase activity," Biological Psychiatry, vol. 12, no. 1, pp. 75–81, 1977.
21. H. Goldenberg and A. Fernandez, "Simplified method for the estimation of inorganic phosphorus in body fluids," Clinical Chemistry, vol. 12, no. 12, pp. 871–882, 1966.
22. O. H. Lowry, N. J. Rosenbrough, A. L. Farr, and R. J. Randall, "Protein measurment Folin with the fend reagent," The Journal of Biological Chemistry, vol. 193, pp. 256–267, 1951.

23. D. E. Atkinson, "The energy charge of the adenylate pool as a regulatory parameter. Interaction with feedback modifiers," Biochemistry, vol. 7, no. 11, pp. 4030–4034, 1968.
24. B. Dbski, "The effect of training and physical exercise on the energetic metabolism of equine erythrocytes," Zentralblatt für Veterinärmedizin. Reihe A, vol. 32, no. 3, pp. 190–195, 1985.
25. A. Miseta, P. Bogner, E. Berenyi, et al., "Relationship between cellular ATP, potassium, sodium and magnesium concentrations in mammalian and avian erythrocytes," Biochimica et Biophysica Acta, vol. 1175, no. 2, pp. 133–139, 1993.
26. W. Stankiewicz, Veterinary Haematology, PZWiL, Warszawa, Poland, 1972.
27. W. Leyko, G. Bartosz, W. Duda, Z. Wojtkowiak, and A. Kołtaj, "The content of nucleotides in erythrocytes of different breeds of cattle," Genetica Polonica, vol. 15, no. 1-2, pp. 91–96, 1974.
28. J. W. Harvey and J. J. Kaneko, "Glucose metabolism of mammalian erythrocytes," Journal of Cellular Physiology, vol. 89, no. 2, pp. 219–223, 1976.
29. S. Fujii and E. Beutler, "High glucose concentrations partially release hexokinase from inhibition by glucose 6-phosphate," Proceedings of the National Academy of Sciences of the United States of America, vol. 82, no. 5, pp. 1552–1554, 1985.
30. M. Janiak, M. Suska, W. Dudziska, and E. Skotnicka, "Blood glutathione status and activity of glutathione-metabolizing antioxidant enzymes in erythrocytes of young trotters in basic training,"Journal of Animal Physiology and Animal Nutrition. In press.
31. R. J. Zeleznikar, P. P. Dzeja, and N. D. Goldberg, "Adenylate kinase-catalyzed phosphoryl transfer couples ATP utilization with its generation by glycolysis in intact muscle," The Journal of Biological Chemistry, vol. 270, no. 13, pp. 7311–7319, 1995.
32. J. M. Ramsey and S. W. Pipoly Jr., "Response of erythrocytic 2,3-diphosphoglycerate to strenuous exercise," European Journal of Applied Physiology and Occupational Physiology, vol. 40, no. 4, pp. 227–233, 1979.
33. K. V. Fokina, M. B. Dainyak, N. K. Nagradova, and V. I. Muronetz, "A study on the complexes between human erythrocyte enzymes

participating in the conversions of 1,3-diphosphoglycerate," Archives of Biochemistry and Biophysics, vol. 345, no. 2, pp. 185–192, 1997.
34. P. J. Mulquiney, W. A. Bubb, and P. W. Kuchel, "Model of 2,3-bisphosphoglycerate metabolism in the human erythrocyte based on detailed enzyme kinetic equations: in vivo kinetic characterization of 2,3-bisphosphoglycerate synthase/ phosphatase using 13C and 31P NMR," Biochemical Journal, vol. 342, no. 3, pp. 567–580, 1999.
35. N. Lasker, L. Hopp, S. Grossman, R. Bamforth, and A. Aviv, "Race and sex differences in erythrocyteNa+, K+, and Na+-K+-adenosine triphosphatase," The Journal of Clinical Investigation, vol. 75, no. 6, pp. 1813–1820, 1985.
36. F. Canestrari, F. Galli, S. Boschi, et al., "Erythrocyte Na+,K+-ATPase properties and adenylate energy charge in normotensives and in essential hypertensives," Clinica Chimica Acta, vol. 224, no. 2, pp. 167–179, 1994.
37. H.-J. Apell, M. T. Nelson, M. M. Marcus, and P. Lauger, "Effects of the ATP, ADP and inorganic phosphate on the transport rate of the Na+,K+-pump," Biochimica et Biophysica Acta, vol. 857, no. 1, pp. 105–115, 1986.
38. G. N. Ling, "Explaining on request a correlation between membrane Na+,K+-ATPase and K+ content in erythrocytes and other findings in the preceding paper," Physiological Chemistry and Physics and Medical NMR, vol. 30, no. 1, pp. 89–97, 1998.
39. P. L. Pedersen, "Transport ATPases in biological systems and relationship to human disease: a brief overview," Journal of Bioenergetics and Biomembranes, vol. 34, no. 5, pp. 327–332, 2002.
40. M. Udziela, "Sodium and potassium concentrations in erythrocytes and blood plasma of young women in differential physiological state," Wiadomosci Lekarskie, vol. 21, no. 21, pp. 1905–1908, 1968 (Polish).

Chapter 10

Scrotal Circumference and Its Relationship with Testicular Growth, Age, and Body Weight in Tho Tho (Bos indicus) Bulls

P. Perumal

Animal Reproduction Laboratory, National Research Centre on Mithun (ICAR), Jharnapani, Nagaland 797 106, India

ABSTRACT

The present study was undertaken to assess the relationship between the scrotal circumference and testicular parameters with body weight and age in Tho Tho bulls (Bos indicus), which were maintained at around the villages of National Research Centre on Mithun (ICAR), Jharnapani,

Nagaland, India. A total of 32 Tho Tho bulls were selected and divided into four groups according to their age and each group consisted of 8 bulls, namely, Group I: 18–24 months (n=8), Group II: 25–36 months (n=8), Group III: 37–48 months (n=8), and Group IV: 49 months and above (n=8). The scrotal circumference and testicular parameters were measured with caliper and tape and age of animals was calculated with dental formula. The body weight of bulls was estimated with Shaeffer's formula. Result revealed that the scrotal circumference was highly correlated with testicular parameters and body weight compared to age. Compared to exotic cattle (Bos taurus), Tho Tho bull's testicular parameters and scrotal circumference were lower. The results of the present study in Tho Tho bulls revealed that scrotal circumference is a useful indicator and is an important selection criterion to determine the testicular development and breeding soundness in young bulls as it is highly correlated with tesicular parameters.

INTRODUCTION

Tho Tho cattle (Bos indicus) is a local indigenous bovine species of North Eastern Hilly (NEH) region especially in Nagaland state of India. It is rearing under semi-intensive system. The bull is half of the herd in animal husbandry, which indicates that the sire is one of the parents of all the calves in the herd. Since the bull has more genetic influence (80–90%) of calves it sires, fertile bull selection can be the most powerful method for improvement of the herd. The demand for sperm from outstanding sires has increased with the development of frozen semen technology and the growth of large artificial breeding organizations. Methods to predict sperm production potential and particularly to identify the bulls with high sperm output potential at an early age are important, which is related with testicular parameters and scrotal circumference. Traditionally, Tho Tho bulls have been selected on the basis of growth, rather than on reproductive traits. However, reproduction is one of the most important factors for the economics of livestock production. Generally, testicular measurements at early ages are very useful in selection of breeding sire to collect semen for artificial insemination or breeding purpose. The most important parameters are testicular diameter, testicular length, testicular volume, and scrotal circumference. The males with bigger testes produce more sperm than the males with smaller testes [1]. Regression equations have revealed that testicular size was positively related to body weight and age [2]. Positive correlations between prepubertal male hormone levels and subsequent testes size and mating frequency have also been reported [3]. These are the potentially useful indicators of reproductive traits and have been used to compose selection indices for Tho Tho bulls to use in breeding purpose. These traits are easily measured and correlated with body weight and reproductive performance [4–6]. Testicular weight and body growth of large number of dairy bulls were measured to develop techniques which would give repeatable results and to determine which one was most highly correlated with scrotal circumference. This study also was designed to provide the basis for investigation of parameters useful in predicting future reproductive performance and in establishing the extent to which differences in these parameters are varied.

Measurement of scrotal circumference and testicular parameters is an essential part of breeding soundness evaluation of breeding bulls. Measurement of these parameters especially scrotal circumference has a great value on onset of puberty, total semen production, semen quality, pathological conditions of reproductive system, and the fertility or infertility status of breeding bulls [7]. Moreover, testicular measurements have been utilized as the indicators for reproductive capabilities in the postpubertal period of bulls [8]. Scrotal circumference is highly correlated with body weight and age [9] and it is highly correlated with testis weight [10] and testicular consistency is correlated with fertility [11]. Scrotal circumference and testicular parameters have a direct relationship with sperm production. Testis size and body weight provides idea about the physical and physiological maturity of the bulls, its sperm output, and birth weight of its young ones [12]. There are various reports on the testicular growth and related to semen attributes in matured dairy bulls [13–18], buffaloes [19–21], ram [22], and mithun bulls [23]. If these reproductive traits are to be incorporated into management and breeding programs, it is desirable that their relationships to other traits are to be understood. There are various factors involved in influencing scrotal circumference and testicular measurements such as age, breed of the bulls [24], and season of the year [25].

Studies associating with body weight, testicular measurements, and scrotal circumference obtained during the different phases of growth of

Tho Tho bovine species are scarce. In this respect, it is not only necessary to determine how these traits respond to selection at different ages, but also to determine the magnitude of correlation between these traits. Therefore, the present study was designed to estimate the testicular parameters at different ages and correlate with body weight and age in Tho Tho bulls to provide data for the definite selection of Tho Tho bulls for future breeding purpose and conservation of this precious indigenous bovine species.

MATERIALS AND METHODS

Experimental Animals

A total of thirty-two apparently healthy Tho Tho bulls with different age groups were selected from the herd of villages at around the National Research Centre on Mithun (ICAR), Nagaland, India. The study area lies between 25°54'30" North latitude and 93°44'15" East longitude and at an altitude range of 250–300 mean sea levels. The animals were maintained under semi-intensive condition of grazing in the forest during day time and ting them in shed during night time. The experimental animals in shed were fed daily with ad libitum quantity of locally available forages without providing concentrate. Fresh water was available throughout the day.

Age of the bulls was determined using their dental formula. The body weight of each bull was calculated according to Shaeffer's formula [25]: $L \times G^2/300 \times 2.2$, where L = body length in inch and G = girth in inch. According to their age, the experimental bulls were equally divided into four groups, each of 8 bulls, namely, Group I: 18–24 months (n=8), Group II: 25–36 months (n=8), Group III: 37–48 months (n=8), and Group IV: 49 months and above (n=8).

Testicular Measurement

Testicular parameters and scrotal circumference were measured with a caliper (Mitutoya Digimatic Caliper) and a tape after restraining the bull in the chute [26]. Testicular length was measured by placing the fixed arm of the caliper at the proximal end and the sliding arm at the distal end of the testes. Care was taken to exclude the epididymides. Thickness or depth was measured by placing the fixed arm of the caliper at the anterior aspect and the sliding arm at the posterior aspect of the each testis, at the point of maximum depth. Width of each testis was measured by sliding the other testes up in the scrotum and placing one arm of the caliper at the medial aspect and the other at the lateral aspect, at the point of maximum width. For measurement of scrotal circumference, the testicle was pushed firmly into the bottom of the scrotum by placing the thumb and fingers laterally on the side of the neck of the scrotum and pushed ventrally. A flexible cloth tape was formed into a loop and slipped over the scrotum and scrotal circumference was measured in centimeters by pulling the tape snugly around its greatest diameter [26]. Testes volume was calculated by using the formula for volume of an ellipsoid, that is, $4/3\pi abc$, where a = thickness/2, b = width/2, and c = length/2 (Love et al. 1991). Weight of the testes was measured by multiplying volume with 1.038 which is the approximate density of testicular tissue in cattle [27].

Statistical Analyses

The results were analyzed statistically and expressed as the mean ± S.E.M. Means were analyzed by one way analysis of variance between the different age groups of Tho Tho bulls, followed by Tukey's post hoc test to determine significant differences between the groups using the SPSS/PC computer program (version 15.0; SPSS, Chicago, IL). Differences with values of $P<0.05$ were considered to be statistically significant. Correlation coefficient was estimated among the testicular parameters, scrotal circumference, age, and body weight of the bulls. Differences at $P<0.05$ and $P<0.01$were considered to be statistically significant.

RESULTS

The results of different testicular parameters, scrotal circumference, and body weight at different age of Tho Tho bulls were presented in Table 1, which indicated that these parameters were significantly ($P<0.05$) different between the age groups. It has been reported that the average estimated testicular weight was 18.50, 40.20, and 51.25% greater in bulls aged 25–36, 37–48, and >49 months of age than in 18–24-month-old bulls. Similarly the average estimated testicular volume was 15.50, 28.69, and 33.85% greater in bulls aged 25–36, 37–48, and >49 months of age than in 18–24-month-old bulls. In case of scrotal circumference, the average estimated value was 6.76, 10.58, and 13.35% greater in bulls aged 25–36, 37–48, and >49 months of age than in 18–24-month-old bulls. Correlations between the different measurements for the 32 bulls are shown in Table 2. Similarly as expected, various measurements of the testis were highly correlated with each other (P<0.01) as in exotic cattle [18], buffalo [21], and mithun [23]. Body weight was more highly correlated with the various testicular measurements than age. But also according to age, the testicular parameters were increased significantly (P<0.05) in Tho Tho cattle bulls. Moreover age (Figure 1), testis weight (Figure 2), and body weight (Figure3) of Tho Tho cattle bulls were highly correlated with scrotal circumference. Scrotal circumference was highly correlated with other testicular measurements as well as testicular volume. Scrotal circumference was a simple measurement to obtain; maximum circumference is reached at 5-6 years of age and remains relatively constant thereafter. These results indicate that scrotal circumference is a useful indicator and is an important selection criterion to determine the testicular development in young bulls and it has highly correlation with testicular parameters.

Table 1: Scrotal circumference, testicular, and seminal parameters of Tho Tho (Bos indicus) bulls at different ages (mean ± S.E.)

Scrotal and testicular characters	18–24 months (n=8)	25–36 months (n=8)	37–48 months (n=8)	49 months and above (n=8)
Age	20.83 ± 1.52a	30.50 ± 2.12b	42.50 ± 2.24c	55.33 ± 2.08d
Body weight (Kg)	219.33 ± 4.31a	282.83 ± 4.01b	323.17 ± 5.47c	423.83 ± 5.56d
Scrotal circumference (cm)	27.97 ± 1.18a	30.00 ± 1.05b	31.28 ± 0.98bc	32.27 ± 1.22c

Left testes length (cm)	8.84 ± 0.68a	9.63 ± 0.59b	9.63 ± 0.66b	9.78 ± 0.60b
Left testes width (cm)	5.72 ± 0.52a	5.77 ± 0.54a	6.58 ± 0.44b	6.82 ± 0.38b
Left testes thickness (cm)	5.88 ± 0.61a	6.23 ± 0.38b	6.45 ± 0.37bc	6.87 ± 0.40c
Left testes volume (cm3)	146.53 ± 4.12a	181.46 ± 4.68b	213.80 ± 4.23c	239.05 ± 4.64d
Left testes estimated weight (gm)	152.09 ± 4.20a	188.35 ± 4.74b	221.93 ± 4.20c	248.13 ± 4.38d
Right testes length (cm)	9.74 ± 0.69a	10.03 ± 0.61ab	10.40 ± 0.77b	10.25 ± 0.60ab
Right testes width (cm)	6.11 ± 0.52a	6.26 ± 0.49a	6.99 ± 0.41b	7.19 ± 0.37b
Right testes thickness (cm)	6.21 ± 0.48a	6.67 ± 0.50b	6.85 ± 0.53bc	7.12 ± 0.43c
Right testes volume (cm3)	191.66 ± 5.78a	219.25 ± 4.56a	260.37 ± 5.26b	272.48 ± 4.12b
Right testes estimated weight (gm)	198.95 ± 5.42a	227.58 ± 4.98a	270.26 ± 5.09b	282.83 ± 4.20b
Total volume (cm3)	338.19 ± 6.59a	400.71 ± 6.75b	474.17 ± 6.29c	511.53 ± 5.24c
Total weight (gm)	351.04 ± 6.71a	415.94 ± 6.88b	492.19 ± 6.40c	530.97 ± 5.32c

Figures in parenthesis indicate number (n) of Tho Tho cattle bulls.

Figures with same superscript (a, b, c, and d) do not differ significantly in rows.

Table 2: Correlation coefficients between scrotal circumferences, age, body weight, and various testicular measurements in Tho Tho (Bos indicus) bulls

Number	Measurement	2	3	4	5	6	7	8	9	10	11	12	13	14	15
1	Age	0.82**	0.90**	0.56**	0.91**	0.86**	0.88**	0.88**	0.62**	0.92**	0.90**	0.94**	0.94**	0.93**	0.93**
2	Body weight		0.89**	0.52**	0.86**	0.85**	0.85**	0.85**	0.62**	0.87**	0.88**	0.91**	0.91**	0.89**	0.98**
3	Scrotal circumference			0.70**	0.88**	0.93**	0.93**	0.93**	0.70**	0.86**	0.92**	0.93**	0.93**	0.94**	0.94**
4	Right testes length				0.61**	0.72**	0.82**	0.82**	0.72**	0.54**	0.64**	0.68**	0.67**	0.76**	0.76**
5	Right testes width					0.86**	0.93**	0.93**	0.57**	0.95**	0.86**	0.92**	0.92**	0.94**	0.94**
6	Right testes thickness						0.95**	0.96**	0.77**	0.83**	0.92**	0.93**	0.93**	0.96**	0.95**
7	Right testes volume							0.98**	0.75**	0.88**	0.88**	0.95**	0.93**	0.97**	0.96**
8	Right testes weight								0.76**	0.87**	0.89**	0.94**	0.94**	0.98**	0.94**
9	Left testes length									0.55**	0.64**	0.76**	0.76**	0.76**	0.76**
10	Left testes width										0.87**	0.95**	0.93**	0.92**	0.93**
11	Left testes thickness											0.94**	0.95**	0.93**	0.93**
12	Left testes volume												0.98**	0.98**	0.96**

13	Left testes weight													0.99**	0.97**
14	Total testes volume														0.98**
15	Total testes weight														1.00

**Correlation coefficient was highly significant, P<0.01.

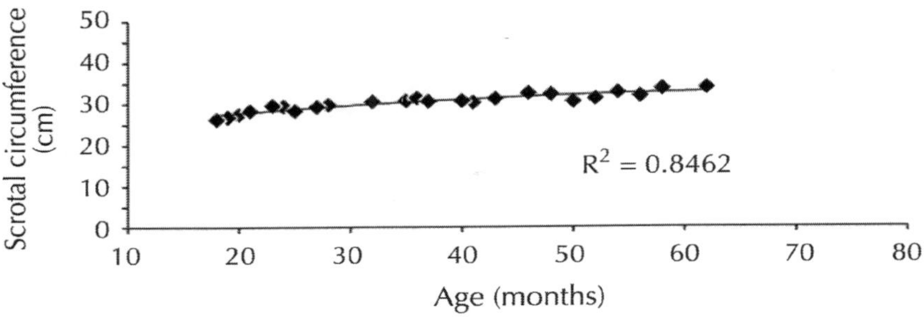

Figure 1: Relationship between scrotal circumference and age in Tho Tho (Bos indicus) bulls.

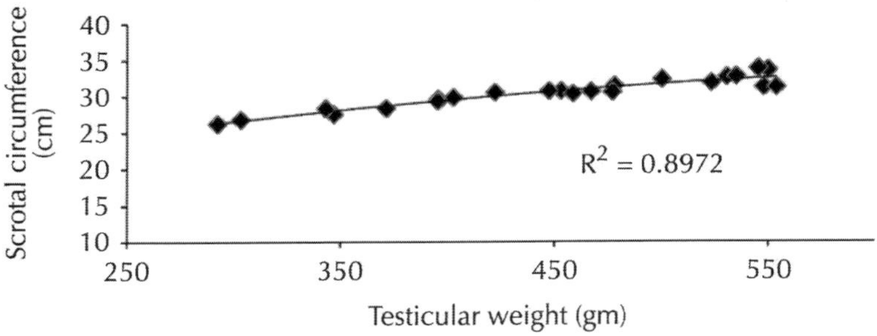

Figure 2: Relationship between scrotal circumference and testis weight in Tho Tho (Bos indicus) bulls.

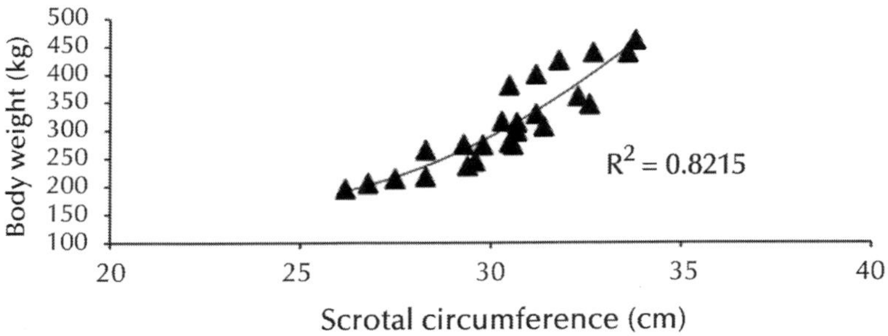

Figure 3: Relationship between scrotal circumference and body weight in Tho Tho (Bos indicus) bulls.

DISCUSSION

In the present study, the results revealed that scrotal circumference of Tho Tho bulls have been highly correlated with other testicular parameters. Thus, measurement of scrotal circumference in Tho Tho bulls is very useful to predict the testicular parameters and can be used in breeding centre to select suitable breeding male for artificial breeding purpose.

There was no report on effect of scrotal circumference on testicular parameters in Tho Tho cattle and, to the best of our knowledge, this is the first report on the effect of scrotal circumference on testicular parameters in Tho Tho bulls. Analysis of various testicular parameters such as testis length, width, thickness, volume, and weight is important for extensive selection of Tho Tho bulls for future breeding and conservation program in the NEH region especially in Nagaland state.

Correlation coefficients measured among the different testicular measurements and scrotal circumference for the 32 bulls were presented in Table 2. Body weight was somewhat more highly correlated with the various testicular measurements than with age. As would be expected the various measurements of testis size were highly correlated with each other. All correlation coefficients were highly significant ($P<0.01$). Circumference of the testes was highly correlated with other testicular measurements (Table 2); it was highly repeatable (Table1) and it was a simple measurement to obtain and easy to interpret. The correlations among this trait and other testicular measurements on a within-age group basis are not given, but they remained high. The correlation of 0.94 between scrotal circumference and testis weight is similar to the values of 0.90 to 0.96 reported by other researchers [28] for various comparisons between testicular dimensions and weight. Since circumference of the testes was easy to measure, the measurement had high repeatability and it was highly correlated with testis weight and volume and this measurement subsequently was taken on all bulls examined.

In the present study, the correlation among the various testicular measurements were in agreement with the study in Nigerian indigenous bulls [29], Bangladesh indigenous bulls [30], Sahiwal bulls [28], buffalo [19], and Mithun bulls [23], but are at variance with another report on other bulls in which testes volume and length were not correlated with age and body weight [20]. In our experience, Tho Tho bulls are indigenous animals, maintained under semi-intensive system and were sensitive to handle the testes and other reproductive organs. So that it was difficult to take measurement accurately. Also in the earlier study of other cattle bulls, testicular volume was calculated by multiplying mean values for length, thickness, and total width of the testes [19]. In our experiment, in this procedure, results were in higher side than those obtained by using the formula for estimating the volume of an ellipsoid which has a very high accuracy [31].

Interestingly, in the present study, within each age group, the testicular measurement of Tho Tho bulls were lower than those reported for Holstein bulls and higher than buffalo bulls [21], but maximum scrotal circumferences was reached at nearly the same age [18]. Nevertheless, there appears to be ample scope for selecting Tho Tho bulls with large scrotal circumference since about 60 to 70% of bulls, within each age group had a scrotal circumference greater than the mean scrotal circumference for that age group. In young dairy and beef bulls, scrotal circumference and testes size were highly correlated [18, 32] and bulls designated questionable or unsatisfactory potential breeders have smaller scrotal circumference measurements [7]. But the reports in other species like bubaline [21] and bovine [16] species showed that the spermatogenesis was higher in younger than older age. So that further studies with semen collection and more number of animals will help to pinpoint the exact age at which the mature rate of spermatogenesis is attained.

In the present study, the mean value of scrotal circumference in Group II (25–36 months) was significantly ($p<0.05$) higher than Group I (18–24 months) and Group IV higher value than the other three groups. It has been observed in the present study that SC was increased rapidly in young bulls and gradually in mature bulls. But it has been reported that in old age this parameter is decreased due to senile atrophy [33]. In the present study also, the proportion of increasing the scrotal circumference and testicular parameters was low in older bulls than in growing younger bulls. Based on our results on the mean testicular circumference of 32 Tho Tho bulls, we recommend that, for optimum breeding potential and possible higher fertility, Tho Tho cattle bulls with a mean scrotal circumference of ≥27.97, 30.00, 31.28, and 32.27 cm in the age groups of 18–24, 25–36, 37–48, and >48 months, respectively, should be selected as the breeding sires.

Scrotal circumference (Table 1) was increased with age and following a pattern similar with BW (Figure 1), but testes tended to reach mature size more rapidly, as indicated by the linear relationship between SC and BW (Figure 2). This is consistent with an earlier report [24].

High correlation was observed between testis size and scrotal circumference and based on this collective information, testicular diameter along with scrotal circumference are excellent indicators of spermatogenic function [33] and this can be used for breeding soundness evaluation in Tho Tho bulls [34]. In conclusion, present results indicate that as in exotic cattle [18] and buffalo [21] and Mithun [23] bulls, scrotal circumference in the Tho Tho bulls is a useful indicator of breeding soundness and should be used as an important criterion for selection of young bulls for breeding purpose. However, estimates of changes in testicular development can be considerably improved by following the same bulls at different ages to avoid confounding between bulls and ages. Future, semen collection and the seminal parameters will be correlated with testicular and scrotal parameters are warranted to confirm the present findings.

REFERENCES

1. M. Kaymakci, C. Sarican, and O. Karaca, "Investigations on the testis characteristics in Acıpayam male lambs," Ege Üniversitesi Ziraat Fakültesi, vol. 25, pp. 109–123, 1988.
2. S. A. Salhab, M. Zarkawi, M. F. Wardeh, M. R. Al-Masri, and R. Kassem, "Development of testicular dimensions and size, and their relationship to age, body weight and parental size in growing Awassi ram lambs," Small Ruminant Research, vol. 40, no. 2, pp. 187–191, 2001.
3. T. A. Yarney and L. M. Sanford, "Relationship between pre pubertal reproductive-endocrine parameters and post pubescent testicular size and function of rams," in Proceeding of the 10th International Congress on Animal Reproduction and Artificial Insemination, vol. 2, p. 178, Urbana-Champaign, Ill, USA, 1985.
4. C. A. Morris, J. A. Wilson, G. L. Bennett, N. G. Cullen, S. M. Hickey, and J. C. Hunter, "Genetic parameters for growth,

puberty, and beef cow reproductive traits in a puberty selection experiment," The New Zealand Journal of Agricultural Research, vol. 43, no. 1, pp. 83–91, 2000.
5. A. A. Boligon, L. G. Albuquerque, M. E. Z. Mercadante, and R. B. Lôbo, "Models for genetic evaluation of Nelore cattle mature body weight," Journal of Animal Science, vol. 86, no. 11, pp. 2840–2844, 2008.
6. A. A. Boligon, J. A. V. Silva, R. C. Sesana, J. C. Sesana, J. B. Junqueira, and L. G. Albuquerque, "Estimation of genetic parameters for body weights, scrotal circumference, and testicular volume measured at different ages in Nellore cattle," Journal of Animal Science, vol. 88, no. 4, pp. 1215–1219, 2010.
7. R. S. Ott, Breeding Soundness Examination of Bulls, Department of Veterinary Medicine, Urbana, Ill, USA, 1991.
8. N. Ahmad, S. Umair, M. Shahab, and M. Arslan, "Testicular development and establishment of spermatogenesis in Nili-Ravi buffalo bulls," Theriogenology, vol. 73, no. 1, pp. 20–25, 2010.
9. B. Devkota, T. Koseki, M. Matsui et al., "Relationships among age, body weight, scrotal circumference, semen quality and peripheral testosterone and estradiol concentrations in pubertal and postpubertal Holstein bulls," Journal of Veterinary Medical Science, vol. 70, no. 1, pp. 119–121, 2008.
10. G. H. Coulter and R. H. Foote, "Relationship of body weight to testicular size and consistency in growing Holstein bulls," Journal of Animal Science, vol. 44, no. 6, pp. 1076–1079, 1977.
11. C. L. Waldner, R. I. Kennedy, and C. W. Palmer, "A description of the findings from bull breeding soundness evaluations and their association with pregnancy outcomes in a study of western Canadian beef herds," Theriogenology, vol. 74, no. 5, pp. 871–883, 2010.
12. A. C. O. Evans, R. A. Pierson, A. Garcia, L. M. McDougall, F. Hrudka, and N. C. Rawlings, "Changes in circulating hormone concentrations, testes histology and testes ultrasonography during sexual maturation in beef bulls," Theriogenology, vol. 46, no. 2, pp. 345–357, 1996.
13. J. O. Almquist and R. P. Amann, "Reproductive capacity of dairy bulls. II. Gonadal and extragonadal sperm reserves as determined

by direct counts and depletion trials; dimensions and weight of geneitalia,"Journal of Dairy Science, vol. 44, pp. 1668–1678, 1961.

14. R. P. Amann and J. O. Almquist, "Reproductive capacity of dairy bulls. V. Detection of testicular deficiencies and requirements for experimentally evaluating testes function from semen characteristics,"Journal of Dairy Science, vol. 44, no. 12, pp. 2283–2291, 1961.
15. R. P. Amann and J. O. Almquist, "Reproductive capacity of dairy bulls. VI. Effect of unilateral vasectomy and ejaculation frequency on sperm reserves; aspects of epididymal physiology," Journal of Reproduction and Fertility, vol. 3, pp. 260–268, 1962.
16. M. Andersson and M. Alanko, "Relationship between testicular measurements, body weight and semen quality in young dairy bulls," Acta Veterinaria Scandinavica, vol. 33, no. 1, pp. 15–20, 1992.
17. R. H. Foote, G. E. Seidel Jr., J. Hahn, W. E. Berndtson, and G. H. Coulter, "Seminal quality, spermatozoal outpost, and testicular changes in growing Holstein bulls," Journal of Dairy Science, vol. 60, no. 1, pp. 85–88, 1977.
18. J. Hahn, R. H. Foote, and G. E. Seidel Jr., "Testicular growth and related sperm output in dairy bulls,"Journal of Animal Science, vol. 29, no. 1, pp. 41–47, 1969.
19. K. S. Bedi, Studies on genital development and semen quality in buffalo bulls [M.S. thesis], Punjab Agricultural University, Ludhiana, India, 1980.
20. K. S. Heur and M. A. Bajwa, "Selection of Nili Ravi buffalo bulls for artificial insemination," Zuchthyg, vol. 21, pp. 257–262, 1986.
21. H. C. Pant, R. K. Sharma, S. H. Patel et al., "Testicular development and its relationship to semen production in Murrah buffalo bulls," Theriogenology, vol. 60, no. 1, pp. 27–34, 2003.
22. Ö. Elmaz, S. Dikmen, Ü. Cirit, and H. Demir, "Prediction of postpubertal reproductive potential according to prepubertal body weight, testicular size, and testosterone concentration using multiple regression analysis in Kivircik ram lambs," Turkish Journal of Veterinary and Animal Sciences, vol. 32, no. 5, pp. 335–343, 2008.

23. P. Perumal and C. Rajkhowa, "Scrotal circumference and its relationship with testicular growth, age and semen production in mithun bulls," Indian Journal of Animal Sciences, vol. 83, no. 10, pp. 1074–1077, 2013
24. G. H. Coulter, L. L. Larson, and R. H. Foote, "Effect of age on testicular growth and consistency of Holstein and Angus bulls," Journal of Animal Science, vol. 41, no. 5, pp. 1383–1389, 1975.
25. L. F. C. Brito, A. E. D. F. Silva, L. H. Rodrigues, F. V. Vieira, L. A. G. Deragon, and J. P. Kastelic, "Effect of age and genetic group on characteristics of the scrotum, testes and testicular vascular cones, and on sperm production and semen quality in AI bulls in Brazil," Theriogenology, vol. 58, no. 6, pp. 1175–1186, 2002.
26. R. G. Elmore, C. J. Bierschwal, and R. S. Youngquist, "Scrotal circumference measurements in 764 beef bulls," Theriogenology, vol. 6, no. 5, pp. 485–494, 1976.
27. R. P. Amann, "Management of bulls to maximize sperm output," in Proceedings of the 13th Technical Conference on AI Reproduction, pp. 84–91, 1990.
28. E. Ahmad, N. Ahmad, Z. Naseer et al., "Relationship of age to body weight, scrotal circumference, testicular ultrasonograms, and semen quality in Sahiwal bulls," Tropical Animal Health and Production, vol. 43, no. 1, pp. 159–164, 2011.
29. P. A. Addass, A. Midau, M. M. Yahya, and M. A. Tizhe, "Genotype variation, age and body condition score on some paired testes measurements among common indigenous bull cattle breeds in Mubi Adamawa State, Nigeria," Annals of Biological Research, vol. 4, no. 8, pp. 253–256, 2013.
30. M. J. U. Sarder, "Effects of age, body weight, body condition and scrotal circumference on sperm abnormalities of bulls used for artificial insemination (AI) programme in Bangladesh," University Journal of Zoology, Rajshahi University, vol. 27, pp. 73–78, 2008.
31. C. C. Love, M. C. Garcia, F. R. Riera, and R. M. Kenny, "Use of testicular volume to predict sperm output in the stallion," in Proceedings of the Animal Conference of American Association of Equine Practitioners, vol. 36, pp. 15–21, 1991.
32. E. L. Willet and J. I. Ohms, "Measurement of testicular size and its relation to production of spermatozoa by bulls," Journal of Dairy Science, vol. 40, pp. 1559–1569, 1957.

33. J. O. Almquist, R. J. Branas, and K. A. Barber, "Postpuberal changes in semen production of Charolais bulls ejaculated at high frequency and the relation between testicular measurements and sperm output,"Journal of Animal Science, vol. 42, no. 3, pp. 670–676, 1976.

34. G. H. Coulter, "Scrotal circumference-a review," in Proceedings of the Society for Theriogenology, pp. 113–116, 1991.

Chapter 11

Effects of a Commercial Canine Gonadotropin Releasing Hormone Vaccination on Intact Male Llamas and Alpacas

C. E. Donovan[1], J. L. Grossman[2], K. M. Patton[3], S. Lamb[4], G. Bobe[1], and M. A. Kutzler[1]

[1]Department of Animal and Rangeland Sciences, Oregon State University, Corvallis, OR 97331, USA

[2]College of Veterinary Medicine, Oregon State University, Corvallis, OR 97331, USA

[3]Battelle Toxicology Northwest, Richland, WA 99352, USA

[4]Animal Health Diagnostic Center, Endocrinology Laboratory, Cornell University, Ithaca, NY 14853, USA

ABSTRACT

We have investigated the effect of immunization against gonadotropin releasing hormone (GnRH) using a commercial canine GnRH vaccine on testosterone concentration, testicular volume, testicular histology, and intermale behavior in intact male llamas and alpacas. Llamas (n=28) and alpacas (n=20) were either immunized (received 3 mL of vaccine given intramuscularly) or treated as controls (received 3 mL of sterile diluent given intramuscularly) at 0, 3, and 6 weeks. Blood samples and testicular volume measurements were taken at 0, 3, 6, 9, and 12 weeks. Owner surveys grading behavior at 0 and 12 weeks were received for 14 llamas. Two llamas at each time point undergoing the vaccination procedure were also castrated for testicular histological examination. Vaccinated animals elicited a GnRH antibody titer, and there was a significant decrease in testosterone concentration and testicular volume when compared with control animals. Intermale aggressive behavior was also significantly decreased in the surveyed llamas. However, histological examination revealed no significant changes. GnRH immunization using the canine GnRH vaccine may be an effective method for reducing intermale aggression in llamas and alpacas by decreasing circulating testosterone concentrations but cannot be recommended as an immunosterilant because of its lack of efficacy in interrupting spermatogenesis.

INTRODUCTION

The cohousing of intact male llamas and alpacas is a common farm arrangement for camelid owners in the United States, but keeping intact male camelids together frequently results in episodes of intermale aggression to assert territorial and social dominance. Aggressive behaviors include charging other males and forcing body contact, screeching, spitting, mounting, and biting [1]. If these behaviors are frequent, methods implemented by the owner to reduce aggression are necessary. Separating males from a herd can result in further behavioral problems because camelids are a highly social species [2]. Moving males around amongst intermale herds is not ideal either because hierarchal status must be reestablished with each change to the herd or reestablishing hierarchy results in male combat [1].

Castration is a recommended procedure utilized to reduce aggression [3, 4] and is frequently implemented to decrease intermale behavior in many species [2]. Surgical castration is expensive (several hundred dollars per animal) and irreversible. This may not be an ideal solution for owners that do not want the financial burden, want to preserve breeding stock, or want to avoid the risks of surgery. Therefore, there is a need for a cost-effective, reversible, and noninvasive means of reducing intermale aggression in camelids.

The hypothalamic-pituitary-gonadal axis has been a target for developing nonsurgical castration methods. Under normal conditions, hypothalamic gonadotropin releasing hormone (GnRH) stimulates the release of luteinizing hormone (LH) by binding to its receptor on the anterior pituitary. LH secretion is necessary for normal gonadal steroid hormone synthesis in males and females. Following GnRH immunization, GnRH antibodies are produced that block GnRH binding to its receptor on the anterior pituitary. Without this GnRH-GnRH receptor binding, LH is not secreted, and this prevents synthesis of gonadal steroid hormones. In addition to significantly decreasing serum testosterone concentration, GnRH immunization also has been shown to result in testicular atrophy and disruption of normal spermatogenesis in multiple male species [5–8]. The latter effects result specifically from the withdrawal of testosterone as it is required for the maintenance of the seminiferous tubule epithelium in mammals [9].

Many mammalian species have been immunized against GnRH, including horses [5], rats [6], cats [7], sheep [8], swine [11], cattle [12], camels [13], and dogs [14]. To date, immunocastration with a GnRH vaccine is temporary because reproductive activity of immunized animals returns to normal once antibody titers drop off below an inhibitory threshold [15].

There is a GnRH vaccine commercially produced in the US (Canine Gonadotropin Releasing Factor Immunotherapeutic; Pfizer Animal Health, Exton, PA, USA) that is labeled for the treatment of benign prostatic hyperplasia in mature intact male dogs. Benign prostatic hyperplasia (BPH) is an androgen-dependent condition as the presence of androgens is essential for the development and maintenance of BPH [16]. Canine Gonadotropin Releasing Factor Immunotherapeutic is a nonsurgical approach for the treatment of BPH by eliciting GnRH antibodies that ultimately result in diminished testosterone concentration [17]. Earlier investigations in our laboratory using this vaccine have found decreased testosterone concentrations and testicular volume in intact male dogs [18] and decreased frequency of inappropriate urination in neutered male cats [19].

The objective of this study was to determine the humoral and hormonal effects of this canine GnRH vaccine in male llamas and alpacas. We hypothesized that immunizing camelids against GnRH would cause immunocastration (decreased testosterone concentrations, testicular atrophy, and diminished spermatozoa production) and decrease intermale aggressive behavior.

MATERIALS AND METHODS

Preliminary Safety Study

A preliminary safety study was conducted on three mature intact male alpacas to observe any adverse effects following administration of the Canine Gonadotropin Releasing Factor Immunotherapeutic vaccine (Pfizer Animal Health, Exton, PA, USA). One alpaca received a placebo (1.5 mL of a sterile diluent provided by the vaccine manufacturer administered intramuscularly into the left and right semimembranosus muscles for a total of 3 mL), one alpaca received a 1X dose (1.5 mL of the vaccine administered intramuscularly into the left and right semimembranosus muscles for a total of 3 mL), and one alpaca received a 2X dose (3 mL of the vaccine administered intramuscularly into the left and right semimembranosus muscles for a total of 6 mL) administered three times at three-week intervals (at week 0, week 3, and week 6). Serum chemistry panels were determined prior to the first vaccine (week 0) and three weeks following administration of the last vaccine (week 9). Three weeks following the last injection, complete necropsies were performed on these animals to evaluate the potential toxicity of the vaccine.

Animals and Vaccination

Privately owned mature, intact male llamas (n=28, age range 2–17 years) and alpacas (n=20, age range 2–12 years) from Oregon were used in this study. The animals were housed in sex-aggregated groups and were cared for by their owners. Control animals received a placebo (1.5 mL of a sterile diluent provided by the vaccine manufacturer administered intramuscularly into the left and right semimembranosus muscle for a total of 3 mL; n=10 llamas and 6 alpacas) and vaccinated animals received a 1X dose (1.5 mL of the Canine Gonadotropin Releasing Factor Immunotherapeutic vaccine administered intramuscularly into the left and right semimembranosus muscles for a total of 3 mL; n=18 llamas and 14 alpacas). Treatments were administered three-times at three week intervals (at week 0, week 3, and week 6). Animals were closely monitored for adverse reactions for 48 hours following each vaccination. One alpaca developed pyrexia (T=103.4^{0}F), lethargy, and bilateral hind limb lameness within 12 hours following the initial vaccination and was excluded from further vaccinations.

Behavioral Analysis

The owner of fourteen vaccinated llamas was asked to evaluate their social behavior before and after vaccination. These behaviors were classified as follows.

Score 1. (Calm). Quiet demeanor, does not start or participate in fights with other males, is not bothered by females within a visible range.

Score 2. (Moderate). Manageable demeanor, does not start fights with other males but will participate in them, is aware and pays attention to females within a visible range.

Score 3. (Aggressive). Dominant demeanor, starts and participates in fights with other males, focuses obsessively on females within a visible range.

Sample Collection, Scrotal Measurements, Determination of Antibody Titers, and Testosterone Concentrations

Jugular venous blood samples were collected from all animals prior to each injection (0, 3, and 6 weeks) and at 9 and 12 weeks following the initial treatment. All samples were allowed to clot; serum was prepared by centrifugation and stored at −20°C until assayed.

Left and right testes width and length were determined with digital calipers at the time of each blood collection. Each measurement was performed in triplicate by the same investigator to control for variation in measurement technique. Left and right testicular volume for each male was determined according to the formula $V = 4/3\pi ab^2$, where "a" is one-half the length and "b" is one-half the width [20]. A combined total testes volume per animal was determined as the sum of the left and right testes volumes [20].

GnRH antibody titers were determined by ELISA using a technique derived from that previously described [21]. Briefly, 96-well microtiter plates were coated with 100 µL of 2 µg/mL of LH-RH (71447-49-9, Sigma, St. Louis, MO, USA) in sodium bicarbonate buffer (pH 8.0) and incubated at 4°C overnight. After incubation, plates were washed with phosphate-buffered saline containing 0.05% Tween-20 (TPBS) (pH 8.0) and were blocked with StabilCoat (SC05-0100, SurModics, Eden Prairie, MN, USA). After blocking and washing with TPBS, plates were incubated for 1 hour at 20°C with serum samples diluted in a buffer containing 0.5% bovine serum albumin (9048-46-8, Sigma, St. Louis, MO, USA) to yield final serum dilutions ranging from 1 : 16 to 1 : 2048. After another wash with TBPS, antibodies were detected using horseradish peroxidase protein G conjugate (HRP) (10-1223, Invitrogen, Camarillo) diluted at 1 : 2000 in serum dilution buffer for 1 hour at 37°C. After a final wash with TPBS, HRP was visualized with 100 µL of ABTS peroxidase substrate (50-66-01, KPL, Gaithersburg, MD, USA). Absorbances were read at 405 nm using a spectrophotometer (FLUOstar Omega, BMG Labtech Inc., San Francisco, CA, USA), and each serum sample was measured in duplicate. The cutoff for seropositivity, defined in this study as the upper limit of a 95% confidence interval above the mean negative control level, was calculated using the methods of Frey et al. [22]. Serological results are expressed as the reciprocal of the highest twofold serial dilution above the calculated cutoff and normalized using a base-2 logarithmic scale.

Serum samples were also analyzed for testosterone concentration at the Animal Health Diagnostic Center at Cornell University using a Coat-A-Count Total Testosterone radioimmunoassay (Siemens Medical Solutions Diagnostics, Los Angeles, CA, USA) and performed according to the manufacturer's instructions.

Castration and Histological Evaluation

Two llamas at each time point (weeks 0, 3, 6, 9, and 12) undergoing the vaccination procedure outlined previously were castrated using a routine scrotal castration technique. Therefore, the two llamas castrated at week 0 received no vaccinations, the two at week 3 received one vaccination, the two at week 6 received two vaccinations, and the two at weeks 9 and 12 received three vaccinations. Briefly, the llamas were generally anesthetized with a 0.3 mL of a mixture of ketamine (83 mg/mL), xylazine (8 mg/mL), and butorphanol (0.8 mg/mL) [23]. A 2 cm incision was made on either side or parallel to the median raphe along the most ventral aspect of the scrotum [24]. Each testicle was removed and excised using an emasculator. The skin incisions healed by second intention after castration.

Each testis was hemisectioned and fixed, paraffin-embedded, cut into 6 μm sections, and stained with hematoxylin and eosin. Histological evaluation was performed by a veterinary pathologist blinded to the treatment groups. The evaluation included assessment of Leydig cell density and morphology along with the proliferation and maturation of spermatocytes/spermatids. Leydig density was scored on a 0–3 scale: 0 = no cells present; 1 = scattered/few cells present; 2 = moderate number of cells present; 3 = densely packed within the interstitium. Leydig morphology was scored on a 0–3 scale: 0 = normal; 1 = mild changes; 2 = moderate changes; 3 = severe changes. Seminiferous tubules were studied using the Yoshida scoring method, which gives a score of 1–12 according to the presence or absence of germ cells (see Table 1) [10].

Table 1: The criteria used for scoring changes within the seminiferous epithelium of vaccinated llamas at each time point, adapted from Yoshida et al. [10]

Score	Criteria
12	Many late spermatids or spermatozoa (≥10) present
11	Only a few late spermatids or spermatozoa (<10) present
10	No spermatozoa and no late spermatids, but many round spermatids (≥10) present
9	No spermatozoa and no late spermatids, but only a few round spermatids (<10) are present
8	No spermatozoa and no spermatids, but many secondary spermatocytes (≥10) are present
7	No spermatozoa and no spermatids, but only a few secondary spermatocytes (<10) are present
6	No spermatozoa, no spermatids, no secondary spermatocytes, but many primary spermatocytes (≥10) are present
5	No spermatozoa, no spermatids, no secondary spermatocytes, but only a few primary spermatocytes (<10) are present
4	No spermatozoa, no spermatids, no spermatocytes, many spermatogonia (>10) are present
3	Only germ cells present are a few spermatogonia (<10)
2	Absence of germ cells, but Sertoli cells are present
1	Total absence of cells in tubular section

Statistical Analysis

Analyses were carried out using SAS (Version 9.2, SAS Institute Inc., Cary, NC, USA). Antibody titers of GnRH were log-transformed to the base 2 to achieve normalization, testosterone concentrations and testicular volumes were analyzed as percent change from baseline (0 weeks), and these data were analyzed as a repeated measure in time design in PROC MIXED. Fixed effects in the model were vaccination (yes, no), time after first vaccination (3, 6, 9, and 12 weeks), species (llama, alpaca), and the interactions between vaccination and time and between vaccination and species. A first order heterogeneous autoregressive variance-covariance structure was fitted for repeated measurements within animals. Age of animal was not included as fixed effect in the model because the effect was not significant. Behavior scores before and after vaccination were compared using the nonparametric sign test. Histology was evaluated using PROC GLIMMIX for generalized linear mixed models. Significance for all data was defined at $P<0.05$.

RESULTS

Results of the preliminary safety study showed no evidence of biochemical analysis or necropsy of any toxicological effect of the vaccine. There were no significant changes in the serum biochemistry from the beginning to the end of the safety study. The postmortem examinations found the animals to be in good body condition prior to euthanasia. Gross and histopathologic evaluations of all the organs examined were unremarkable with the exception of evidence of intestinal parasitic migration (e.g., fibrous scars present on the diaphragmatic capsular surface of the liver) in the control and in the 2X dose alpacas.

Excluding the alpaca that developed pyrexia, lethargy, and bilateral hind limb lameness following the initial vaccination, mild injection site reactions were observed in six vaccinated llamas and no alpacas. Five llamas experienced swelling at the injection site after the first injection but only one of those five experienced swelling at the injection site after the second injection as well. None of the five experienced a reaction to the third injection. The sixth llama experienced hind limb lameness after the first injection but did not experience a reaction to the second or third injection.

All animals were seronegative for antibodies against GnRH prior to the first vaccination, and there was no significant effect of species on GnRH antibody titer over time ($P=0.1$). Compared to control animals, antibody titers of vaccinated animals were significantly greater at week 6 ($P=0.01$) and week 9 ($P<0.0001$) (Figure 1). Antibody titers of vaccinated animals peaked at 9 weeks after vaccination.

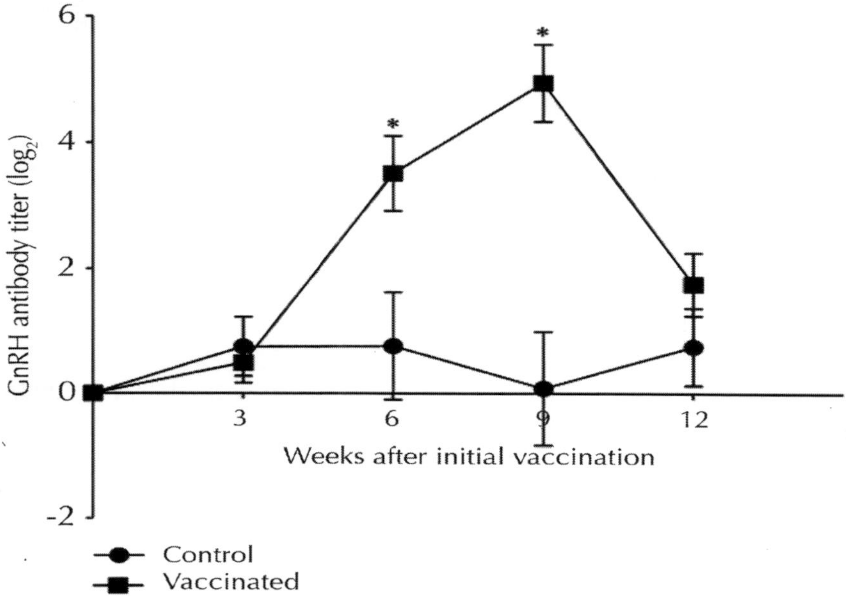

Figure 1: Serum GnRH antibody titer (±SEM) in control (•) and vaccinated (■) animals prior to each injection (0, 3, and 6 weeks) and at weeks 9 and 12 following initial treatment *P<0.05 compared to controls.

There was no significant effect of species on the change in testosterone over time (P=1.0). Compared to controls, testosterone concentrations in vaccinated animals were significantly decreased at week 6 (P<0.0001), week 9 (P<0.0001), and week 12 (P=0.01) (Figure 2). Furthermore, of the fourteen vaccinated llamas evaluated behaviorally, there was a significant decrease in behavior score (P=0.002) following the third vaccination. Of the 8 males identified as being aggressive at the time of vaccination, 5 (62.5%) experienced a marked decrease in aggression, whereas a minimal decrease was seen in 1 male (12.5%) and no change was seen in 2 males (25%) (Figure 3).

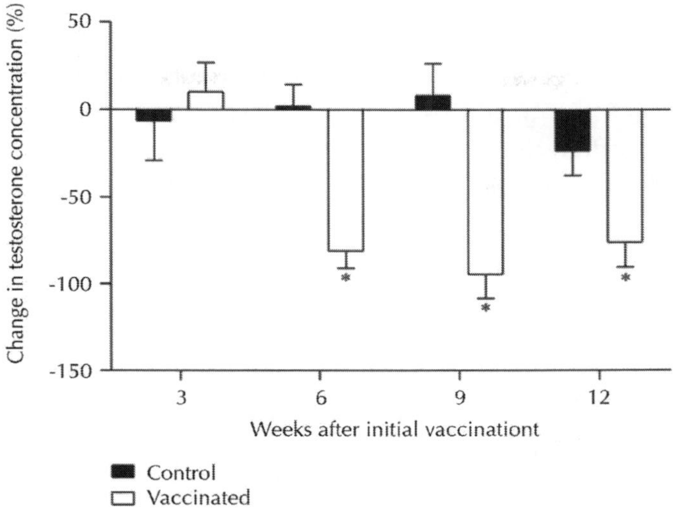

Figure 2: Change in testosterone concentration (%) in control (■) and vaccinated (□) animals prior to each injection (0, 3, and 6 weeks) and at weeks 9 and 12 following initial treatment *P<0.05 compared to controls.

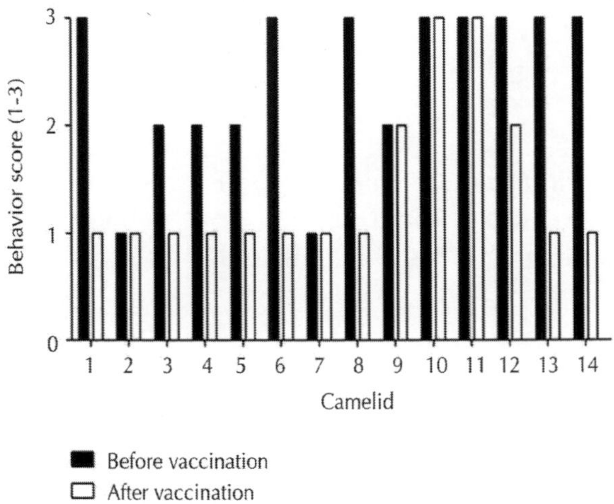

Figure 3: Change in behavior score before initial vaccination (■) and after completion of the vaccination series (□) in 14 llamas. Score 1 = calm, score 2 = moderate, and score 3 = aggressive.

There was no significant effect of species on the change in testicular volume over time (P=0.6). Compared to controls, testicular volumes in vaccinated animals were significantly decreased at week 6 (P=0.04), week 9 (P=0.002), and week 12 (P=0.01) (Figure 4). Unexpectedly, there was no effect of GnRH immunization on spermatogenesis based on seminiferous tubule scoring (P=0.6), Leydig cell morphology (P=0.2), or Leydig cell density (P=0.6) (Figure 5).

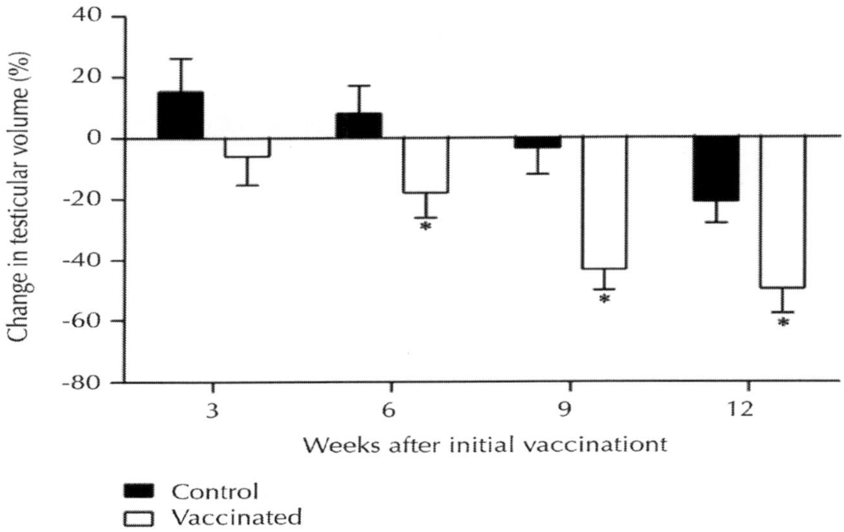

Figure 4: Change in testicular volume (%) in control (■) and vaccinated (□) animals prior to each injection (0, 3, and 6 weeks) and at weeks 9 and 12 following initial treatment *P<0.05 compared to controls.

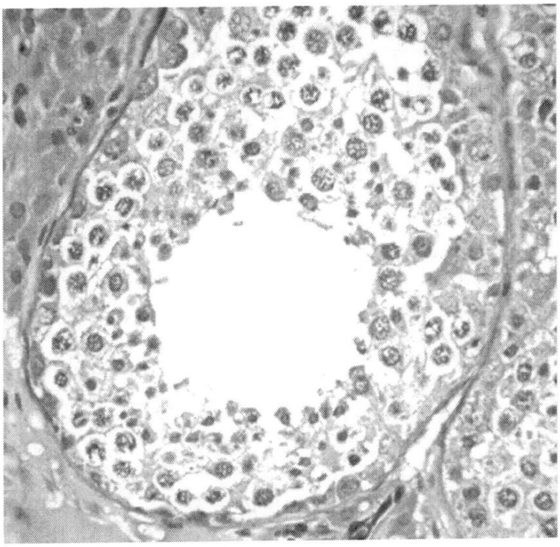

(a)

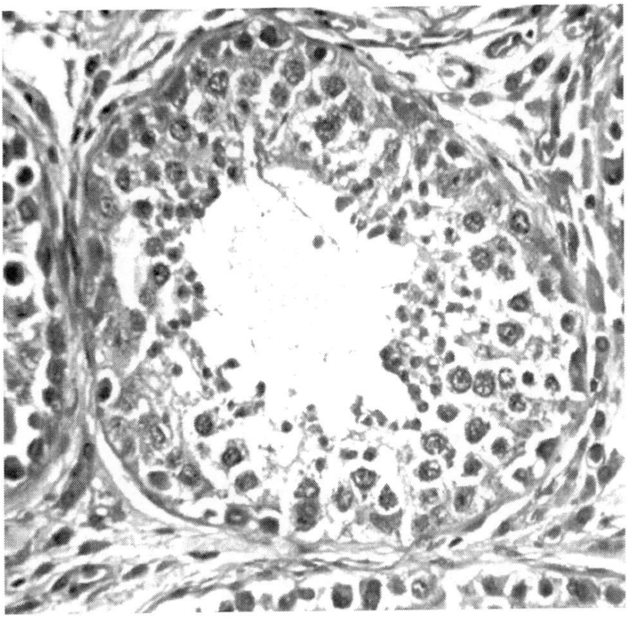

(b)

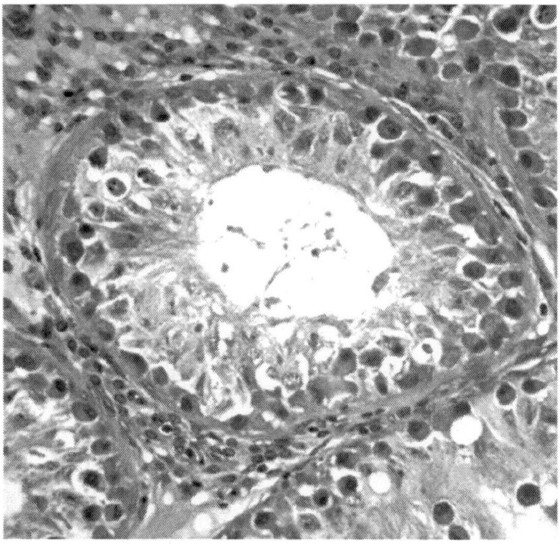

(c)

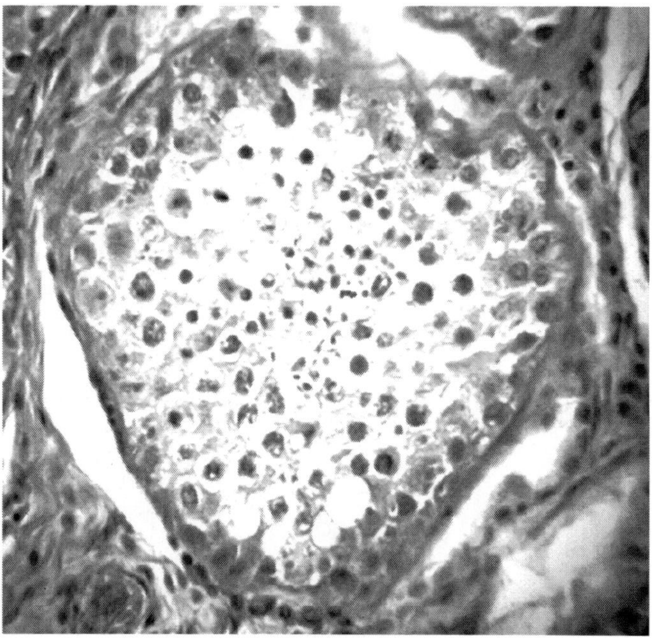

(d)

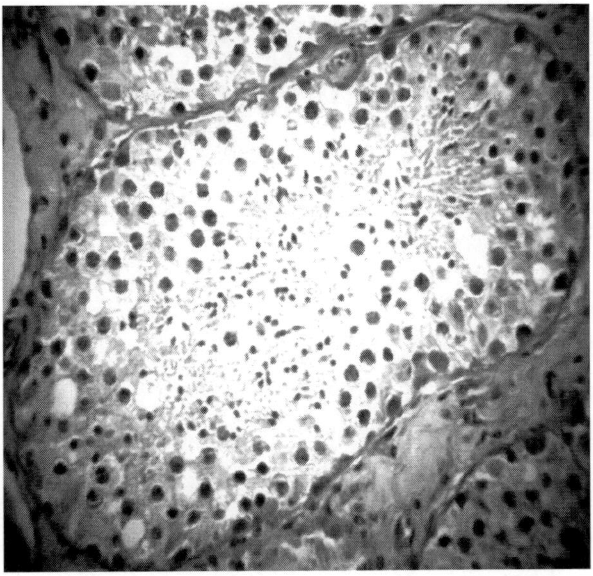

(e)

Figure 5: Cross-sections of testes at 20x magnification from a nonvaccinated llama (a) and vaccinated llamas at week 3 (b), 6 (c), 9 (d), and 12 (e) following initial treatment. There was no effect of GnRH immunization on spermatogenesis at any time point based on seminiferous tubule scoring (P=0.6347) on Leydig cell morphology (P=0.1987) or density (P=0.6256).

DISCUSSION

Immunization against GnRH has been used as an alternative method of castration in various species [5–8, 11–14]. Immunocastration is implemented in order to prevent undesirable effects of androgens, including aggressive behavior. We hypothesized that immunization against GnRH in llamas and alpacas would result in a decrease in serum testosterone concentration, testicular volume, sperm production, and intermale aggression. This is the first study to investigate an alternative means of castrating llamas and alpacas through GnRH immunization.

This study demonstrates that camelids are capable of generating GnRH antibodies following immunization against GnRH, which was correlated with a significant decrease in testosterone concentrations and testicular volume. The average testosterone concentration of vaccinated camelids was <1000 pg/mL, which was below normal parameters reported for adult camelids [25]. It is of interest to note that the control animals showed an apparent fluctuation in testosterone concentration during the study period (Figure 2), which had been previously observed by Bravo et al. [26] in male llamas in the United States from 30 to 50 months of age. Furthermore, in a study conducted in male vicunas where blood samples were taken every 15 minutes for 4–8 hours, testosterone profiles showed high variation among animals and fluctuation throughout the sampling period [27].

Not all participating owners submitted behavior evaluations before and after treatment. However, there was a significant decrease in intermale aggressive behavior in the 14 surveyed llamas, which was correlated with an elevated GnRH antibody titer and reduced testosterone concentration. Furthermore, it is of interest to note that behavior scoring was also performed on two control llamas that were cohoused with the vaccinated llamas. The owner noted that while the behavior of one of the control llamas did not change, the behavior of the other control animal became more aggressive towards the vaccinated males it was cohoused with. This may be the result of the decreased aggressive behavior displayed by the vaccinated males, allowing the control llama to assume a higher hierarchal status. However, further study with a larger subset of animals is necessary to elucidate whether partially vaccinating a herd of co-housed males can alter established herd hierarchies.

While the change in testicular volume decreased significantly more in vaccinated animals compared to controls, there was also an apparent decrease in testicular volume in the controls over time (Figure 3). This study took place during the summer in the USA, so it is possible that season could have affected testicular volume. In male vicunas, seasonal variation was found to affect testes size [27]. However, the mechanism regarding seasonality in male camelids is poorly studied [25] and further research on seasonality in male camelids with respect to geographic location and management practices is necessary to determine whether season can affect testicular volume.

Even though there was a significant change in testicular volume in vaccinated animals compared to controls, there was no significant difference in seminiferous tubule score, Leydig cell density, or Leydig cell morphology between the different groups of castrated llamas. It is generally accepted that testosterone is required to maintain spermatogenesis in the adult. However, normal spermatogenesis can be maintained despite up to 80% reduction in intratesticular testosterone concentrations in rats [28, 29]. It is also important to note that intratesticular testosterone concentration is much higher (approximately 50 ng/mL) compared to circulating testosterone concentration (1-2 ng/mL) [30]. This suggests that spermatogenesis in camelids could be maintained despite circulating testosterone concentration below the limits of detection, which is what we observed in the current study. Further study is needed in camelids to compare circulating testosterone concentration to intratesticular testosterone concentration in GnRH vaccinated males.

In conclusion, GnRH immunization using the canine GnRH vaccine may be an effective method for temporarily reducing intermale aggression amongst co-housed male camelids by decreasing circulating testosterone concentrations. However, further investigation is needed before GnRH immunization using the canine GnRH vaccine can be recommended as an immunosterilant because of the lack of efficacy in interrupting spermatogenesis that was observed in this study.

ACKNOWLEDGMENTS

The authors sincerely appreciate Merck Merial Veterinary Student Scholars for supporting this project and Pfizer Animal Health for product donation. They thank Dr. Timothy Hazzard and Bernadette Stang for their assistance in validating the ELISA and Niki Fadden for assistance with paper preparation. They also thank the llama and alpaca owners within the Willamette Valley for making their animals available to them.

REFERENCES

1. M. E. Fowler, "Llama and alpaca behaviour: a clue to illness detection," Journal of Camel Practice and Research, vol. 6, no. 2, pp. 135–152, 1999.
2. S. Nickolmann, S. Hoy, and M. Gauly, "Effects of the castration of male llamas (Lama glama) on their behavior, the testosterone

and serum thyroid horomone level," in Proceedings of the 3rd European Symposium and Supreme European Seminar on Progress in South American Camelids Research, pp. 75–78, Gottingen, Germany, 1999.

3. J. L. Grossman and M. A. Kutzler, "Effects of castration in male llamas (Lama glama) on human-directed aggression," Theriogenology, vol. 68, p. 511, 2007.
4. M. E. Fowler, "Castration," in Medicine and Surgery of South American Camelids, pp. 135–137, Iowa State University Press, Ames, Iowa, USA, 1998.
5. F. Janett, R. Stump, D. Burger, and R. Thun, "Suppression of testicular function and sexual behavior by vaccination against GnRH (Equity) in the adult stallion," Animal Reproduction Science, vol. 115, no. 1–4, pp. 88–102, 2009. · ·
6. T. Peirouvi and S. Salami, "GnRH agonist induces apoptosis in seminiferous tubules of immature rats: direct gonadal action," Andrologia, vol. 42, no. 4, pp. 231–235, 2010. · ·
7. J. K. Levy, L. A. Miller, P. C. Crawford, J. W. Ritchey, M. K. Ross, and K. A. Fagerstone, "GnRH immunocontraception of male cats," Theriogenology, vol. 62, no. 6, pp. 1116–1130, 2004. · ·
8. Z. Kiyma, T. E. Adams, B. W. Hess, M. L. Riley, W. J. Murdoch, and G. E. Moss, "Gonadal function, sexual behavior, feedlot performance, and carcass traits of ram lambs actively immunized against GnRH," Journal of Animal Science, vol. 78, no. 9, pp. 2237–2243, 2000.
9. R. P. Amann and B. D. Schanbacher, "Physiology of male reproduction," Journal of Animal Science, vol. 57, pp. 380–403, 1983.
10. A. Yoshida, K. Miura, and M. Shirai, "Evaluation of seminiferous tubule scores obtained through testicular biopsy examinations of nonobstructive azoospermic men," Fertility and Sterility, vol. 68, no. 3, pp. 514–518, 1997. · ·
11. G. Zamaratskaia, L. Rydhmer, H. K. Andersson et al., "Long-term effect of vaccination against gonadotropin-releasing hormone, using Improvac, on hormonal profile and behaviour of male pigs,"Animal Reproduction Science, vol. 108, no. 1-2, pp. 37–48, 2008. · ·

12. R. B. Cook, J. D. Popp, J. P. Kastelic, S. Robbins, and R. Harland, "The effects of active immunization against GnRH on testicular development, feedlot performance, and carcass characteristics of beef bulls," Journal of Animal Science, vol. 78, no. 11, pp. 2778–2783, 2000.
13. I. M. Ghoneim, M. M. Waheed, M. M. Al-Eknah, and S. M. El-Bahr, "Immunization against GnRH in the male camel (Camelus dromedaries): effects on sexual behavior, testicular volume, semen characteristics and serum testosterone concentrations," Theriogenology, vol. 78, no. 5, pp. 1102–1109, 2012.
14. J. Walker, S. Ghosh, J. Pagnon et al., "Totally synthetic peptide-based immunocontraceptive vaccines show activity in dogs of different breeds," Vaccine, vol. 25, no. 41, pp. 7111–7119, 2007. · ·
15. C. A. Herbert and T. E. Trigg, "Applications of GnRH in the control and management of fertility in female animals," Animal Reproduction Science, vol. 88, no. 1-2, pp. 141–153, 2005. · ·
16. J. Trachtenberg, L. L. Hicks, and P. C. Walsh, "Androgen- and estrogen-receptor content in spontaneous and experimentally induced canine prostatic hyperplasia," Journal of Clinical Investigation, vol. 65, no. 5, pp. 1051–1059, 1980.
17. Pfizer Animal Health, "Canine gonadotropin releasing factor immunotherapeutic," Vaccine Package Insert, Exton, Pa, USA.
18. C. E. Donovan, M. Greer, and M. A. Kutzler, "Physiologic responses following gonadotropin-releasing hormone immunization in intact male dogs," Reproduction in Domestic Animals, vol. 47, no. 6, pp. 403–405, 2012. ·
19. M. Greer and M. Kutzler, "Use of a canine GnRH vaccine for behavior modification in cats," Clinical Theriogenology, vol. 4, no. 3, p. 422, 2012.
20. R. M. Harrison, G. J. Domingue, P. M. Heidger, J. A. Roberts, and J. U. Schlegel, "Vasectomy in rhesus monkeys. I. Surgical techniques and gross observations," Urology, vol. 9, no. 6, pp. 639–644, 1977.
21. M. Elhay, A. Newbold, A. Britton, P. Turley, K. Dowsett, and J. Walker, "Suppression of behavioural and physiological oestrus in the mare by vaccination against GnRH," Australian Veterinary Journal, vol. 85, no. 1-2, pp. 39–45, 2007. · ·

22. A. Frey, J. Di Canzio, and D. Zurakowski, "A statistically defined endpoint titer determination method for immunoassays," Journal of Immunological Methods, vol. 221, no. 1-2, pp. 35–41, 1998. · ·

23. B. A. Valentine, T. W. Riebold, P. L. Wolff, and A. L. Sanchez, "Cerebral injury from intracarotid injection in an alpaca (Vicugna pacos)," Journal of Veterinary Diagnostic Investigation, vol. 21, no. 1, pp. 149–152, 2009.

24. A. N. Baird, D. G. Pugh, J. G. W. Wenzel, and H. C. Lin, "Comparison of two techniques for castration of llamas," Journal of the American Veterinary Medical Association, vol. 208, no. 2, pp. 261–262, 1996.

25. A. Tibary and J. Vaughan, "Reproductive physiology and infertility in male South American camelids: a review and clinical observations," Small Ruminant Research, vol. 61, no. 2-3, pp. 283–298, 2006. · ·

26. P. W. Bravo, M. E. Fowler, G. H. Stabenfeldt, B. L. Lasley, and R. Frey, "Testis growth and testosterone concentrations in the male llama," in Proceedings of the 12th International Congress on Animal Reproduction, vol. 3, p. 789, 1992.

27. B. Urquieta, R. Cepeda, J. E. Céceres, L. A. Raggi, and J. R. Rojas, "Seasonal variation in some reproductive parameters of male vicuña in the High Andes of northern Chile," Journal of Arid Environments, vol. 26, no. 1, pp. 79–87, 1994. · ·

28. G. R. Cunningham and C. Huckins, "Persistence of complete spermatogenesis in the presence of low intratesticular concentrations of testosterone," Endocrinology, vol. 105, no. 1, pp. 177–186, 1979.

29. B. R. Zirkin, R. Santulli, C. A. Awoniyi, and L. L. Ewing, "Maintenance of advanced spermatogenic cells in the adult rat testis: quantitative relationship to testosterone concentration within the testis,"Endocrinology, vol. 124, no. 6, pp. 3043–3049, 1989.

30. T. T. Turner, C. E. Jones, and S. S. Howards, "On the androgen microenvironment of maturing spermatozoa," Endocrinology, vol. 115, no. 5, pp. 1925–1932, 1984.

Chapter 12

Single Layer Centrifugation with Androcoll-P Can be Scaled-Up to Process Larger Volumes of Boar Semen

Marjet van Wienen[1,2], Anders Johannisson[3], Margareta Wallgren[1,4], Joyce Parlevliet[2] and Jane M. Morrell[1]

[1]Division of Reproduction, Department of Clinical Sciences, Swedish University of Agricultural Sciences—SLU, P. O. Box 7054, 75007 Uppsala, Sweden

[2]Faculty of Veterinary Medicine, 3508TD Utrecht, the Netherlands

[3]Institute of Anatomy, Physiology and Biochemistry, Swedish University of Agricultural Sciences, P. O. Box 7011, 75007 Uppsala, Sweden

[4]Quality Genetics, Hörby, Sweden

ABSTRACT

The objective of this study was to scale-up the procedure for Single Layer Centrifugation (SLC) through Androcoll™-P, as a preliminary step towords processing the whole ejaculate. The first experiment compared Single Layer Centrifugation using 4.5 mL and 15 mL extended ejaculate (SLC-4.5 and SLC-15, resp.), assessing sperm quality by objective motility analysis, morphology, viability, and the production of reactive oxygen species (ROS). In the second experiment, SLC-4.5 was compared to Single Layer Centrifugation with 25 mL extended ejaculate (SLC-25) using motility analysis and morphology. In both experiments, normal morphology and linear motility were significantly higher in the SLC-selected samples than in the uncentrifuged controls (P <. 0 0 1), whereas total motility and membrane integrity were unchanged. Although ROS production was higher in the SLC-selected samples than in the controls (P <. 0 1), this might have been due to the presence of antioxidants in seminal plasma in the latter. In conclusion, there was no difference in sperm quality between SLC-4.5 and SLC-15 samples, or between SLC-4.5 and SLC-25 samples, indicating that the SLC method can be scaled-up successfully.

INTRODUCTION

A technique for improving sperm quality is considered desirable in many domestic species, for example, cattle and horses, where sperm quality is related to pregnancy rates after artificial insemination (AI). In cattle, pregnancy rate is correlated with increasing sperm motility in the sperm dose, whereas in the boar, increasing motility over 60%–70% is not reflected in increased pregnancy rates [1, 2]. Similarly, stallion sperm morphology is highly correlated to pregnancy rate, whereas the correlation is lower in the boar [3]. Selection of boars as breeding sires is usually based on genetics for production characteristics rather than on semen quality, since the high sperm doses used in AI (three billion motile spermatozoa) are thought to compensate for the presence of defective spermatozoa [4, 5].

Nevertheless, a method that selects the most robust spermatozoa from an ejaculate could have many advantages for the boar AI industry, either by reducing the sperm number used for AI [5], potentially enhancing sperm survival during cryopreservation, or by removing pathogens in the ejaculate such as bacteria [6] and viruses [7]. Such a selection method would have a cost benefit for the pig industry, depending on the value of the boar, the actual price of semen doses, and the perceived need to increase biosecurity and reduce antibiotic usage.

Single layer centrifugation (SLC) using a silane-coated silica-based formulation optimised for stallion spermatozoa (Androcoll-E) has been shown to select spermatozoa with the best motility, normal morphology, and chromatin integrity [8–10]. Preliminary results with boar spermatozoa indicated that SLC with a boar-specific colloid formulation, Androcoll-P, selects the most highly motile boar spermatozoa [11]. However, the volume used (1.5 mL of a sperm suspension at 100×10^6 spermatozoa/mL) was considered to be impractical for processing large volumes of ejaculate. Recently, the SLC method was scaled up to allow 15–18 mL of stallion ejaculate to be processed through Androcoll-E per 50-mL centrifuge tube [12]. Therefore, the aims of this study were to scale up the SLC procedure through a silane-coated silica colloid (Androcoll-P) to allow larger volumes of extended boar ejaculate to be processed, as a preliminary step for further increases.

MATERIALS AND METHODS

Ejaculates were available from 6 mature boars (Swedish Yorkshire, Norwegian Landrace, and Swedish Landrace), 1–4 years old, housed at the Division of Clinical Sciences, Swedish University of Agricultural Sciences (SLU), Uppsala, Sweden. All boars were fed and housed according to Swedish husbandry standards [13] and were provided with water ad libitum. The experimental protocol had previously been reviewed and approved by the Ethical Committee for Experimentation with Animals, Uppsala, Sweden.

Semen Collection

The sperm-rich fraction (SRF) of ejaculates was collected using the gloved-hand technique into a plastic bag in a prewarmed thermos flask. The semen was immediately extended 1:1 (v/v) in warm (35°C) Beltsville Thawing Solution (BTS; [14]).

Media

BTS consisted of 200 mL deionised water, 7.4 g glucose, 1.2 g trisodium citrate, 0.26 g sodium bicarbonate, 0.26 g sodium ethylene diamine tetraacetic acid (EDTA), and 0.16 g potassium chloride. The BTS was prepared on the day of semen collection.

Androcoll-P and Androcoll-P-Large (SLU, Uppsala, Sweden) are a ready-to-use glycidoxypropyltrimethoxysilane-coated silica colloid in a species-specific buffered salt solution. No preparation is required other than equilibration to room temperature (22–23°C) before use.

Sperm Concentration

Sperm concentration was measured using a Nucleocounter-SP100 (Chemometec, Allerød, Denmark), according to the manufacturer's instructions [15]. The sperm concentration in the extended ejaculates was adjusted to 100×10^6 spermatozoa/mL with BTS for SLC. The sperm concentration in the SLC-selected samples was also measured, to allow the yield obtained to be calculated.

Single Layer Centrifugation

Aliquots of the extended semen were layered on top of a single layer of Androcoll-P, using different volumes according to the experimental design (see below).

After centrifuging at 300 g for 20 min, the resulting sperm pellets were resuspended in BTS containing either 1.25 mg/mL bovine serum albumin (BSA; Bovine Serum Albumin Fraction V, Sigma, Stockholm) (Experiment 1) or 5.0 mg/mL BSA (Experiment 2). All sperm samples were subsequently stored in a Climate Box (Unitron, Tørring, Denmark) at a temperature of 16 to 18°C. Aliquots of unselected and SLC-selected samples were taken for various analyses as described below.

Computer-Assisted Sperm Motility Analysis (CASA)

Sperm motility in all samples was assessed after incubating in a water bath at 38°C for 30 min. An aliquot (5 µL) of the sample in a prewarmed Makler counting chamber (Sefi Medical Instruments, Haifa, Israel) was placed on the warm (38°C) microscope stage of a phase-contrast microscope and analyzed by CASA using a Mika Cell Motion Analyser (CMA) (MTM Medical Technologies Montreux, Switzerland). The software settings, which had been previously determined to be optimal [16], were as follows: 32 frames per sequence, a minimum of 15 frames per object, minimum area for objects = 25 pix, velocity limit for immobile objects = 10 µm/s, and velocity limit for locally motile objects = 25 µm/s. Motile spermatozoa were classified in three categories: linear (spermatozoa deviating less than 10% from a straight line), circular (spermatozoa moving in a circle with a radius less than 25 µm), and nonlinear, the latter being spermatozoa falling into neither of the first two categories [16]. At least 200 spermatozoa were analyzed for each sample. The software reports proportions of immotile, locally motile, and motile spermatozoa, with the latter being further classified as circular, nonlinear, and linear motile populations, in addition to other parameters. For the purposes of this report, only the proportion of motile spermatozoa and the three subclasses (circular, nonlinear, and linear motile) were considered for analysis.

Morphology

Aliquots for morphology analysis were taken on Day 0. The methods have been described in detail previously [8]. Briefly, aliquots of the fresh extended ejaculates and centrifuged sperm preparations were used to prepare air-dried slides for assessment of sperm head shape of 500 spermatozoa at X1000 magnification. The following abnormalities were assessed: proximal cytoplasmic droplets, detached heads, acrosome defects, nuclear pouches, midpiece defects, and tail defects (bent, coiled, or double bend). The proportions were used to calculate the total pathological heads and the number of morphologically normal spermatozoa. In addition, aliquots were fixed in formol-saline for counting of 200 spermatozoa on wet smears (X1000) [17], focussing on the following: pear-shaped heads, and heads narrow at the base, heads with abnormal contour, undeveloped heads, detached heads, narrow (tapering) heads, heads of variable size. The mean proportion of morphologically normal spermatozoa was estimated as the remaining proportion left from total abnormal spermatozoa, including those spermatozoa with distal cytoplasmic droplets which were considered to be normal. Since the number of specific abnormalities was low in most cases (<1%), they have been classified as head and tail abnormalities in this study. As the total incidence of cytoplasmic droplets and midpiece defects was greater than 5% in the uncentrifuged ejaculates, these two types were considered separately from the other abnormalities. Morphology evaluation was carried out by skilled personnel according to the standard protocol in the Swedish Sperm Reference Laboratory at SLU.

Plasma Membrane Integrity

Aliquots from the unselected and selected samples were extended to a concentration of approximately 5 × 1 0^6sperm cells/ mL using BTS. Each sample was evaluated using a BD LSR flow cytometer (Beckon Dickinson, San José, CA, USA). Excitation was with an argon-ion laser (488 nm). Green fluorescence was detected with a FL1 band-pass filter (530/30 nm) while red fluorescence was measured using a FL3 long-pass filter (>670 nm). A total of 50,000 sperm-specific events were evaluated and calculated as percentages.

Assessment of plasma membrane integrity (PMI) was made using the procedure described by Johannisson et al. [18]. Briefly, 1000 µL of each sample was stained with 1 µL of SYBR-14 (final stain concentration 0.02 µM) followed by 5 µL of PI (final stain concentration 12 µM) (Live-Dead Sperm Viability Lit L-7011; Invitrogen, Eugene, OR, USA). After incubating at 38°C for 10 minutes, the fluorescence was measured using the FC. The cells were classified as: living (SYBR14-positive/PI-negative), dead (SYBR14-negative/PI-positive), or dying (SYBR14-positive/PI-positive).

Reactive Oxygen Species (ROS)

Aliquots from the unselected and selected samples were extended to a concentration of approximately 5 × 1 0^6 sperm cells/mL using BTS and were stained as follows: an aliquot of 300 μL from the extended samples was mixed with 3 μL of Hoechst 33258 (HO) (final stain concentration 0.4 μM), 3 μL of hydroethidine (HE) (final stain concentration 0,4 μM), and 3 μL of dichlorodihydrofluorescein diacetate (DCFDA) (final stain concentration 20 μM). HO was purchased from Sigma, Stockholm, while HE and DCFDA where purchased from Invitrogen Molecular Probes, Eugene, OR, USA. The samples were incubated at 38°C for 30 minutes before being analyzed by flow cytometry (FC). The method is a modification of that described previously [19], the modification being the use of HO as an independent analysis of living spermatozoa. Each sample was evaluated using a BD LSR flow cytometer. Excitation was with an argon-ion laser (488 nm) and a HeCd laser (325 nm). Detection of green fluorescence was with a FL1 band pass filter (530/30 nm), red fluorescence was measured using a FL3 long-pass filter (>670 nm), and blue fluorescence was detected in FL4 with a band-pass filter (510/20 nm). A total of 30,000 sperm-specific events were evaluated and calculated as percentages. The cells were classified as ROS-negative living, ROS-positive living, or dead in the HE-HO dotplot, after gating for sperm cells in the FSC-SSC-dotplot (Figure 1). The DCFDA fluorescence was not used for evaluation, since it was always highly correlated with the HE fluorescence.

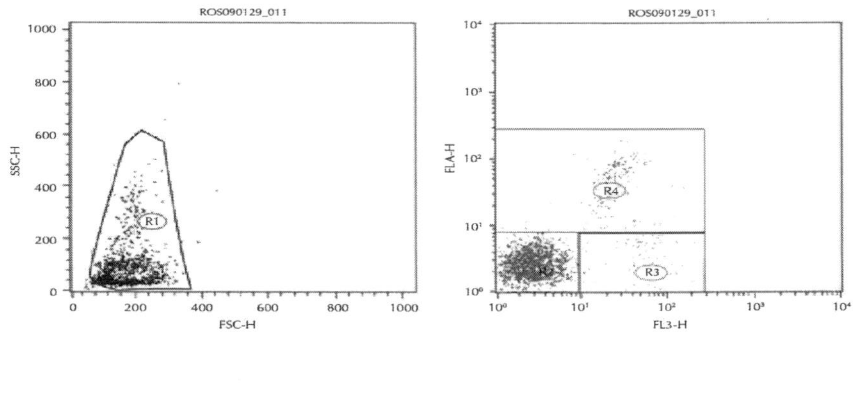

(a)

					Region Statistics				
File:ROS090129.011					Log date units: linear values				
Sample ID: 87 50 wed					Patient ID:				
Tube:					Panel:				
Acquisition date 29-jan-09					Gate:G1				
Gated events: 28729					Total events: 30000				
X parameter: FL3-H(Log)					Y parameter: FL3-H(Log)				
Region	Events	%Gated	%Total	X mean	X Geo mean	Y mean	Y Geo mean	P x, P y
R1	28729	100.00	95.76	8.81	4.00	8.40	3.45	1,2
R2	23877	83.11	79.59	3.00	2.67	2.69	2.45	7,5
R3	1449	5.04	4.83	60.79	50.09	3.73	3.28	7,5
R4	3340	11.63	11.13	27.46	23.36	51.22	40.00	7,5

Figure 1: Flow cytometric analysis of boar spermatozoa stained with hydroethidine and dichlorodihydrofluorescein diacetate. Note: (left) R1 = total gated; (right) R2 = ROS-negative living; R3 = ROS-positive living; R4 = dead.

Experimental Design

Experiment 1. Ejaculates (n = 5) were obtained from each of four boars (total sample size n = 2 0). A comparison was made of two volumes: SLC-4.5: 4 mL of Androcoll-P plus 4.5 mL of extended semen in a 12-mL conical centrifuge tube (12 mL centrifuge tube; Sarstedt, Landskrona, Sweden) and SLC-15: 15 mL of Androcoll-P-Large plus 15 mL semen in a 50-mL Falcon centrifuge tube. The control samples consisted of aliquots of uncentrifuged extended semen. Aliquots from three ejaculates per boar were taken for morphology evaluation and analysis of viability and ROS production on the day of semen collection (Day 0), whereas aliquots from all sperm samples were used for sperm motility assessment on Day 0, after 24 h storage (Day 1) and 72 h storage (Day 3) at 16–18°C.

Experiment 2. Ejaculates (n = 3 per boar) were collected from two of the boars from Experiment 1 and from other two (total sample size n = 1 2). For this experiment, SLC-4.5 (as above) was compared with SLC-25 (20 mL Androcoll-P plus 25 mL extended semen in a 100-mL glass centrifuge tube). The control samples were as described above. Morphology and motility evaluations were carried out as for Experiment 1.

Statistical Analysis

The statistical analyses were performed using the SAS software (Ver. 9, SAS Institute Inc., Cary, NC, USA). Variables were analyzed using analysis of variance (PROC MIXED). The statistical model included the fixed effects: boars, treatments (three: 4.5, 15, UN for Experiment 1; 4.5, 25, UN for Experiment 2) and the interaction between treatment and boar. Least squares means were calculated for each level of the fixed effect, and levels of significance were estimated for differences between least squares means.

RESULTS

Sperm Motility

In both experiments, there were no significant differences among treatments for total motility (Table 1), although there were significant differences in the proportions of linear and nonlinear motility between treatments and time, as shown in Figures 2 and 3 for Experiments 1 and 2, respectively, ($P < .001$). The variation between boars was not significant.

Table 1: Mean (±SD) motility in boar sperm samples with and without single layer centrifugation through Androcoll-P in SLC-4.5 and SLC-15 (n = 20)

	Uncent. (%)	SLC-4.5 (%)	[redacted]
Day 0	75 ± 16	78 ± 11	73 ± 17
Day 1	66 ± 21	63 ± 19	65 ± 19
Day 3	67 ± 21	47 ± 24	47 ± 13

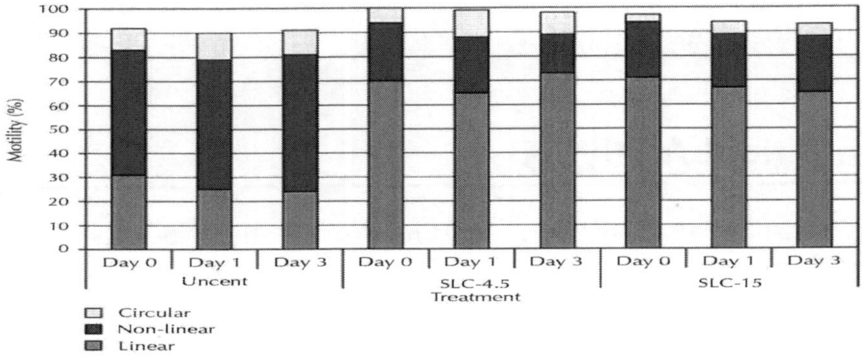

Figure 2: Motility patterns in SLC-selected spermatozoa (SLC-4.5 and SLC-25) and nonselected controls, showing the increase in linear motility and concomitant decrease in nonlinear motility in the SLC samples (n = 2 0).

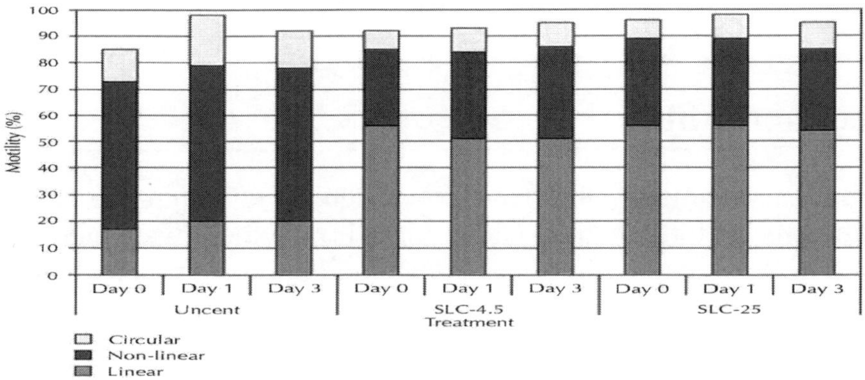

Figure 3: Motility patterns in SLC-selected spermatozoa (SLC-4.5 and SLC-25) and nonselected controls, showing the increase in linear motility and concomitant decrease in nonlinear motility in the SLC samples (n = 1 2).

Yield after SLC

There was no difference in the mean yields for the different SLC treatments in either experiment (Experiment 1: SLC-4.5 6 6 . 5 ± 1 8 %; SLC-15 5 8 ± 1 9 %, NS; Experiment 2: SLC-4.5 4 0 ± 1 6 %; SLC-25 3 9 ± 2 0 %, NS). There was significant within-boar variation (*P* <. 0 0 1).

Sperm Morphology

In both experiments, the proportion of morphologically normal spermatozoa (Tables 2 and 3) was significantly higher in the SLC samples than in the untreated samples ($P < .001$ in both experiments). There were fewer tail defects in the SLC-selected samples compared to the nonselected controls ($P < .01$ and $P < .001$ for Experiments1 and 2, resp.), while in Experiment 2 there was also a trend towards fewer total head abnormalities in the SLC-selected samples compared to the nonselected controls ($P < .054$). There were no differences for other morphological abnormalities, which appeared with a prevalence of less than 1%, apart from proximal drops, and have not been included in the statistical analysis. Variation between boars was not significant.

Table 2: Percentage of spermatozoa with normal morphology (%) (mean ± SD) in boar sperm samples before and after Single layer centrifugation (n = 12 ejaculates)

Group	Unselected (%)	SLC-4.5 (%)	SLC-15 (%)
Normal morphology	83.6 ± 13.6a	96.5 ± 3.6a	94.0 ± 5.1a
Abnormal heads	4 ± 0.9	4 ± 1.1	4 ± 1.2
Tail defects	9.4 ± 10.9b c	0.4 ± 0.5b	1.6 ± 2.6c

Note: superscript letter denotes significant difference in the SLC samples than in the non-SLC-selected samples, $^{a}P < .001$, $^{b}P < .01$, $^{c}P < .05$.

Table 3: Effect of Single layer centrifugation on boar sperm morphology in Experiment 2 ($n = 12$)

	Uncent. (%)	SLC-4.5 (%)	SLC-25 (%)
Normal morphology	82 ± 14a b	97 ± 1.4a	97 ± 2b
Abnormal heads	3.15 ± 1.3c	2.3 ± 0.8c	2.3 ± 0.7c
Abnormal tails	7.0 ± 10.4c	0.2 ± 0.2c	0.3 ± 0.5c

Note: superscript letter denotes significant difference in the SLC samples than in the non-SLC-selected (uncentrifuged) samples, $^{a}P < .001$, $^{b}P < .01$, $^{c}P < .05$.

Sperm Membrane Integrity

Mean values (±SD) for living, dying, and dead spermatozoa for the different treatments in Experiment 1 are shown in Table 4. There were no significant differences between the unselected and SLC-selected samples or between the two SLC treatments.

Table 4: Proportion (%) (mean ± SD) of living, ROS producing, dead, and dying boar spermatozoa measured 24 h after semen collection and SLC (n = 1 6 ejaculates)

Parameter	Classification	Unselected (%)	SLC-4.5 (%)	SLC-15 (%)
	Living	9 4 ± 2. 7	9 2. 8 ± 3. 2	9 4. 4 ± 2. 5
SYBR14/PI	Dying	4. 7 ± 2. 3	5. 6 ± 2. 4	4. 2 ± 1. 8
	Dead	1. 3 ± 0. 6	1. 4 ± 0. 7	1. 2 ± 0. 8
	Living ROS −ve	8 5. 1 ± 3. 6a c	6 7. 9 ± 1 3. 1a	7 2. 1 ± 1 6. 6c
ROS	Living ROS +ve	4. 8 ± 1. 7b c	8. 4 ± 3. 5b	8. 6 ± 5. 7c
	Dead	9. 6 ± 2. 6a	2 3. 1 ± 9. 5a	1 8. 9 ± 1 0. 9b

Note: ROS = reactive oxygen species; SYBR14/PI staining for membrane integrity. ^{a}P<. 0 0 1; ^{b}P<. 0 1; ^{c}P <. 0 5. For viability (SYBR14/PI), there were no statistically significant differences among treatments.

ROS Production

Table 4 shows mean (±SD) sperm viability measured with Hoechst 33258 in the ROS assay compared with the overall means for living spermatozoa from the SYBR14/PI staining. There was a difference in % living spermatozoa in all treatments between the ROS-staining method and the SYBR14-PI-staining method, with % living being higher in the SYBR14/PI assay. Regression analysis showed only a weak relationship between the two methods with a trend towards significance (R^2= 0 .

3 1 2; $P < .058$). There were fewer ROS-positive spermatozoa and fewer dead spermatozoa in the unselected samples than in the selected samples ($P < .01$), although there were significant differences between boars ($P < .001$). There were more ROS-negative spermatozoa in the uncentrifuged samples than in both SLC 4.5 and SLC 15 mL samples ($P < .01$ for uncentrifuged versus SLC 4.5 mL, $P < .001$ for uncentrifuged versus SLC 15 mL).

DISCUSSION

The objective of this paper was to scale up the original SLC method to allow larger volumes of ejaculate to be processed. The parameters of sperm quality assessed were sperm motility, morphology, membrane integrity and ROS production for Experiment 1 (scaling up to 4.5 ml and 15 mL), whereas in Experiment 2 (scaling up to 25 mL) only sperm motility and morphology were evaluated.

The proportions of motile spermatozoa were not different between the different treatments, in contrast to previous results where subjective motility assessment was used [11] However, in the present study, less BSA (1.25 mg/mL) was added to the BTS in Experiment 1 compared to previous studies, which resulted in spermatozoa adhering to the microscope slide, thus not being included in the CASA motility analysis, and also might have contributed to decreased sperm survival. Furthermore, the boars were older in the experiment reported here than in the previous study [11] which might have affected sperm quality. In Experiment 2 in the present study, 5.0 mg/mL BSA was added to the BTS, that is, the same concentration as was added in the previously reported study [11] which might have improved sperm survival in the SLC-selected samples, although some sperm aggregation was observed as a result. Again, these aggregated sperm clumps were ignored by the CASA analysis. Therefore, on the basis of these observations, it would appear that CASA is not helpful for analyzing motility in SLC-selected samples if BTS is used to resuspend the sperm pellets.

Although the proportion of motile spermatozoa was not different between treatments, the motility patterns did differ, with SLC-selected spermatozoa showing more linear motility and less nonlinear motility than the unselected controls (Figures 2 and 3). The difference was less marked for the SLC-4.5 and SLC-25 treatments in Experiment 2 than that in Experiment 1, which might have been due to the increased content of BSA in the BTS, but nevertheless was significant ($P < .001$).

Normal morphology was significantly improved in all the SLC treatments compared to the nonselected controls. There was no difference between the different SLC-treatments for these parameters, or for sperm yield, indicating that scaling up the SLC method did not have a detrimental effect on sperm quality. These findings are consistent with previous observations made on stallion spermatozoa [9, 10] and preliminary observations on boar spermatozoa [11].

SLC treatment did not improve boar sperm viability, according to the SYBR-14/PI results (which was why it was excluded from Experiment 2). This observation is in contrast to results with stallion spermatozoa where viability was improved by SLC selection [20]. One explanation for this finding could be that the viability in the samples was already high and, therefore, hard to improve significantly. This result is in agreement with previous work on bull spermatozoa where there was no change in viability after density gradient centrifugation (DGC) where semen from animals of high fertility was used, although there was an improvement when semen from bulls of low fertility was subjected to DGC [21]. Previously, values for "living" spermatozoa determined by SYBR14-PI staining were 80%–90% for boars [22, 23]. In the study reported here, a higher percentage of living spermatozoa (up to 95%) were found, possibly because the concentration of the stain and/or the concentration of protein in the extender were not optimal. The SYBR14/PI staining method has been validated previously for bull spermatozoa [24]; similar staining patterns were subsequently found for the spermatozoa of other species [23].

The observation that there was less ROS production in the untreated samples than in the SLC-selected samples was, at first, surprising, since DGC has been shown to reduce ROS production in boar sperm samples. Previously, a concentration of less than 4% of ROS production was found [19], while in the current study it was around 6%. However, the SLC samples apparently contained a higher proportion of dead spermatozoa than in the non-SLC-selected samples, which might have been a source of ROS. Furthermore, different proportions of living spermatozoa were detected for the ROS staining method and the SYBR14-PI staining method, despite the analyses being performed on the same day, indicating that one of the staining procedures was not optimal for boar semen. Alternatively, the different incubation times for stained samples for the two techniques (10 min for SYBR/PI versus 30 min for HO/HE/DCFDA) might have contributed to the difference. Since the uncentrifuged samples contained seminal plasma, some ROS might have been removed by antioxidants present in the seminal plasma whereas no seminal plasma, and therefore no antioxidant activity were present in the SLC-samples. Previously, it has been suggested that some ROS production is necessary to obtain fertilization in IVF. In a preliminary IVF experiment with one of the boars, the oocytes fertilized with SLC-selected spermatozoa showed a 35% rate of development to blastocysts, compared with 19% for the non-SLC-selected sample (Gonzalez Herrero et al., unpublished observations).

One parameter of sperm quality not evaluated in this study is chromatin integrity. Previous experiments with stallion spermatozoa showed that SLC selects spermatozoa with good chromatin integrity [10]. However, unlike stallions, boars generally have very good chromatin integrity in the unselected ejaculate [25]. SCSA was done on ejaculates from the four boars used in Experiment 1 on another occasion: although the mean DFI values were2 ± 1 % for uncentrifuged and 0 . 7 ± 0 . 6 % for SLC-selected spermatozoa, these values lie within the interassay variation for our flow cytometer and therefore do not necessarily represent selection for spermatozoa with good chromatin integrity (Morrell & Johannisson, unpublished data).

For most of the parameters measured, there were no significant differences between either the 4.5 mL-SLC and 15 mL SLC-treatments, or the SLC-4.5 and SLC-25 treatments indicating that the SLC can be scaled up to 4.5 mL, 15 mL, or 25 mL without reducing sperm quality in the resulting samples. These results confirm earlier observations with stallion spermatozoa [11], where 15 mL extended semen was used on 15 mL Androcoll-E-Large. The SLC-25 protocol would be feasible for producing AI doses from very valuable boars since approximately 1 5 0 0 × 1 0^6 spermatozoa could be obtained per SLC-25, that is, half a normal AI dose. However, the relevance of the technique would depend on the boar: when the SLU boars were compared with Hampshire boars on a commercial boar station, there were considerable among group differences for all parameters of sperm quality (P < . 0 0 1; data not shown). Further adjustments are required to scale up the technique to a larger volume and to investigate among boar variation. However, overall these results are very promising in that it seems to be possible to improve some aspects of sperm quality, such as normal morphology and progressive motility, in boar semen samples with SLC and that sufficient sperm numbers could be obtained for AI doses with the larger volumes from some boars. SLC-selected spermatozoa showed normal functionality in the IVF study referred to previously, which is in agreement with fertility data from bulls [26] and stallions [27], respectively.

In conclusion, SLC can be used to enhance the quality of boar sperm samples, particularly for normal morphology and linear motility. Furthermore, the technique could be scaled-up to process 15 mL or 25 ml extended ejaculate per tube without compromising in vitro assessed sperm quality in the selected samples. These results are encouraging as preliminary steps to a further scale up procedure, to enable large volumes of ejaculate to be processed for the swine insemination industry.

ACKNOWLEDGMENTS

The authors thank the animal husbandry staff of the Division for their excellent care of the boars at SLU and the laboratory staff (Annika Rikberg and Karin Selin-Wretling) for their skulled morphology analysis. The project was supported by the Swedish Farmers' Foundation for Research in Agriculture (SLF), Stockholm, Sweden (V7050239). In addition, M. van Wienen received an Erasmus Scholarship to undertake her student project in Sweden.

REFERENCES

1. W. L. Flowers, "Management of boars for efficient semen production," Journal of Reproduction and Fertility, vol. 52, supplement, pp. 67–78, 1997.
2. J. M. Morrell and H. Rodriguez-Martinez, "Biomimetic techniques for improving sperm quality in animal breeding: a review," The Open Andrology Journal, vol. 1, pp. 1–9, 2009.
3. X. Xu, S. Pommier, T. Arbov, B. Hatchings, W. Sotto, and G. R. Foxcroft, "In vitro maturation and fertilization techniques used

for assessment of semen quality and boar fertility," Journal of Animal Science, vol. 76, no. 12, pp. 3079–3089, 1998.

4. W. L. Flowers, "Selection for boar fertility and semen quality—the way ahead," Society of Reproduction and Fertility, vol. 66, supplement, pp. 67–78, 2009.
5. R. G. Saacke, "Sperm morphology: its relevance to compensable and uncompensable traits in semen,"Theriogenology, vol. 70, no. 3, pp. 473–478, 2008.
6. M. Wallgren, H. Rodriguez-Martinez, and J. M. Morrell, "Single LayerCentrifugation with AndrocollTM-P removes, or substantially reduces, bacterial contamination in boar sperm samples," in Proceedings of the 11th International Symposium on Spermatology, Okinawa, Japan, 2010.
7. J. M. Morrell and R. M. Geraghty, "Effective removal of equine arteritis virus from stallion semen," Equine Veterinary Journal, vol. 38, no. 3, pp. 224–229, 2006.
8. J. M. Morrell, A.-M. Dalin, and H. Rodriguez-Martinez, "Prolongation of stallion sperm survival by centrifugation through coated silica colloids: a preliminary study," Animal Reproduction, vol. 5, pp. 121–126, 2008.
9. J. M. Morrell, A. M. Dalin, and H. Rodriguez-Martinez, "Comparison of density gradient and single layer centrifugation of stallion spermatozoa: yield, motility and survival," Equine Veterinary Journal, vol. 41, no. 1, pp. 53–58, 2009.
10. J. M. Morrell, A. Johannisson, A. M. Dalin, and H. Rodriguez-Martinez, "Morphology and chromatin integrity of stallion spermatozoa prepared by density gradient and single layer centrifugation through silica colloids," Reproduction in Domestic Animals, vol. 44, no. 3, pp. 512–517, 2009.
11. J. M. Morrell, F. Saravia, M. van Wienen, M. Wallgren, and H. Rodriguez-Martinez, "Selection of boar spermatozoa using centrifugation on a glycidoxypropyltrimethoxysilane-coated silica colloid," Journal of Reproduction and Development, vol. 55, no. 5, pp. 547–552, 2009.
12. J. M. Morrell, A. Johannisson, A. M. Dalin, and H. Rodriguez-Martinez, "Single layer centrifugation with Androcoll-E can be scaled up to allow large volumes of stallion ejaculate to be

processed easily,"Theriogenology, vol. 72, no. 6, pp. 879–884, 2009.

13. A. Simonsson, "Näringsrekommendationer och fodermedelstabeller till svin (Nutritional recommendations and feedstuffs for swine)," Swedish University of Agricultural Sciences, Uppsala, Sweden, 1994.
14. V. G. Pursel and L. A. Johnson, "Freezing of boar spermatozoa: fertilizing capacity with concentrated semen and a new thawing procedure," Journal of Animal Science, vol. 40, no. 1, pp. 99–102, 1975.
15. C. Hansen, T. Vermeiden, J. P. W. Vermeiden, C. Simmet, B. C. Day, and H. Feitsma, "Comparison of FACSCount AF system, improved Neubauer hemocyometer, Corning 254 photometer, SpermVision, Ulitmate and Nucleocounter SP-100 for determination of sperm concentration of boar semen,"Theriogenology, vol. 66, no. 9, pp. 2188–2194, 2006.
16. B. M. Eriksson, J. M. Vazquez, E. A. Martinez, J. Roca, X. Lucas, and H. Rodriguez-Martinez, "Effects of holding time during cooling and of type of package on plasma membrane integrity, motility and in vitro oocyte penetration ability of frozen-thawed boar spermatozoa," Theriogenology, vol. 55, no. 8, pp. 1593–1605, 2001.
17. N. Lagerlöf, "Morphological studies on the change in sperm structure and in the testes of bulls with decreased or abolished fertility," Acta Pathologica et Microbiologica Scandinavica, vol. 19, supplement, pp. 254–267, 1934.
18. A. Johannisson, J. M. Morrell, J. Thorén, M. Jonsson, A. M. Dalin, and H. Rodriguez-Martinez, "Colloidal centrifugation with AndrocollTM prolongs stallion sperm motility, viability and chromatin integrity,"Animal Reproduction Science, vol. 116, no. 1-2, pp. 119–128, 2009.
19. H. D. Guthrie and G. R. Welch, "Determination of intracellular reactive oxygen species and high mitochondrial membrane potential in Percoll-treated viable boar sperm using fluorescence-activated flow cytometry," Journal of Animal Science, vol. 84, no. 8, pp. 2089–2100, 2006.
20. J. M. Morrell and M. Wallgren, "Androcoll-P-Large selects boar spermatozoa with good membrane integrity from the sperm-rich fraction of the ejaculate," Animal Reproduction. In press.

21. H. Rodriguez-Martinez, B. Larsson, and H. Pertoft, "Evaluation of sperm damage and techniques for sperm clean-up," Reproduction, Fertility and Development, vol. 9, no. 3, pp. 297–308, 1997.
22. W. M. C. Maxwell, L. A. Johnson, and S. T. Mortimer, "Evaluation of morphology and function of frozen-thawed boar spermatozoa in vitro," Boar Semen Preservation, Allen Press, Beltsville, Md, USA, 2000.
23. D. L. Garner and L. A. Johnson, "Viability assessment of mammalian sperm using SYBR-14 and propidium iodide," Biology of Reproduction, vol. 53, no. 2, pp. 276–284, 1995.
24. D. L. Garner, L. A. Johnson, S. T. Yue, B. L. Roth, and R. P. Haugland, "Dual DNA staining assessment of bovine sperm viability using SYBR-14 and propidium iodide," Journal of Andrology, vol. 15, no. 6, pp. 620–629, 1994. View at Scopus
25. D. P. Evenson and R. Wixon, "Clinical aspects of sperm DNA fragmentation detection and male infertility," Theriogenology, vol. 65, no. 5, pp. 979–991, 2006.
26. M. Thys, L. Vandaele, J. M. Morrell et al., "In vitro fertilizing capacity of frozen-thawed bull spermatozoa selected by single layer (Glycidoxypropyltrimethoxysilane) silane-coated silica colloidal centrifugation,"Reproduction in Domestic Animals, vol. 44, no. 3, pp. 390–394, 2009.
27. G. Mari, E Iacono, G. Kutvölgyi, B. Mislei, H. Rodriguez-Martinez, and J. M. Morrell, "Stallion spermatozoa prepared by Single Layer Centrifugation with Androcoll-E are capable of fertilisation in vivo," Reproduction in Domestic Animals. In press.

Citations

CHAPTER 1

Stefania Dall Olio, Luca Fontanesi, Leonardo Nanni Costa, Marco Tassinari, Laura Minieri, and Adalberto Falaschini, "Analysis of Horse Myostatin Gene and Identification of Single Nucleotide Polymorphisms in Breeds of Different Morphological Types," , vol. 2010, doi:10.1155/2010/542945.

CHAPTER 2

Terttu Katila, Tiina Reilas, Kaisa Nivola, Terttu Peltonen, and Anna-Maija Virtala, A 15-Year Survey of Reproductive Efficiency of Standardbred and Finnhorse Trotters in Finland - Descriptive Results, doi:10.1186/1751-0147-52-40.

CHAPTER 3

Filipa Paiva Brandão Deslandes Heitor and Luís António Matos Vicente, "Stallion Mate Choice and Mare Sexual Behaviour in a Herd of Sorraia Horses (Equus caballus)," ISRN Zoology, vol. 2011, Article ID 705790, 9 pages, 2011. doi:10.5402/2011/705790.

CHAPTER 4

Lidia Gil, Iván Galindo-Cardiel, C. Malo, N. González, and C. Álvarez, "Effect of Cholesterol and Equex-STM Addition to an Egg Yolk Extender on Pure Spanish Stallion Cryopreserved Sperm," ISRN Veterinary Science, vol. 2013, Article ID 280143, 6 pages, 2013. doi:10.1155/2013/280143.

CHAPTER 5

Rubens Paes de Arruda, Daniela Franco da Silva, Maria Augusta Alonso, André Furugen Cesar de Andrade, Juliana Nascimento, Andres Mejia Gallego, Simone Maria Massami Kitamura Martins, and Thaís Marques Granato, Nutraceuticals in reproduction of bulls and stallions, doi: 10.1590/S1516-35982010001300043.

CHAPTER 6

P Kuisma, M Andersson, E Koskinen, and T Katila, fertility of frozen-thawed stallion semen cannot be predicted by the currently used laboratory methods, doi: 10.1186/1751-0147-48-14.

CHAPTER 7

Véronique A. Lacombe, "Expression and Regulation of Facilitative Glucose Transporters in Equine Insulin-Sensitive Tissue: From Physiology to Pathology," ISRN Veterinary Science, vol. 2014, Article ID 409547, 15 pages, 2014. doi:10.1155/2014/409547.

CHAPTER 8

Basil Alexander, Gabriela Mastromonaco, and W. Allan King, Recent Advances in Reproductive Biotechnologies in Sheep and Goat, doi:10.4172/2157-7579.1000101.

CHAPTER 9

Maria Suska and Ewa Skotnicka, "Changes in Adenylate Nucleotides Concentration and Na+, K+-ATPase Activities in Erythrocytes of Horses in Function of Breed and Sex," Veterinary Medicine International, vol. 2010, Article ID 987309, 8 pages, 2010. doi:10.4061/2010/987309.

CHAPTER 10

P. Perumal, "Scrotal Circumference and Its Relationship with Testicular Growth, Age, and Body Weight in Tho Tho (Bos indicus) Bulls," International Scholarly Research Notices, vol. 2014, Article ID 249537, 6 pages, 2014. doi:10.1155/2014/249537.

CHAPTER 11

C. E. Donovan, J. L. Grossman, K. M. Patton, S. Lamb, G. Bobe, and M. A. Kutzler, "Effects of a Commercial Canine Gonadotropin Releasing Hormone Vaccination on Intact Male Llamas and Alpacas," Journal of Vaccines, vol. 2013, Article ID 181834, 7 pages, 2013. doi:10.1155/2013/181834.

CHAPTER 12

Marjet van Wienen, Anders Johannisson, Margareta Wallgren, Joyce Parlevliet, and Jane M. Morrell, "Single Layer Centrifugation with Androcoll-P Can Be Scaled-Up to Process Larger Volumes of Boar Semen," ISRN Veterinary Science, vol. 2011, Article ID 548385, 8 pages, 2011. doi:10.5402/2011/548385.

Index

D

E

F

G

H

I

L

M